Investigating Animal Abuse Crime Scenes

Animal abuse is well established as a gateway crime linked to other forms of antisocial behaviors and broader criminal violence. Increased awareness of the link between animal abuse and criminal behavior has led many states to mandate cross-reporting between agencies overseeing the welfare of families and of animals.

Investigating Animal Abuse Crime Scenes: A Field Guide is designed for first responders—such as animal control officers and police officers—as well as forensic scientists, other criminal justice and veterinary professionals who are tasked with processing and analyzing animal crime scenes and evidence.

The book addresses the key areas that must be considered in a thorough investigation of an animal abuse crime. This starts with general crime scene procedures that include securing and releasing the scene, search and seizure issues, chain of custody, documentation, searching for evidence, and the use of enhancement technologies. While many readers may already be familiar with such concepts, they are addressed in the context of unique factors relating to animals and animal abuse cases. The book then addresses the recognition, collection and preservation of different types of evidence that may be located at animal abuse scenes, with examples of the most important evidence for specific case types.

The critical role of the veterinarian, and the key aspects of veterinary forensic medicine, receives in-depth consideration. This includes issues such as examining animal victims of crime; determining cause of injury or death through the forensic clinical exam or necropsy; and techniques for evidence documentation, collection, and preservation. The physical and emotional abuse of animals is outlined throughout a series of chapters focused on specific types of animal abuse. Finally, report writing and testimony, from the perspectives of both the crime scene investigator and forensic veterinarian, are addressed. Further, three appendices provide useful checklists and templates for all animal abuse crime scene responders and veterinarians.

Investigating Animal Abuse Crime Scenes fills the growing need for a handy, comprehensive field reference that specifically focuses on the crime scene processing, investigation, analysis of evidence, and the subsequent adjudication of animal abuse cases within the court system.

Virginia M. Maxwell is a Professor in the Forensic Science Department at the University of New Haven. She has over 30 years of experience in Forensic Science as both a practitioner in the State of Connecticut Forensic Science Laboratory and at the University of New Haven, CT.

Martha Smith-Blackmore is a forensic veterinarian and president of a private veterinary forensic consulting firm, Forensic Veterinary Investigations, LLC. She frequently called as an expert witness in criminal and civil matters involving animals and is adjunct faculty at the Cummings School of Veterinary Medicine at Tufts University in North Grafton, MA.

Investigating Animal Abuse Crime Scenes
A Field Guide

Virginia M. Maxwell
Martha Smith-Blackmore

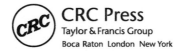

CRC Press
Taylor & Francis Group
Boca Raton London New York

CRC Press is an imprint of the
Taylor & Francis Group, an **informa** business

Designed cover image: With permission, and courtesy of, ACO Shayla Howe

First Edition published 2024
by CRC Press
6000 Broken Sound Parkway NW, Suite 300, Boca Raton, FL 33487-2742

and by CRC Press
4 Park Square, Milton Park, Abingdon, Oxon, OX14 4RN

CRC Press is an imprint of Taylor & Francis Group, LLC

© 2024 Taylor & Francis Group, LLC

Library of Congress Cataloging-in-Publication Data
Names: Maxwell, Virginia M., author. | Smith-Blackmore, Martha, author.
Title: Investigating animal abuse crime scenes : a field guide / Virginia
M. Maxwell and Martha Smith-Blackmore.
Identifiers: LCCN 2022055080 (print) | LCCN 2022055081 (ebook) |
ISBN 9780367548278 (hardback) | ISBN 9781032482651 (paperback) |
ISBN 9781003090762 (ebook)
Subjects: LCSH: Animal welfare. | Crime scenes. | Criminal investigation.
Classification: LCC HV4708 .M38319 2023 (print) | LCC HV4708 (ebook) |
DDC 636.08/32–dc23/eng/20230130
LC record available at https://lccn.loc.gov/2022055080
LC ebook record available at https://lccn.loc.gov/2022055081

ISBN: 978-0-367-54827-8 (hbk)
ISBN: 978-1-032-48265-1 (pbk)
ISBN: 978-1-003-09076-2 (ebk)

DOI: 10.4324/9781003090762

Typeset in Minion Pro
by codeMantra

To all the unknown, unloved, and abused animals everywhere.
Dedicated especially to Puppy Doe, who illuminated the way.

Contents

9   Animal Abuse Involving Large Animals   91

MARTHA SMITH-BLACKMORE

10   Releasing the Scene   99

VIRGINIA M. MAXWELL

11   Biological Evidence   103

VIRGINIA M. MAXWELL

12   Trace and Chemical Evidence   121

VIRGINIA M. MAXWELL

13   Pattern Evidence   135

VIRGINIA M. MAXWELL

14   Drugs and Controlled Substances   151

VIRGINIA M. MAXWELL

15   Digital Evidence   159

VIRGINIA M. MAXWELL

Authors

Virginia M. Maxwell is a Professor in the Forensic Science Department and the Henry C. Lee Endowed Chair of Forensic Science at the University of New Haven. She has over 30 years of experience in Forensic Science as both a practitioner in the State of Connecticut Forensic Science Laboratory and at the University of New Haven. As a practitioner, Dr. Maxwell specialized in trace evidence, examining cases ranging from property crimes to multiple homicides; she has provided expert testimony in criminal cases at both the state and federal level. Dr. Maxwell is the director of the MS Forensic Science and Assistant Chair of the Forensic Science Department. She teaches Forensic Investigation of Animal Cruelty and has created a graduate certificate in Animal Cruelty Investigation at the University. She also teaches Law and Forensic Science at the University of Connecticut School of Law. As part of the Collaboration for investigation of Animal Maltreatment with the University of Connecticut School of Law, she has developed Animal Cruelty Investigation trainings for animal control officers and other first responders. Dr. Maxwell's research focuses on physical evidence issues in animal cruelty investigations, environmental degradation of pattern evidence and farm animal welfare. Dr. Maxwell is a member of the American Academy of Forensic Science, the Animals and Society Institute, the Dairy Cattle Welfare Council and the American Dairy Science Association. She holds a Doctorate in Physical Chemistry from Oxford University and Bachelor of Science in Chemistry from Liverpool University. She has published extensively on crime scene investigation, physical evidence, and trace and transfer evidence.

Martha Smith-Blackmore is a forensic veterinarian and president of a private veterinary forensic consulting firm, Forensic Veterinary Investigations, LLC. She frequently called as an expert witness in criminal and civil matters involving animals and is a faculty fellow of the Center for Animals & Public Policy at the Cummings School of Veterinary Medicine at Tufts University in North Grafton, MA, teaching *Veterinary Forensics*, and *Law & Veterinary Medicine*. She is a recent Visiting Fellow in the Brooks McCormick Jr. Animal Law & Policy Program at Harvard Law School. She is an associate member of the American Academy of Forensic Sciences, the National Association of Medical Examiners, the National Sheriffs Association, and the International Association of Chiefs of Police, appointed to their forensic science committee. She serves on the National Institute of Science and Technologies Organization of Scientific Area Committees in the Crime Scene Investigation and Reconstruction subcommittee.

Her forensics career has included working with a variety of police departments, animal control departments and attorneys. She trained for one year at the Massachusetts Office of Chief Medical Examiner in Boston. She has contributed her veterinary forensics expertise to the prosecution of cases of simple animal abuse, intentional abuse & torture, animal sexual abuse and animal fighting and she has also worked as a consulting expert witness for defense teams throughout the country.

Contributors

Amanda Fitch
American Society for the Prevention of
  Cruelty to Animals
New York, New York

Leigh Anne Wilson
American Society for the Prevention of
  Cruelty to Animals
New York, New York

Acknowledgments

With gratitude to the supportive colleagues who have enriched our professional lives and to our friends and families who make everything worthwhile.

Introduction

The investigation of suspected animal abuse scenes requires the same attention to detail as any other potential crime scenes, and it can be complicated by scarce investigative resources, a lack of training and familiarity with animal keeping or behavior. Once warrants are in place, crime scene investigation makes or breaks most cases; animal abuse is no different. The investigative response to crimes with animal victims has both similarities and differences to crimes against people. Physical evidence plays the same vital role; however, the differences in animal and human cases must be fully understood to avoid loss of valuable evidence through an ill-conceived search warrant or lack of appropriate documentation of both scene and victim. In some cases, such as neglect, good scene documentation alone can be sufficient to support an investigation. The first responders to many animal-related crime scenes are specialized animal control or animal protection officers who often do not have the support and training of a typical law enforcement crime scene unit or detective bureau. Without specialized training, critical documentation may be omitted, or valuable evidence not recognized and collected appropriately. The underlying complexity of animal cruelty laws and their jurisdiction brings similar confusion to the crime scene in terms of assignment of responsibility and subsequent execution.

Where sworn law enforcement personnel are involved in the response, their academy training and subsequent in-service training rarely include animal abuse-specific modules. The nuances of cruelty cases, both small- and large-scale, have little overlap with the types of cases seen on a regular basis, and important evidence and observations are easily overlooked. Indeed, even when living, animal victims cannot give a witness statement, thus there is no opportunity to compensate when omissions or mistakes occur. First responders must also be aware of the important role of forensic veterinarians both at the crime scene and beyond; whether this is for establishing probable cause, evidence collection, necropsy, examination or determination of pain and suffering.

We anticipate that this field guide will be of use to the seasoned CSI faced with the need to investigate a potential crime scene involving animals, and for the animal control officer or veterinarian less familiar with crime scene investigative techniques. Keep in mind that the harmed animal is simultaneously considered a crime scene, evidence, property and victim; investigators must not only maintain a chain of custody on the victim, but also may need to juggle the logistics of caring for over 100 suffering animals in some cases, while also having regard for owner's property rights.

Crimes against animals are considered by the FBI and the Department of Justice as crimes against society, and for good reason. Every state has legal prohibitions against harming animals – animals deserve protection from criminal activity that causes them injury or suffering, and sometimes criminal prosecution is the only pathway to releasing animals from the circumstances where they are being maltreated.

Equally important is the recognition that there is a known association between hurting animals and interpersonal violence. Animal cruelty can be a "red flag" event that signals the potential for future egregious acts. This is not to say that every animal abuser will become the next school shooter or serial killer, but the willingness to harm vulnerable animals signals a potential to be violent with people as well. In order to have public safety, it is vital that animal cruelty investigations are conducted with the same care and urgency as other violent crimes.

In less obviously violent circumstances, animals can be experiencing prolonged suffering from a lack of adequate nutrition, shelter or sanitation. In these scenes, there are frequently human victims as well, juveniles, elders or disabled persons who are unable to escape the same conditions. Intervening for animals brings the potential for the relief of human suffering too.

This text covers the basics of crime scene investigation, grounded in the realities of animal cruelty laws in the US. There is guidance on detecting, documenting, and collecting evidence, and documenting scenes, as well as advice on conduct of complex multianimal scenes such as animal-hoarding and animal-fighting scenes. The reader will learn about the collection of live animals and deceased animal evidence as well as what to do in cases of specific types of harm such as animal sexual abuse. In addition, different classes of evidence, both physical and digital, are addressed in separate chapters covering their use, limitations and specific collection and preservation issues.

The intent is that this book can be read from start to finish or can be used as a "just in time" resource to guide the investigator facing a particular scene involving crimes against animals. We hope that this field guide helps the investigator to be confident in their work documenting scenes where animals are thought to have been maltreated.

The Role of the Animal Control Officer and First Responders

LEIGH ANNE WILSON

Introduction

As of 2014, all 50 states and the District of Columbia have both misdemeanor and felony animal cruelty laws designed to punish those who commit acts of cruelty against animals. Each state law, however, differs in the specific acts that are prohibited and which species are protected. Violation of animal laws can carry significant sentences. For this reason, judges and juries expect to see the same protocols of crime scene processing and evidence handling that would be applied in human cases. While forensic procedures used in human crime scenes may also pertain to animal crime scenes, many prosecutors, investigators, and crime scene analysts are unfamiliar with evidence processing related to animal crimes, including the animals themselves (National District Attorney's Association). Animal Control Officers/Investigators have specific training and experience, which make them an essential partner in the investigation, crime scene documentation and prosecution of animal related crimes. In this chapter, we will discuss the animal welfare enforcement sector and how it differs from region to region, the subject matter expertise animal cruelty investigators bring to cruelty investigations, and best practices for the delineation of roles and responsibilities on crime scenes.

Understanding the Animal Welfare Enforcement Sector Structure

The structure and organization of traditional law enforcement agencies are largely consistent, whereas animal welfare and animal cruelty enforcement operate under a variety of structures throughout the country. There are arrays of organizations and individuals who can provide animal services to a community – some located within government agencies and others affiliated with nonprofit or for-profit organizations. Government agencies that oversee animal services may include public safety, code compliance, public health, health and human services, environmental or agricultural

DOI: 10.4324/9781003090762-1

agencies, animal services/control or public works. Nonprofit organizations may include an animal welfare league, humane society, a Society for the Prevention of Cruelty to Animals (SPCA) or an animal rescue. Examples of for-profit organizations may include a veterinary clinic, local business or a private animal control contractor (Alley Cat Allies). Understanding which agency or authority enforces animal cruelty statutes from location to location will be important in determining who to contact when faced with an animal cruelty case. See for a state-by-state comparison of agencies or authorities that enforce animal cruelty statutes, how the system is set up and how the system is funded (Vermont Humane, 2015).

Many are authorized to enforce cruelty laws, whereas others have more limited authority in terms of the laws they are authorized to enforce (National Link Coalition). Some jurisdictions have more than one agency that specifically enforces laws and ordinances, while others have none. For example, the State of Pennsylvania has humane police officers (nonprofit), as well as Dog Law officers, also known as Dog Wardens. Humane society police officers are trained and court-appointed to enforce the cruelty-to-animals section of the Pennsylvania Crimes Code. They investigate cases of animal cruelty, neglect and dog fighting, as well as rescue animals that are abandoned or mistreated, and testify in court to assist in the prosecution of animal abusers. The Bureau of Dog Law Enforcement, which is housed within the Pennsylvania Department of Agriculture, oversees annual licensing of dogs and rabies vaccinations, but it is also responsible for "ensuring the welfare of breeding dogs and puppies in commercial kennels and regulates dogs that are classified as dangerous" (Hook, 2018). Wardens do not oversee or have jurisdiction over animal cruelty; however, they receive humane officer training, so if cruelty is suspected, the warden will refer the case to a humane society police officer or a police officer for official investigation (ibid). For reference, the National Link Coalition website provides a National Directory of Abuse Investigation Agencies with links to individual states.

Other common titles of animal cruelty officers include, but are not limited to, Animal Control Officers, Animal Services Officers, Humane Officers, Humane Law Enforcement Officers, Animal Welfare Officers, and the like. For purposes of this chapter, the term "Animal Control Officer" will be used and refers to officers who perform animal cruelty investigations, but who do not have full law enforcement authority.

Animal Control Officers as Essential Partners

The role of Animal Control Officers (ACOs) has significantly evolved over the past 20 years. Whereas ACOs were once referred to as dogcatchers, their roles and responsibilities have expanded to more complex issues requiring specialized training, experience, and subject matter expertise, which law enforcement officers and other first responders may not routinely experience in their day-to-day job activities. ACO responsibilities may range from issuing citations and removing animals dangerous to humans to investigating complex animal cruelty cases including, but not limited to, animal fighting ventures, hoarding, breeding mills, nonaccidental injury, zoophilia and animal victims of satanic rituals. Responsibilities are wholly dependent on the jurisdiction in which the ACO serves.

Jurisdiction also dictates the training, experience and certification requirements of each ACO. Some jurisdictions simply require a high school diploma (or GED) and some experience in handling animals, whereas others have laws requiring successful completion of a 40-hour Basic Animal Control Officer Certification Course prior to issuing citations and annual continuing education (Leon County Animal Control Division). Basic certification courses include topics such as investigations, preparing search warrants and affidavits, breed identification and behavior, animal handling and perceptional safety, basic nutrition, federal laws for controlled substances, animal first aid and disease recognition, control and prevention (NACA). Some animal cruelty investigators receive additional certifications in advanced animal first aid, Chemical Immobilization Technician Certification, national certification in cruelty investigations and specialized certifications in horse abuse investigations and general animal cruelty investigations. While training prepares animal cruelty investigators for the multitude of situations they may face each day, field experience helps builds a unique subject matter expertise, making a well-trained ACO an essential partner to law enforcement where animal crimes are involved.

Animal cruelty investigations require specific levels of expertise and support to obtain the required facts of the crime. A study by the American Society for the Prevention of Cruelty to Animals (ASPCA) revealed that "only 19 percent of law enforcement officers stated they received formal animal cruelty training. Forty-one percent said they are familiar with animal cruelty laws in their jurisdiction, but fewer – 30 percent – admitted being familiar with the penalties" (ASPCA). In other words, first responders are not required to know everything about a crime but should know that there are resources available to support them.

Working with animals daily allows ACOs to become familiar with different animal species, including their behavior. They typically have experience and/or training about how to remain safe around potentially fractious animals and how to keep others safe as well. They may also have some familiarity with common ailments and injuries and know how to use appropriate handling techniques for animals that may be sick, injured or simply overwhelmed. Likewise, they learn to recognize symptoms and behaviors associated with diseases such as rabies, distemper, parvo, upper respiratory infections, parasites and zoonotic diseases for which they may recommend quarantining populations of animals to lessen the likelihood of disease transmission. Most importantly, ACOs gain subject matter expertise in the identification and documentation of cruelty-related conditions (Roufa, 2019).

The Role of First Responders and Other Key Partners in Animal Crime Scenes

Animal crimes may be discovered in a variety of ways. Oftentimes, law enforcement and/or ACOs will receive a complaint from a concerned citizen or because of a report by a veterinarian. Other times, cruelty is discovered through routine welfare checks at a home. In some cases, cruelty is the primary focus of a long-term investigation, and in others, it may be discovered in connection with another crime such as domestic violence or drugs. Regardless, law enforcement will more than likely be the first on scene and ultimately responsible for the case presented against the offender; however, success in animal cruelty cases often comes when multiagency collaboration and communication occurs.

One best practice is to ensure that key partners are contacted to assist with crime scenes so that crucial animal evidence is captured and documented before any alterations are made. For example, in cases of animal neglect where animals may be in poor body condition due to a lack of food and water, first responders may feel compelled to provide immediate care by offering needed sustenance to alleviate hunger and thirst. However, offering an animal food or water can significantly alter medical and behavioral evidence necessary to support probable cause for criminal charges. The neglect to which the animals are subjected must first be documented, animals identified with evidence numbers, and photographed *before* any changes to the animal's condition are made. Depending on the jurisdiction, ACOs may have training and experience in this area and, therefore, may be an essential resource in the identification and documentation of animal evidence. It should be noted that there are exceptions to providing animal care before a crime scene is fully documented. One exception involves animals found in a state of "exigency", thus requiring immediate medical care. In animal cases, exigency has an imminent life-threatening component. While first responders may feel an animal is in a life-threatening circumstance, the court may not always agree. Having veterinary exams conducted immediately is critical to show rapid intervention and removal was necessary. As such, veterinarians are another essential key resource that law enforcement should consider having on-scene.

　　While roles and responsibilities of the various disciplines may often overlap, each one is equally important in the success of an animal crimes investigation. Key partners and the roles in which they may assist are as follows:

- Law enforcement: Investigation, obtain warrants; scene control; collect and preserve physical and animal evidence; scene documentation including photographs, video, sketch, administrative paperwork; witness and subject interviews; evidence custodian; chain of custody; work with prosecutor to identify appropriate charges; court testimony.
- Animal Control Officer/National Animal Welfare Groups: Animal handling; investigation; crime scene consultation; animal documentation; evidence collection; evidence custodian; witness and subject interviews; transportation; court testimony.
- Forensic veterinarian: Conduct on-scene and postscene forensic exams; determine if animals require immediate medical care; necropsies; medical documentation; court testimony.
- Health certification veterinarian: Animals being transported across state lines require vaccinations and Certificates of Veterinary Inspection.
- Prosecutors: Determine criminal charges and prosecute criminal cases (and may or may not become involved in related civil proceedings depending on the jurisdiction).
- Local rescues and shelters: Transportation; sheltering; daily animal care.

Animal crimes such as hoarding may have mental and physical health/safety components for which other agency resources may be needed. Likewise, it is not uncommon for violence against animals to intersect with violence toward humans, thus requiring expertise and services provided by domestic violence organizations. As such, law enforcement may consider incorporating the following agencies into the investigative process:

- Department of Health and Social Services: Provide services where needed in cases such as hoarding
- Domestic violence support partners: Provide services in animal cruelty cases that also involve domestic violence
- Building inspectors: May condemn a dwelling if found unsafe in cases such as hoarding

This list is not exhaustive, but since animal cruelty crosses many spectrums, the cases may require a multiagency approach. These organizations have a specialized role in supporting animal cruelty cases. The public often expects positive outcomes for the animals as well as accountability for those who harmed them. Cross-coordinating teams like these for open communication create a positive response for an organization by addressing the human and animal elements of these crimes.

Conclusion

First responders should remember that animal cruelty is a dynamic and dimensional issue. Animal cruelty investigations require specific levels of expertise and support to obtain the required facts of the crime and ensure successful prosecution. Bringing in teams and agencies to help assist with an act of cruelty is a best practice for ensuring the best outcome.

Bibliography

Alley Cat Allies. Understanding your local government and animal control. https://www.alleycat.org/resources/guide-to-local-government-animal-control/.

ASPCA. ASPCA announces groundbreaking research study underscoring importance of animal cruelty law enforcement. 2010. https://www.aspca.org/about-us/press-releases/aspca-announces-groundbreaking-research-study-underscoring-importance-animal.

Hook J. Should you call an animal cruelty officer, or the dog warden? They're not the same. 2018. www.publicopiniononline.com/story/news/local/2018/08/16/dog-wardens-and-humane-officers-not-the-same-pennsylvania/991754002/.

Leon County Animal Control Division. Frequently asked questions. https://cms.leoncountyfl.gov/Home/Departments/Office-of-Public-Safety/Animal-Control/Frequently-Asked-Questions.

National District Attorney's Association. Unique aspects of processing animal crime scenes. https://ndaa.org/resource/unique-aspects-of-processing-animal-crime-scenes/.

National Link Coalition. How do I report suspected abuse? https://nationallinkcoalition.org/how-do-i-report-suspected-abuse.

Roufa T. What does a Humane Law Enforcement Officer (HLEO) do? 2019. https://www.thebalancecareers.com/humane-law-enforcement-officer-career-profile-974829.

Vermont Humane. State comparison. 2015. https://www.vermonthumane.org/wp-content/uploads/2015/08/State-by-State-comparison_FINAL.pdf.

Securing the Scene and First Actions

2

VIRGINIA M. MAXWELL

Introduction

The initial steps taken in the response to any reported incident will set the stage for a thorough and successful investigation supported by admissible physical and digital evidence. A crime scene processed incorrectly or not supported by adequate documentation will jeopardize any case, no matter how strong the evidence. While every case and every scene are unique in their own way, a standard methodical approach provides a strong foundation and maximizes the likelihood of thorough collection of evidence without compromising or contaminating that evidence. However, the need for flexibility with all crime scene investigations is important as information developed or evidence located can quickly change the direction of the investigation with changing priorities and additional scenes that may temporarily be of higher importance than the initial scene. Flexibility is the key to a good investigation.

Initial Response and Preliminary Scene Evaluation

The first responder to a scene has the responsibility for the early critical steps in the case investigation and the crime scene response. In animal cruelty cases, this individual might be an animal control officer or a police officer. These first steps set the groundwork for the investigation and must be undertaken in a methodical manner to ensure no important information is lost. Upon arrival at the scene, the lead investigator will undertake a preliminary scene evaluation.

The following sections address the important first steps to a crime scene response.

1. Information received
   Once a report of a potential scene has been received, the first responder should note the date, time, location of the scene and any additional information that is supplied, such as the type of incident, type of location, e.g., house, number of people or animals involved, any apparent need for emergency medical or veterinary care, etc.

DOI: 10.4324/9781003090762-2

2. Identify and establish boundaries

A comprehensive crime scene investigation requires that scene boundaries are identified and established correctly prior to scene processing commencing. During the initial phase of a scene response, information is constantly being received or developed. Rushing to set initial boundaries can leave areas subsequently determined to be of importance outside the established boundaries. The integrity of evidence obtained from these excluded areas will always be in question and likely unusable. It is better to set wider boundaries than initially thought necessary than to inadvertently omit important areas of the scene. The scope of the boundary can be determined by starting at the main location of the incident and expanding outward. Some scenes have natural boundaries, such as an interior scene, but others, such as a dog fighting operation, could ultimately be more extensive than initially realized.

A physical barrier should be set up at the primary boundary which should encompass the following:

i.   The location(s) at which the crime is believed to have occurred.

ii. Any locations to which a victim may have been moved or pursued.

iii. Any locations to which evidence may have been moved or possibly concealed.

iv. Any locations at which clean up may have occurred.

v.   Any locations at which deceased animals are thought to have been buried.

vi. Any points of entry or exit and the pathways to those points.

In addition to the primary boundaries for evidence search and collection, a secondary secure area should be established to allow for the staging of the scene personnel, evidence packaging and administrative tasks that is outside the primary boundary, but it is still a restricted entry and secure area. This secondary area may not be necessary in the case of small scenes with a limited number of responders.

3. Secure and protect boundaries

Once boundaries have been established, they must be secured and protected by designated personnel. Absolutely nothing inside the boundaries should be altered at this time; this includes moving any item, handling and replacing any items, using bathrooms, adjusting thermostats, opening or closing windows, etc. All people entering and leaving the scene must sign in and out along with the date and time of entry and exit. If primary and secondary boundaries are deemed necessary and established, both must be protected, but only those people with a designated role or purpose should be permitted beyond the primary boundary and into the active crime scene. This must be enforced regardless of the rank of the individual.

4. Initiate documentation and observations

Documentation begins at the moment the initial report of a possible crime is received with the fundamental details of the incident including the first description of the event, though this may be subject to amendments as the case develops. Early scene documentation should include location (GPS coordinate readings should be used if no street address is appropriate), date, time and any transient conditions such as the weather, temperature, smells, noises, etc., as well as initial impressions of the first responders and investigators. Nothing should be dismissed as too insignificant to document because it may become important as further information is gathered. As the scene is processed, and in particular when animals are removed from the scene, some of these early conditions will change. Reliance upon memory is not only imprudent but can appear unprofessional and may give the impression that information is being concealed.

5. Establish personnel roles

Every scene, no matter the size, must be processed in a methodical manner to ensure that all the documentation is complete, and thorough evidence collection and packaging occurs in a manner that minimizes the risk of contamination and establishes the chain of custody. Though some small scenes only require a single investigator, when multiple personnel are involved, roles must be assigned before entering the scene for the first time. If all personnel do not clearly know and understand their designated role prior to the inception of scene processing, the chances of an important step or component of scene processing being missed increase significantly. It is easy to assume that someone else will be responsible for a specific aspect of scene processing only to find that the task fell through the cracks and cannot be performed at a later date. Once the first person enters the scene, it has been changed and can never be returned to its initial state. If multiple personnel are processing the scene, then one person must be designated as the primary investigator who shall be responsible for the initial walk-through, final walk-through, and scene release. This individual should also manage the investigative response to the scene and delegate individual responsibilities.

6. Safety concerns

Upon arrival at the scene, the first responder should approach cautiously and begin an initial assessment of any possible safety concerns before proceeding further. Vigilance regarding any potential threats to themselves or other responders is important. These could include hazardous materials as well as potentially dangerous people or animals. Aside from obvious safety issues, further safety concerns might be indicated by sight, sound or unusual odors.

7. Need for emergency care

The first responder should identify whether any people or animals are in need of emergency medical care and call for appropriate assistance if necessary. Developing working relationships with veterinarians, in particular mobile veterinarians, can be useful when a scene response is needed. Any decedents, human or animal, should be left in place with no covering placed over them. Medical and veterinary personnel should be made aware of any important physical evidence that has been identified, as this might assist them in rendering appropriate aid to the sick and injured. Once aid is complete, medical and veterinary responders should leave all material or waste at the scene and make no cleanup efforts before leaving. Names and contact information for these responders should be recorded for both scene integrity and future contact for the purpose of collecting exemplar samples if needed. Information regarding the transportation and destination of any individuals requiring further care should be obtained. First responders should be aware that animals' legal status as property means any animal victims are considered evidence and should be treated as such, and consent may be required for nonemergency treatment. Prior to the departure and treatment of animals, they should be documented using photography and video so that their initial condition at the scene prior to any veterinary care is memorialized.

8. Control of live individuals or animals

Any living people at the scene should be removed as soon as possible to prevent any alteration of the scene or evidence either deliberately or accidentally. Similarly, any loose animals should also be removed and controlled. In the case of large-scale scenes with large numbers of animals, careful planning is needed prior to initiating the scene response. Plans can be developed ahead of time in case of such a situation; however, the logistics involved in the documentation, removal, transportation, veterinary examination, and subsequent housing of live animals must be in place prior to entering the scene. See Chapter 8 for a more detailed discussion of large-scale scenes.

9. Preliminary scene evaluation

All scene observations and documentation from first responders made prior to the arrival of investigators should be collected for evaluation. This may include information from the first report and that acquired during the initial steps such as live animal logistics, personal safety, etc. Prior to the entry of any scene processing personnel, the lead investigator must determine any search and seizure issues and is responsible for obtaining either consent or, in the absence of consent, a search warrant. No entry into the scene or search for, and collection of, evidence should take place without a warrant unless it has been unequivocally determined that a warrant is not necessary. The lead investigator should consult with the relevant prosecutor if any doubts exist as to the necessity of a warrant. While exigent circumstances are grounds for warrantless search, they are limited in scope and should never be relied upon as a means of avoiding the process of obtaining a valid search warrant.

10. Personal safety

All personnel entering the active crime scene should be wearing personal protective equipment (PPE) both for their own safety and to prevent contamination of the scene. PPE available should consist of masks, gloves, Tyvek suits, booties, hair coverings and even beard coverings, if necessary. In the case of suspected clandestine laboratories or hoarding scenes, full respirators should be considered as chemicals and bioaerosols may be present at toxic levels in the air. Due to other significant dangers, only personnel with appropriate training should process clandestine laboratory scenes. Personnel should never eat, drink, smoke or chew gum within the crime scene boundaries and should avoid touching their faces, eyes or mouths both inside the crime scene boundaries and prior to the removal of all PPE with subsequent thorough hand washing. Pens, notepads, phones and other similar items should be considered as potential sources of chemicals or biohazards if touched with gloved hands or taken inside the scene boundaries. If controlled substances are suspected, additional caution should be exercised as these may be absorbed through the skin and mucous membranes, and even low exposures can be toxic.

11. Live animals

If live animals are to be removed, legal possession (ownership) must be determined, and consent and voluntary surrender should be obtained from that entity (see Chapter 3). This consent must be written, witnessed and voluntarily made. Unborn animals must be considered and included when drafting documents for surrender; otherwise they must be considered property of the original party and ordered to be returned once born. If live animals are thought to require veterinary care, the lead investigator should arrange for transportation and veterinary assistance prior to entry. If any victims must be removed for emergency treatment, investigators should immediately ensure appropriate documentation is executed and transportation/destination details are recorded.

Initial Walk-Through

Once all initial scene assessment and external documentation are complete, the lead investigator should perform an initial walk-through of the scene. The purpose of the walk-through is to identify any transient or fragile evidence within the scene that should be prioritized for documentation and collection purposes. Further, this walk-through is a time to note any important scene conditions that may become important at a later stage in the investigation. These include things such as whether lights are on or off, doors are open or closed, signs of forced entry, signs of struggle, thermostat settings, whether security cameras have been disabled and many other such details. While they may seem insignificant in the early stages, once suspect and witness statements are gathered, they can provide important contradictions to information provided. In addition to specific evidence issues, the investigator should determine if an area of the scene requires particular attention or prioritization over the remainder of the scene.

A suitable pathway for entry and exit of the scene for all authorized personnel must be identified to prevent inadvertent destruction or contamination of evidence. Ideally, this path would not be an important part of the crime scene but should still be thoroughly checked for any evidence prior to use. The lead investigator may be accompanied on the initial walk-through by other scene personnel but anyone taking part should ensure that they do not alter or compromise the scene in any way during this process. Initial documentation, preliminary photographs and video may be taken during the walk-through so that, upon completion of the walk-through, all personnel can assess and determine processing strategy and prioritization. Any photographs and notes should be preserved as part of the case record as these represent the scene as first observed.

Preventing Contamination

Critical to the success of any scene investigation is maintaining the integrity of any seized evidence. This requires that all possible steps are taken to prevent contamination from the initial arrival at the scene to the release of the scene. Every interaction of investigators or other individuals with the scene is an opportunity for contamination to occur. Thus, it is critical that all personnel are aware of, and following, the standard procedures to minimize the potential for contamination. Scene access must be limited to only those personnel who are involved in processing. No individual should be admitted solely for the purpose of curiosity; maintaining and enforcing a written record of those entering the scene often helps to prevent unnecessary visitors.

Once a designated pathway of entry and exit is established, that should be the only route followed into and out of the scene. Outside of the search, documentation and evidence seizure, all other crime scene activities should take place in the secure staging area established when the scene boundaries were determined. This area can also be used for the storage of supplies, field instrumentation and trash containment.

Safety Issues

1. Crime scenes can pose numerous hazards to an unwary or unprotected individual. These consist of biological, physical and chemical hazards, and investigators must be vigilant as they work. Carelessly reaching into a pocket or drawer can result in an injury from a dirty needle exposing the investigator to both biological and drug hazards.
2. PPE must always be worn when working in a crime scene. While the initial walk-through is a time for preliminary identification of safety issues, it cannot always identify every hazard the investigator might encounter. In addition, when encountering blood, it will be handled before it has been determined whether it is human or animal in origin and the investigator might never know what pathogens it contains. Thus, all biological materials should be considered to be infectious and handled as such. Biological hazards in animal cruelty crime scenes can go beyond the typical ones considered such as blood-borne pathogens like HIV and Hepatitis C. Zoonotic hazards and parasites are rarely encountered in crimes against people but are a potential danger in animal abuse scenes. Investigators must remain aware of this and treat animal abuse scenes with the same attention to safety as any case involving human biological material.
3. Certain types of animal abuse cases are commonly associated with illicit substances, whether they are given to animals, or their abuse may co-occur with the animal abuse. Some controlled substances, such as fentanyl and LSD, can be highly toxic in very low doses and can also penetrate the skin. Investigators should consider double gloving and always replace any protective equipment that gets punctured or torn immediately. Care must also be taken to avoid touching the face, eyes or mouth with gloved hands, as well as items such as pens that might be subsequently handled with bare skin.
4. Respiratory hazards are usually present in hoarding scenes and suspected clandestine laboratories. While clandestine laboratories are processed by specialized teams, initial entry might be made while responding to an animal abuse report. The level of ammonia and

other chemicals is an important piece of information in scenes containing large numbers of animals such as hoarding or puppy mill cases, and those scenes should not be aired out before readings can be taken. All investigators entering the scene during the early stages should wear respirators until the atmosphere can be made safe.

Final Thoughts

The early steps in any crime scene investigation, no matter the size or scope, must be undertaken methodically and regarded as no less important than the actual search and collection of evidence. Rushing or omitting some early steps can jeopardize the investigation through loss or contamination of evidence, or rendering it inadmissible at the trial stage. Further, it can lead to an overall impression of sloppiness and unprofessional work that can also taint an investigation.

Search and Seizure

3

VIRGINIA M. MAXWELL

Introduction

All search and seizure actions of a crime scene investigation must be lawful and in compliance with the Fourth Amendment rights of an individual. This states that "The right of the people to be secure in their persons, houses, papers and effects against unreasonable searches and seizures shall not be violated". Thus, "reasonable" search and seizure is permitted, and it is people, rather than places, that are protected. While there are specific circumstances under which a search can take place without a warrant, it is cleaner and eliminates many possible future challenges if search and seizure is done with a legal search warrant whenever possible. If it is not clear that a warrantless search is permitted, then investigators should always err on the side of caution and get a warrant. In some cases, exigent circumstances will permit initial entry to be warrantless, but once the issues that required exigency have been addressed, no further search and seizure should take place without procuring a legal search warrant. Examples might include animals in critical condition or evidence that is likely to be destroyed.

Further complicating search and seizure issues in animal cruelty cases is the legal status of animals who are considered to be property. Thus, in the absence of exigent circumstances such as imminent danger to the animal, animals must be voluntarily surrendered, or legally seized with a warrant. When seeking consent to seize an animal, the right of the individual to provide the consent must be established, e.g., legal ownership.

The Fruit of the Poisonous Tree doctrine subjects all evidence and analytical results derived from unlawful search and seizure to inadmissibility challenges regardless of their significance to a case. If evidence is unlawfully seized, as far as the Court is concerned, it does not exist, nor does any evidence or information derived from it. It may not be used to confront the accused in the case. Investigators should always obtain a search warrant unless it is absolutely clear that exigent circumstances or a warrantless search applies, keeping in mind that exigent circumstances may not cover a full search before obtaining a warrant becomes necessary.

While a full discussion of the Fourth Amendment as it applies to animal maltreatment is beyond the scope of this book, this chapter will address potential pitfalls and the scope of search warrants.

DOI: 10.4324/9781003090762-3

Warrantless Search and Other Special Cases

The Supreme Court ruled that warrantless search may comply with the Fourth Amendment as long as it is reasonable under the circumstances. While some of the specified conditions determined might apply to an animal cruelty case, most will not. It is worth considering that many animal-fighting cases are discovered through other criminal activity, thus some warrantless searches for other reasons might reveal evidence related to animal fighting. In this case, it would be advisable to consult with a prosecutor and determine whether a warrant is required to address evidence specifically related to animal fighting.

In regard to animal cruelty, the situations in which warrantless search is permitted are as follows:

1. Consent: Police may conduct a search without a search warrant if they obtain consent. Consent must be freely and voluntarily given by a person with a reasonable expectation of privacy in the area or property to be searched. When seizing animals, legal possession should be determined for the purposes of obtaining consent. Consent should be obtained without duress, in writing and witnessed. Consent may be withdrawn at any time.
2. Plain view: Evidence may be seized without a warrant if an investigator is lawfully at a location, the evidence of a crime is found in plain view and the investigator did not have probable cause to believe that the evidence was there. However, plain view does not extend to picking up or moving items to see what they may conceal; no manipulation of any object to reveal information (such as a serial number) or another item is permissible. Plain view also does not extend beyond the location in which the investigator is lawfully allowed to be, e.g., another room or area into which the person has not been invited. In regard to animals, it must be visibly apparent that the animal has been subjected to abuse; the animal may not be handled to make this determination.
3. Evictions: If an individual has been legally evicted from premises and has left animals behind at that location, those animals may be seized without a warrant. It is advisable to ensure that the eviction was legal. If the individuals have vacated the premises prior to legal eviction, abandoned animals may still be lawfully seized. Other abandoned property is addressed below.
4. Free of restraint: When an animal is legally required to be restrained in some manner, such as by a leash or a fence, and is roaming free, then the animal may be seized. This does not generally apply to cats unless other circumstances apply, such as an injury to the cat.

5. Open fields: The Supreme Court ruled that the Fourth Amendment does not cover open fields thus searches of areas like pastures, woodlands, open water and vacant lots do not comply with the requirements of probable cause and warrants. If a location is clearly posted as "No Trespassing", then seek advice before entering as there may be jurisdictional variation on whether a warrant is required.

6. Exigent circumstances: Impoundment of an animal without a warrant is always permissible when exigent circumstances are present. Exigent circumstances in animal abuse cases would be those in which immediate action must be taken to ensure the safety and well-being of the animal. Examples of exigent circumstances as they pertain to an animal include heatstroke, downed livestock, animal is unresponsive, extreme weather and lack of shelter, animal tangled in a restraint in a dangerous manner, etc. Exigent circumstances may also include a situation where the owner is not home, but the animal requires immediate assistance. It is important that exigent circumstances are determined objectively, and witnessed or photo/video documented, as claiming exigent circumstances existed when they did not will result in loss of evidence from the investigation. For example, an animal with a limp does not trigger exigent circumstances, nor does an underweight animal or one that is already dead. Courts may apply a "reasonable person" approach to exigent circumstances; a reasonable and objective person would conclude that the animal's life is in danger if not rescued. If exigent circumstances are used as the reason to seize an animal without a warrant, then that animal must be taken to a veterinarian immediately; otherwise it can be inferred that the situation was not urgent, and the animal would have survived if the investigator had taken the time to get a legal warrant.

Exigent circumstances may also exist if there is a real danger of evidence being lost or destroyed during the time needed to obtain a warrant, for example, deliberate destruction by the suspect or loss of transient evidence. However, with digital technology available to obtain warrants, this time frame is now significantly reduced, thus if possible, a search warrant should be obtained ahead of time if the possibility of evidence destruction or danger to the animal victims is suspected.

Scope of the Search

In preparing the search warrant, investigators must ensure that it comprehensively covers the scope of search required both in terms of physical locations and evidence sought. While warrants for animal cruelty cases have many similarities to those used in other cases, there are nuances that must be considered to ensure that a thorough search is possible and minimize the need to reapply for a more comprehensive warrant. These include the following:

1. Animals
   The warrant should comprehensively include all animals, living or dead, as well as unborn animals. If unborn animals are omitted from the warrant, they must be returned upon birth. Animals should be included regardless of whether they are specifically contained or free roaming.
2. Locations
   All places that animals, or their remains, can be confined, sheltered, hidden or buried must be on the warrant. This can include houses, outbuildings, sheds, cars, car trunks, cages, crates, appliances, such as refrigerators, attics, basements, crawl spaces, and any other places that an animal, living or dead, can be hidden. Specifically stating that the search must include above and below ground will permit excavation of animal remains, or other buried evidence. Fenced pastures and gated fields should also be specifically included, as should both attached and unattached structures.
3. Records
   Records pertaining to the animals can include proof of ownership, veterinary records, sales receipts, pedigree certificates, training records, prescriptions, food bills, intake or export records, boarding receipts or contracts and any photos/videos of communications relating to the animals. These records may be in both hard copy and digital format; thus the warrant must include all digital devices, media and storage devices. Access to cloud storage should be verified as this may be permissible if undertaken via devices lawfully seized rather than via subpoena from the cloud host. However, ownership of data uploaded to the cloud may be a contentious area as some data are uploaded voluntarily but other data are collected involuntarily.
   In addition to specific records related to the animals, any records that pertain to ownership or occupancy of the location, vehicles and other places evidence may be located should also be included.
4. Transportation
   Any items used for transportation of animals including vehicles, trailers, blankets, beds, crates and carriers.
5. Training and control
   Any items and equipment used for breeding, training or control of animals

6. Medical supplies
   Any veterinary supplies, including paraphernalia, regardless of the species or specific animal listed on any labeling.
7. Miscellaneous
   Cleaning supplies and other chemicals, food and water containers including samples of contents, dirt or other material that may have absorbed chemicals, blood or any other substance of interest.

Special Considerations

1. Personnel
   When compiling a search warrant, all non law enforcement personnel who will be assisting in the execution of the warrant should be listed on the warrant. These personnel might include veterinarians, shelter personnel responsible for transportation of the animals and any other volunteers who will be assisting with the animals. No unlisted people can be involved in the execution of the warrant. Bringing media representatives and other unnamed parties is considered to be a violation of the Fourth Amendment.
2. Curtilage
   Curtilage is the area immediately surrounding a residential building where privacy is presumed. There is no exact distance defined; however, it is dependent upon the proximity to the building, such as areas where a visitor might enter, and the seclusion from public pathways. When determining if an item is located within a dwelling's curtilage, courts will typically consider: the proximity of the item to the dwelling, whether the item is within an enclosure surrounding the home, what the item is used for and what steps, if any, an individual took to protect the item from people passing by.
3. Mail Carrier Rule
   The "Mail Carrier Rule" is sometimes used when determining where investigators may lawfully enter. This rule allows a person to enter into areas not considered curtilage and where anybody else, including mail carriers, might legally enter, keeping in mind that they should take a direct route to the most obvious main entrance of the domicile. Once there, they may take enforcement action in regard to any activity that is in plain view. Agencies should seek guidance before using this approach.
4. Use of drones and aircraft
   In some cases, preliminary surveillance of suspected illegal activity is undertaken with the use of aircraft or drones. Caution should be exercised when surveilling a property this way as, even when illegal activity is visible from these aircraft, any entry must still be lawful

within the constraints of a search warrant. In prior cases in which surveillance drones showed illegal material, such as marijuana plants, and entry was made without a search warrant, the evidence was ruled inadmissible. In any situation where the use of a drone is considered, it is advisable to seek guidance regarding the necessity of a warrant.

5. Abandonment

   If property, such as personal items, is abandoned, then the owner no longer has an expectation of privacy in that property. Thus, the police may seize it without a warrant. However, the individual must have voluntarily relinquished the property and therefore have no further expectation of privacy in the property. Abandonment also depends upon the individual's intent which is determined by their actions; if the property is left in a public place, thrown away, or placed in a location where it can no longer be retrieved by that individual, the property is abandoned. This is similar to the "Eviction" category of warrantless searches.

6. Third-party doctrine

   The "third-party doctrine" covers information that is voluntarily given to a third-party, forfeiting the individual's privacy in the facts they have conveyed. This typically relates to phone companies, internet service providers, e-mail servers and banks. While this doctrine removes the search warrant requirement to obtain this information, it does not mean that the information can be obtained in the absence of a subpoena.

Seizing Live Animals

The application of search and seizures laws to live animals will depend upon their need for urgent veterinary treatment. As discussed previously, those animals who require urgent veterinary assistance fall under the exigent circumstance exception to a search warrant, while the remaining animals must be left in place until a valid search warrant or consent of the owner is obtained. Consent requires that two criteria are met to be valid. First, consent must be freely given and should be in writing with a witness present to attest to this fact later if needed. Secondly, the person giving consent must have legal possession of the animal. In some cases, possession is determined as the person providing regular food, water and shelter to the animal, while in others, there is a formal paperwork in place.

If a search warrant is required, the premises should be secured until that warrant is obtained to ensure that no evidence can be lost or removed during the intervening interval. In some cases, veterinary input regarding the need to seize animals should be considered when drafting a search warrant.

Generally, veterinary diagnostic tests (laboratory work, imaging) for the purposes of developing a treatment plan and the alleviation of pain or other suffering are allowed after seizure, without seeking further permission. Treatment of medical conditions is permissible but treatment that will alter the animal, such as spaying or neutering, is generally not allowed. In cases where the animal is suffering a life-threatening condition, emergency treatment is permissible. For cases where an animal is irredeemably suffering, this may include euthanasia. To be safe and if there is time, it is best to seek the advice of the prosecutor before undertaking such actions.

Final Thoughts

When conducting a search for evidence or seizing animals, it is always best to obtain a lawful search warrant before proceeding. This warrant is obtained based on an investigator affidavit and probable cause, and no information should be based on nondefensible statements or exaggerated in order to obtain the warrant. When investigators believe that a warrantless search is permissible, they must be certain that this is the case and ensure that they do not exceed the limits of this search. Whenever doubt exists as to the need for a warrant or in its preparation, investigators should consult a prosecutor or other relevant attorney. If consent is given for a search, thus removing the need for a warrant, this consent must be freely given, and it is prudent to have consent both witnessed and in writing.

Any violations of the Fourth Amendment will trigger the Fruit of the Poisonous Tree doctrine and result in the exclusion of potentially valuable evidence, no matter how important that evidence nor heinous the crime. If in doubt, it is always better to get a warrant.

Bibliography

Bandiero A. *Search & Seizure Survival Guide: A Field Guide for Law Enforcement.* Independently Published. 2021.

Palmore CJ. *The Police Handbook on Searches, Seizures and Arrests. A Law Enforcement Reference Guide.* Teller Books. 2014.

Phillips A, Lockwood R. *Investigating and Prosecuting Animal Abuse.* National District Attorneys Association. 2013. https://www.sheriffs.org/publications/NDAA-Link-Monograph.pdf.

Documenting the Crime Scene

4

VIRGINIA M. MAXWELL

Introduction

From the first call for assistance to the final release of a crime scene, thorough and continuous documentation in different forms is a hallmark of a well-executed crime scene investigation. It is often said that "if it isn't written down it never happened", and this should be at the front of every scene investigator's mind as they go about their assigned tasks. While specific individuals may have overall responsibility for different aspects of documentation, other investigators should still take notes as they go about their work. However, as a note of caution, while every smartphone puts high-quality photography in our pockets, using these devices for crime scene photography renders them available for discovery at trial. Regardless, there will always be times when there is no option but to use a phone if no other camera is available, and the benefits of documentation outweigh the limitations of discovery.

One particular nuance of animal cruelty cases is the need for documentation to continue far beyond the time of crime scene processing to document an animal's recovery. In cases in which live animals are removed from the scene to shelters or veterinary care, the condition and appearance of these animals will not remain static and will change, and improve, as time passes between scene response and the judicial phase of the investigation. The court will not be able to picture the healthy, well-fed dog they might see in recent photographs placed in front of them as a frightened, neglected, emaciated animal found at a hoarding scene unless photographs, video and notes are carefully taken at the time of discovery, removal of the animal from the scene and throughout the recovery period. It is also important to ensure that animals are documented from all aspects (from both sides, front and back, from the top and the underside, if possible) to clearly show their condition and recovery. Neglect cases in some form comprise the highest percentage of animal abuse cases, and the physical changes in an animal over time can be dramatic. Thorough documentation in all its forms can significantly improve the chances of an animal abuse case reaching trial; in fact, there is no easier way to stall a case, or cause it to be dismissed, than inadequate documentation.

Complete scene documentation will encompass different forms including notes, photographs, sketches and video. It is recommended that all are

DOI: 10.4324/9781003090762-4

used extensively in animal abuse cases both at the time of scene process-ing and throughout the recovery of the animal(s). Because victims in animal abuse cases cannot be interviewed or testify, video should be freely used to memorialize the appearance, movement, responses to food, water or people and vocalizations of the animal victims of these cases.

Crime Scene Notes

The written record of a crime scene investigation begins the moment that the first call for assistance is received. From this point forward, a meticu-lous record of dates, times, personnel, observations and information received should be maintained and placed in the case file. Notes must be recorded chronologically as the investigation unfolds and actions are taken, not from recollection afterward. A phone log should be maintained in which each call should be noted with the date and time, the participants (including who initi-ated the call) and notes of the conversation.

Notes may be grouped according to the different stages of the investiga-tion such as the initial report, scene briefing and allocation of duties, scene walk-through with initial observations, scene processing (including screen-ing tests and evidence location), collection and packaging of evidence, final walk-through and release of scene. When multiple scenes are involved, then each scene should be addressed separately. While the existence of multiple scenes may be known in advance, in complex cases, these scenes might be uncovered as the case proceeds. Regardless, each scene should have a sepa-rate set of notes.

Notes are the primary mechanism by which observations are recorded and their scope should not be limited to just visual observations. Any tran-sient observations such as temperature, weather, smell, sound and touch/feel should also be included as these may become important and not all of these can be effectively recorded in other ways. All notes must be legible to eliminate the possibility of misinterpretation at a later date both by the note-taker or others that may rely upon them for information, including if they are subject to a discovery request at trial. If any corrections need to be made during note-taking, the note should be crossed out with a single line, initialed, and the date and time clearly written. Notes should never be obliterated. Blank spaces should not be left, and if any remain on a page, they should also have a line put diagonally through them, with initials, date and time. If any information needs to be added to the scene notes, it should be done clearly with the initials of the person, the date and the time. Once scene processing is complete, a formal crime scene report must be generated and maintained with other reports relating to the case.

All notes should be maintained in the case file for future use and review, even after the final report is complete.

When confronted with the challenges of a large-scale scene, such as animal fighting, puppy mills or hoarding, with the logistics of scene processing, triage, treatment and removal of the animals, it can be easy to lose track of fundamental tasks as the scene progresses. Detailed notes can provide clear and accurate recollection of these complicated situations both as scene decisions are made and at later stages in the investigation. They can also be used for reference during the scene to ensure that all tasks have been assigned and performed.

The following is a list of information that should be recorded at every scene, though note-taking should not be constrained to only these items:

1. Date and time
   a. Note that if the scene processing takes multiple days, then the date/time should be recorded each time scene processing ends and re-commences. Any personnel changes and assignments should also be noted.
2. Location
   a. This might be a street address, a GPS reading or both.
   b. In rural locations, it may not be possible to determine an accurate street address.
   c. In the case of scenes that cover a large area, investigators must remain aware of town, county or state lines as their jurisdiction may not extend to the entire scene.
3. Personnel present
   a. It is appropriate to also list the specific scene tasks assigned to each person.
4. Weather
5. Temperature
6. Transient conditions, e.g., smell, sounds
7. Initial walk-through
8. Location of evidence as it is found
9. Reagents, batch details and results for any chemical testing, including controls
10. Date and time evidence is are located, tested and seized, and by who
11. Date and time of any specific events throughout the crime scene investigation, e.g., final walk-through, release of scene, etc.

Complete and detailed records of the crime scene investigation not only assist investigators but reinforce the investigation as being open and ethical in nature. Gaps in notes, missing pages or obliterated notes can be misinterpreted to mean that information is being withheld. Further, the criminal justice system does not always work quickly, and it can be months, or even years before a case might reach the plea or trial stage. Reliance upon memory for that time period, with many other investigations taking place in the interim, is neither sensible nor appropriate. With the potential for significant lapsed time, a complete record of observations, actions and even decisions taken can assist in any re-investigation of a case or form a solid basis for charging, plea bargaining, testimony and sentencing.

There is no specified format for crime scene notes; however, when taking notes, the date and time of all specific actions, such as screening tests or collecting evidence, must always be recorded. The use of columns in a notepad (or margined paper) is common, with the date/time maintained in the left-hand column or margin and the notes written to the right of this. Some investigators also add an additional column on the right for any additional information such as batch numbers, location, etc. There is no specific correct method to use, as long as the notes are complete and clear.

Some agencies use preprinted note sheets for both general and specific purposes to ensure uniformity in note-taking and to minimize the chance of critical information being inadvertently omitted. These can include, but are not limited to, general notes pages, pages for specific situations such as room searches or vehicle processing, cover sheets for groups of notes, graph paper for sketching and evidence collection sheets.

Other notes that should be maintained as part of the crime scene investigation are phone logs, photo logs, and notes supporting specific decision-making, for example, regarding unusual evidence or additional scenes.

Crime Scene Photography

Visual memorialization of a crime scene, its surroundings and its contents provide investigators and jurors or judges with the ability to see the crime scene and processing unfold. Using photography can quickly illustrate not only the detail of a specific item or animal but also their context within a scene. Some investigators also take overall photographs of those people who observe the processing of crime scenes, as in some cases, the perpetrators of crimes will remain close by and watch how the crime scene develops.

All photographs must be carefully taken in an impartial manner so that they cannot be misinterpreted, and nothing is concealed, artificially enhanced or misrepresented. For example, in the case of neglect, the relative positions of food and water to an animal can easily be visually manipulated if photographs are not taken from multiple and unbiased perspectives, with and without tape measures or yard sticks in the frame. Similarly, lighting must be controlled to ensure that photographs portray an accurate representation of the conditions.

A detailed discussion of specific photographic techniques, such as aperture, f-stop, exposure, alternate light photography, etc., is beyond the scope of this book. However, in order to achieve well-lit, focused photographs, an investigator should ensure they fully understand the operation of their camera, whether through specific photography courses, books or even online videos. In choosing photographic equipment, it is worth considering the differences between smartphone cameras and proper photographic equipment beyond that of discovery issues on personal phones. While point-and-shoot cameras abound, a good DSLR camera with a variety of lenses and a detachable flash is always the best choice for high-quality crime scene documentation. Fortunately, the prices of these have reduced, and compact, high-resolution mirrorless cameras with interchangeable lenses are now available at a reasonable price.

DSLR cameras can be used in fully automatic mode for the less experienced photographer and in fully manual mode for those with more experience, though photographers should be aware of the limitations of the fully automatic mode especially in terms of exposure and focus. The ranges of lenses that should be considered beyond the normal lens are the wide-angle lens, telephoto pens and a macro lens. The macro lens can be used for both closeup work and 1:1 evidentiary quality photography of fingerprint and other pattern evidence. Assembling a comprehensive photography kit that can be taken to each scene is recommended. Apart from the camera, lenses and flash, items such as tripods, filters, spare batteries and memory cards should also be part of a well-stocked kit.

While the use of personal smartphone cameras is strongly discouraged, this is sometimes the only available camera for investigators and must be used in those circumstances. If using a smartphone camera, settings such as high dynamic range (HDR) and other preset formats, such as Portrait mode on iPhones, should be turned off as these will make automatic changes to aperture, exposure and color that may not be apparent to the photographer but will misrepresent the subject of the photograph. Plain, unedited photographs are always best and no post-shoot editing should take place. Smartphone apps, e.g., Camera+, are available that include some of the features of DSLR cameras such as aperture and exposure adjustments. Any settings used should be noted though this is also stored in the metadata of each photograph.

Regardless of the camera equipment, the goal is to obtain well and evenly lit photographs that are both in focus and have a good depth of focus (achieved through a small aperture). Flash photography should be used as appropriate, and photographers should be aware of different flash techniques to ensure even lighting. Photographs should not be edited or enhanced; however, if anything is strictly necessary, then all changes should be noted, or an audit trail maintained in the editing software with the original photo preserved unedited.

Types of Crime Scene Photography

Modern crime scene photography is now primarily digital though there are still some photographers who will shoot some film to supplement the digital, but this is increasingly uncommon and is not required.

When multiple personnel respond to a crime scene, one person must be designated as the photographer and must have the primary responsibility of scene documentation; the approach of having multiple photographers is destined for failure. With more than one photographer, it is easy for the investigators to assume that someone else took important scene and evidence photographs. Further, there is another significant potential pitfall, that of two photographs of the same piece of evidence but with clear discrepancies. Consider a photograph of a bloodstain from which a swab is then taken for a screening test. Later, a second photographer's photograph is taken of the same stain, except now some has been consumed since the initial photograph was taken. There are now two photographs in existence of the same stain in which the stain looks different. Or, one investigator photographs, then picks up an item to examine it but then replaces it in a slightly different location. Photographs by a second investigator would show the difference and create problems. In an ethical investigation, all photographs must be available for examination; the "inconvenient" ones cannot be deleted. Thus, even with a designated photographer, other scene personnel should be cautious of taking casual photographs.

Sequence of Photographs

Beyond documentation of evidence, a key goal of crime scene photographs is to ensure that context can be established for both the scene and for items within the scene. This means that single photographs generally do not suffice; either the shot is too far away to see the subject clearly or too close to establish the context within the overall scene or surrounding objects. The scene should be photographed from multiple angles to ensure that the entire scene may be viewed at a later date, not just small areas. As evidence is located, a standard series of photographs is taken that consists of distance, mid-range and closeup-up photographs, both with and without a scale or other measuring device where appropriate (Figure 4.1).

1. Distance: An overall photograph(s) depicting either the entire scene, if it is relatively contained, or the overall area in which the item of interest is located. These photographs should be taken from multiple angles to capture the entire scene or particular area of the scene. The actual

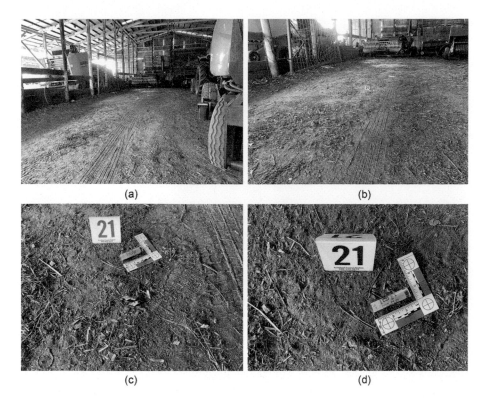

(a)   (b)

(c)   (d)

Figure 4.1 Sequence of photographs that should be taken of any important items or patterns at the scene. (a) Distance for overall context. (b) Mid-range, for context with other objects in the vicinity. (c) Close range to show relationship of item to footwear and tire impressions. (d) Closeup to show the specific item of interest.

item may not be clearly visible in this photograph, but the general area should be clear when viewed in conjunction with the mid-range shot.

2. Mid-range: A photograph that shows the specific area in which an item is located. Unless the item is actually concealed, it will be visible in this photograph but any details on the object may not be apparent.
3. Close range: A photograph showing only the item of interest or even just a portion of it (in which case there must be a photograph of the object in its entirety).

Use of Scales

It is important to use some kind of appropriately sized measuring device such as a scale, ruler or tape measure in crime scene photography. Other than the overall scene photographs, which may depict an area that is simply too large, some form of measurement should be used to provide an

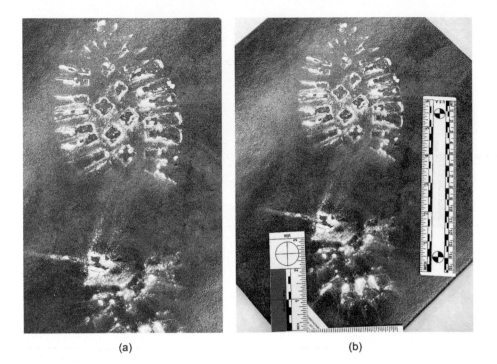

(a)   (b)

Figure 4.2 Photo documentation of a footwear imprint in a white powder (a) without a scale and (b) with a scale.

accurate representation of size and relative positions of items or patterns. It is customary to take photographs both with and without a scale (Figure 4.2a and b). Scales in photographs need to be clearly visible scales and may be purchased in several different colors to ensure maximum contrast is possible. Scales are also available in both a linear and L-shaped configuration, as measurements in two axes are useful especially when photographing patterns. For clarity, case numbers and item numbers may be written directly onto scales to ensure they are clearly visible in all photos.

As a word of caution, contamination issues must be considered when using non-disposable scales. If the same scale is going to be used throughout the scene, then it should be cleaned after each use with either ethanol or 10% bleach. Alternatively disposable self-adhesive scales are widely available. Further, when documenting wet stains, care must be taken to avoid smearing.

Evidence Markers

Evidence markers are used at crime scenes to designate the location of items of evidence as they are found (Figure 4.3). Photographs should be taken both before and after evidence markers are placed and added to the crime scene.

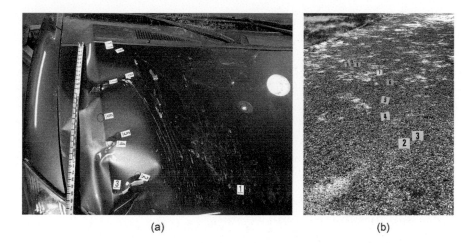

(a)   (b)

Figure 4.3 Use of evidence markers to highlight the location of evidence. (a) Small adhesive markers to indicate evidence on the hood of a vehicle that struck a victim. (b) Yellow markers to show the location of spent casings from a shooting.

It is a better practice to take photographs prior to the placement of markers rather than pick them up and then replace them to ensure continuity and avoid slight changes in position in different photographs. Though the standard color of evidence marker is yellow, other colors may be purchased (or printed on colored cardstock) for use at complex or large-scale scenes if differentiating between types or sources of evidence is useful for clarity.

Photo Log

A photo log may be maintained recording each photograph taken at the scene. If maintained, it should include the date, time, location and photographer, as well as a very brief note of the subject in each photo, e.g., overall living room or west wall of kitchen. When photographing scenes containing hundreds of animals, resulting in thousands of photographs, photo logs may not be used by some agencies, who instead rely on the sequential numbering of the photos derived from the camera. When taking digital photographs, the camera settings used are generally recorded in the metadata of each photograph; however, the specific equipment used should be noted, including the serial number, if desired. If used, the completed photo log should be maintained in the case file.

Drone Photography

Overall photographs of large scenes used to require the use of aerial photography from a small plane, or the use of cranes, both of which were prohibitively expensive for most agencies. The widespread availability of drones with photographic capabilities has now made aerial photography accessible to most agencies. Scenes that are large and fully, or partly, outdoors should always now be considered candidates for an overall aerial view using drones. In addition to regular photography, forward-looking infra-red (FLIR) photography is now available on drones which may help in identifying live evidence and other thermal information. It should be noted that the downdraft from a drone can displace valuable evidence so caution must be exercised when drones are used.

Examination-Quality Photographs

Taking examination-quality photographs is common for some types of physical evidence and is highly recommended when enhancement, lifting or casting techniques have the potential to damage the actual evidence. Examination-quality photographs are those which can be used at a later date for measurements or comparisons to known samples, and from which conclusions will be drawn. They are not taken for the sole purpose of scene documentation and these photographs are shot with care. The types of evidence for which these photographs are recommended include footwear and tire imprints/impressions, latent prints, questioned documents and blood spatter patterns. When shooting examination-quality photographs, care must be taken to ensure that the subject is evenly lit and the camera is precisely perpendicular to the subject, as any deviation from this will cause apparent elongation or shortening of the subject. Thus, the use of tripods and plumb lines or levels is recommended (Figure 4.4). Further, a scale must always be included in the photographs to ensure printed photographs are 1:1 in size. Special 1:1 lenses are available for most DSLR cameras.

Video

Video is an integral part of crime scene documentation and serves many purposes in memorializing the scene for investigators and for presentation at trial. Video can be taken during the initial walk-through of the scene to highlight any problem or important areas and for use in team briefings before scene processing begins. The accompanying audio can capture the initial sounds of the scene prior to entry and removal of animals. Though video is an integral part of all crime scene investigation, it can play a larger and more important role in animal cruelty cases, providing video and audio documentation of not only the crime scene but also the condition of the animals themselves.

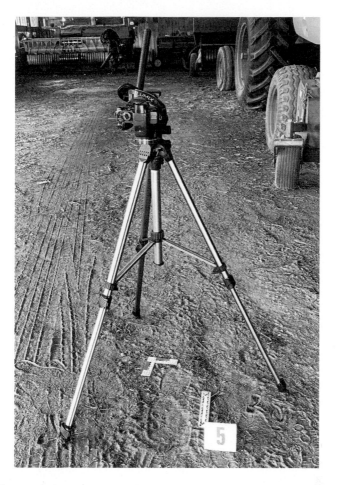

Figure 4.4 Typical set up to produce an examination-quality photograph of a footwear impression in dirt. Note the scales, evidence marker and the tripod (with built-in spririt [bubble] level) to ensure that the photograph is perpendicular to the impression.

Use of Video in Animal Cruelty Cases

Animal cruelty cases are often likened to homicides; in both instances, the victims cannot be interviewed. Animals cannot provide a statement describing the actions taken by their abuser; however, video can provide invaluable information regarding their condition, injuries and behavior that indicate pain or fear. Further, when confronted with a suspect who denies maltreatment of the animal or provides excuses as to the condition of the animal, video can be used to provide affirmation or contradiction of their statements. For example, audio can capture sounds of animals in pain or distress, and with a victim that cannot speak, this is invaluable for veterinarians and also illustrates the conditions and the animals at trial. A photograph cannot show if an animal is limping, whether their gait indicates previous injuries or whether they are fearful, but all are clearly seen with video. When the owner of a neglected companion animal says that they are emaciated because they won't eat, video can show how that same animal responds when given food and water. Video also captures the response of an animal to a particular person, whether they are fearful or aggressive. The use of video in animal cruelty cases extends far beyond the videos of regular crime scenes and regular follow-up video of the animal victims can be taken over time to document their recovery. Thus, the additional uses of video in animal cruelty can include the following:

1. Audio: Sounds of animals in distress or sounds of aggression.
2. Gait: The movement of the animal in a way that indicates injury or weakness.
3. Injuries: The presence of visible injuries on the animal and whether the animal can stand unaided.
4. Response to people: Whether the animal shows fear toward certain people.
5. Response to food and water: Whether an emaciated animal will eat or drink when provided with good food and clean water.
6. Change in animal with time once it is removed from the owner and/or the scene and provided with regular food, water and veterinary care.
7. Location and condition of food and water at scene, whether they are accessible to the animals and whether any tethered animal can reach them.
8. To document humane handling by individuals collecting animals, to refute future claims that injuries were inflicted by the responders capturing animals.

Other Sources of Video

While video of animals taken at the crime scene will show the condition of animals at the time the animals are seized, other sources of video can be used to show how the condition of an animal deteriorated with time, the sequence of events at the scene, sources of injuries or even specific acts of cruelty taking place. Indeed, seized videos can even launch new paths of investigation and other, previously unknown, victims are discovered. These videos can be obtained from many other sources such as home security cameras, computers, cell phones and CCTVs. These will be covered in more detail as digital evidence in Chapter 15, but investigators should not overlook them as valuable sources of information as to the changing condition of animals with time, or the source of injuries and other actions.

Note of Caution

When recording video, the microphone on the device should be enabled, thus any background noise, including casual conversations, will also be recorded. However, as scene videos should not be edited, these conversations cannot be deleted without placing the veracity of the video into doubt. Microphones are now remarkably sensitive, so it is a good practice to have all nonessential personnel relocate to the staging area while the crime scene video is being recorded. Cell phones and other audible electronics should be placed on silent mode anytime video is being recorded.

Sketching

Sketches are used to produce a scale presentation of the scene showing the location of victims and evidence. While new technology is available to assist in this process and to produce high-quality finished sketches, there is still no replacement for pen and paper in making rough sketches and recording measurements during scene processing. Traditionally, there are two types of sketch; the rough sketch made in real time during crime scene processing and the final sketch that is made at a later date with the rough sketch as the basis. If the scene is large and complex, there may be several sketches consisting of an overall diagram to show the overall scene and position of relevant areas, as well as sketches of each of these areas and the items, or victims, contained within them.

Rough Sketches

Rough sketches are made in real time by a designated investigator at the scene. They are hand-drawn representations of the scene and location of victims, major or immovable objects and items of evidence and are not drawn to scale. They are used to record measurements taken for the purposes of producing a final scale drawing. The general process is to start with general location, e.g., room outline, and then fill in the larger objects before adding items of evidence, or patterns, as they are located. All measurements used to plot the location of an item on the sketch must be triangulated, i.e., the measurements must be taken from two fixed points that should be identified on the sketch. This process has been facilitated by the use of accurate laser measurement devices that are now readily available for a reasonable cost. All objects in the sketch should be identified in some way to ensure that the final sketch will be accurately labeled. If annotations on the actual sketch are not possible due to space constraints, a legend should be created to detail all labels and symbols. The rough sketch should also have case and location-specific information recorded including:

Date and Time
Case Number or Identifier
Investigator
Location of the scene whether street address or GPS location
Compass North
Legend, if needed

The rough sketch should be thoroughly checked for completeness prior to the release of the scene to ensure that all items and measurements are recorded.

Finished Sketch

A final finished sketch is produced from the rough sketch, though both sketches should be maintained in case records. The final sketch can be produced either by hand (with appropriate drafting tools) or using widely available computer software or apps. The final sketch should be drawn to scale with all major objects and items of evidence included on the sketch. A legend identifying any symbols, numerical labeling or abbreviations and a compass identifying north should also be present. The finished sketch must also be labeled with the same scene and case-specific information as the rough sketch.

New Technology for Documentation

Technological advances have brought new products that create visual renditions of crime scenes to the market. These can produce highly accurate measurements for incorporation into computer-assisted diagrams (CAD) of the scene and, in some cases, automated 3-D renderings of specific areas of the scene. While the cost of these products may be prohibitive for smaller agencies, larger agencies may already have these available. Examples of these technologies include Total Station˚ (Leica) and FARO˚.

Total Station˚ is a tool that was originally developed for surveyors which has now moved into widespread use by law enforcement. It accurately measures horizontal distances, slope distances, angles, height differences and 3D coordinates. These are then downloaded into diagramming software to produce scaled 2D and 3D diagrams.

FARO˚ is an example of a 3D scanner. These devices can be placed in the scene and remotely controlled to scan the scene and to produce a 3D rendering via the accompanying software. They can be attached to tablet computers as well as regular desktop and laptop computers.

At a far lower price point is the use of handheld laser measuring devices, such as Leica DISTO, that can sync with smartphone and tablet apps, either free or low cost, to produce sketches as the investigator takes measurements.

Final Thoughts

"If it isn't written down it never happened" is the mantra that all scene investigators should remember as they take notes and photo document the crime scene and investigator actions. Thorough documentation of all scenes is important, but in the case of animal cruelty scenes, this documentation must extend after the scene investigation is complete and the scene has been released to ensure that the initial condition and recovery of an animal victim are clearly shown.

While all investigators can, and should, make notes as they go about their work, care must be taken in regard to photographs. Having numerous photographers at a scene can lead to slight discrepancies in photographs which can lead to challenges in court and sabotage a case.

Bibliography

Edelman GJ, et al. Infrared imaging of the crime scene: Possibilities and pitfalls. *Journal of Forensic Sciences.* 2013;58(5):1156–1162.

FARO. Forensic analysis and pre-incident planning solutions. https://www.faro.com/en/Application/Forensic-Analysis-and-Pre-incident-Planning.

Gardner R. 2018. *Practical Crime Scene Processing and Investigation,* 3rd Edition. Boca Raton, FL: CRC Press.

National Forensic Science Technology Center (NFSTC). Crime scene investigation: A guide for law enforcement. 2013. https://www.nist.gov/system/files/documents/forensics/Crime-Scene-Investigation.pdf.

Robinson E. 2016. *Crime Scene Photography,* 3rd Edition. Cambridge, MA: Academic Press.

Scientific Working Group on Digital Evidence. General photography guidelines for the documentation of evidence items in the laboratory. 2019. https://drive.google.com/file/d/1L2WSneV7XM68qodTeCZjkticeLV8uWOB/view.

Locating Physical Evidence

5

VIRGINIA M. MAXWELL

The goal of a well-executed crime scene investigation is the location, iden-tification, collection and packaging of evidence to support and provide important linkages in a case investigation. While some evidence is obvious and clearly visible, other evidence is more subtle and only found through a well-planned, systematic and methodical search. Further, investigators must keep an open mind about the evidence they might encounter, not look only for items that support information received prior to arrival at the scene. The initial information provided is often fluid as the investiga-tion develops, thus focusing only on evidence that agrees with preconceived ideas can jeopardize the ability to collect items that become significant as more information is gathered. Spending time to consider all possible sce-narios and points of view is more valuable than being focused on only one theory. Considering how people and animals may have interacted and moved around the scene can open up additional areas to search. Also evalu-ating whether items are located in unusual locations, have been moved or are absent, can provide investigative information.

Regardless of the nature of the crime, information received or search pattern chosen, all searches must proceed from the least to the most intru-sive in nature. By following this rule, physical evidence is less likely to be damaged or lost in the search process, especially evidence that is frag-ile or microscopic in nature. For example, a cartridge case is easily seen and robust; there is no urgency to its collection as long as it is safe from accidental displacement. However, a single fiber is easy to overlook or dislodge and should be documented and collected early to ensure it is not lost through other activities. Every entry into, and passage through, the crime scene is an opportunity for evidence to be lost, damaged or contam-inated. Establishing a pathway through the scene for use by investigators is advisable. This pathway should be documented, searched and cleared of evidence before the remainder of the scene is addressed. Investigators must take appropriate precautions at all times to avoid contamination, including the use of Tyvek suits, booties, hair coverings and gloves. If the full protective equipment is not available, then at a minimum, gloves MUST be worn and changed often.

DOI: 10.4324/9781003090762-5

Crime Scene Searches

The initial visual scan to identify potential evidence and locations to search occurs during the initial walk-through, but nothing should be moved at that stage. Based on these observations, an appropriate search pattern can be identified which may be modified for the more intrusive levels of search to follow. Scene processing then progresses with increasing levels of intrusiveness such as moving larger objects, chemical screening or enhancement, fingerprinting, removing evidence and finally fully destructive activities such as cutting out carpets and walls.

Drones can not only be used for the photo and video documentation of a scene, but they are now available with alternate light sources for use in crime scene searches. They are best deployed at large open scenes such as outdoor scenes or large open buildings such as warehouses. They can also be of use in assessing possible risks to investigators prior to their entry into the scene. It is, however, worth noting that drones will produce air disturbances; therefore, investigators must consider what evidence, such as trace materials, might be disturbed by the flight of a drone and whether the benefits of using drones for searching outweigh this issue. The use of a drone may startle some animals, or even cause panic, so a decision on their use should be made in consultation with an expert familiar with the species of animal that may be encountered and the general condition of their containment. The drone should be flown at a height or distance that avoids the risk of being batted out of the air by an energetic animal.

When developing a crime scene search strategy, some information regarding the case will already be known, but regardless the search must be conducted with an open mind to all possible evidence that may ultimately modify the initial information or produce new avenues of investigation. When using any information received, it is important to ensure it is as accurate and objective as possible or, if this is not possible, to keep an open mind as to its possible limitations. Searching with preconceived notions about the evidence sought introduces bias to the search and could ultimately hinder the success of the investigation. Some information is immutable, for example, the victim was shot and therefore firearms evidence will obviously be important, but as the search and investigation progresses, other evidence uncovered might lead to additional searches and scenes. Further, in any crime scene, no area should be ignored with the notion that no evidence could be found there. Hiding areas for valuable, secret or incriminating items are created in the most unlikely places including those made to look like everyday items, such as fake bottles, cans and books.

While interior crime scenes are not subject to weather interferences, this may be a factor in exterior scenes and may modify the order in which the scene is searched and processed. For example, if inclement weather, such as precipitation or high winds, is imminent, then evidence documentation and collection may need to proceed more rapidly than normal, particularly in regard to evidence that might wash or blow away. Thus, the search priorities must change to ensure that evidence is not lost. The use of portable canopies can help under wet conditions but may not provide complete protection.

Available light is an additional factor when planning scene searches, especially exterior searches which can only take place in daylight without the use of additional lighting and power sources for those lights. If supplemental lighting is not available for night searches, the scene must be secured and protected until searching can commence. Unless time is of the essence, it is better to avoid searching using only flashlights as the weaker and less uniform lighting can lead to evidence being missed or even inadvertently destroyed. Searches should employ both visible and alternate light sources as some evidence that is hard to see using regular white light is clearly visible when using different wavelengths such as infrared or ultraviolet light.

When managing large-scale investigations, such as dog fighting, there may be extensive scenes that must be thoroughly processed. Dividing the scene into different areas can make the search process more manageable. However, it is advisable for the lead investigator to create clear assignments and hold regular team updates to ensure that no area gets overlooked.

Search Patterns

The most effective way to search a crime scene is to employ a specific search pattern chosen according to the location in question. Several search patterns are in common usage and with the variety of physical characteristics of crime scenes, e.g., outdoors, indoors, vehicles, etc., some are better suited for specific locations than others. The number of personnel available must also be considered in the choice of pattern, though whenever possible is it best to have at least two people searching as these individuals can search areas separately and then switch areas to ensure that nothing is missed. The common search patterns are spiral, line or strip, grid, ray and zone, described below and shown in Figure 5.1a–e.

1. Spiral search
   As the name suggests, investigators walk in a spiral pattern created by searching in a circular manner with each successive circle getting either bigger or smaller depending on whether the search is from the center to the perimeter or outward; though in moving from the perimeter inward, investigators are going from areas of lower

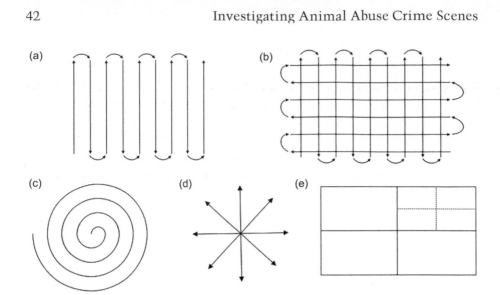

Figure 5.1 Search patterns: (a) strip, (b) grid, (c) spiral, (d) ray and (e) zone.

to higher density of evidence. Although this search pattern can be utilized for both exterior and interior crime scenes, it is most effective when searching a relatively confined area, such as a small, fenced yard versus a large open wooded area. This search pattern can be difficult if there are numerous obstacles and objects within the area. A drawback of this pattern is the difficulty of walking in a perfect spiral which thus evidence can be missed.

2. Line and strip search

    A line search can be used when several investigators are available to search simultaneously. The investigators line up and walk simultaneously in a straight line over the area to be searched. To ensure the search is comprehensive, one other individual, not taking part in the actual search, should be designated as a coordinator to start the search and keep the searchers aligned and searching in the correct direction without deviating from the straight line. A strip search follows the same straight-line approach as a line search, but there is only one investigator. This individual walks in a straight line across the specific area to be searched and then turns and walks back in an adjacent lane. With no coordinator to facilitate the search, the investigator must use care to ensure that no areas, however small, are missed. Both line and strip searches work well with defined boundaries.

3. Grid search

    A grid pattern builds upon the methodology of the strip search, but in this case after completing one full strip search, the investigator turns and repeats the strip pattern in a perpendicular direction.

This is a very thorough search pattern but also works best when there are defined boundaries.

4. Ray search

   A ray search is conducted by gathering the investigators at a set point and then they all walk outward in a straight line. There is a major drawback of this pattern as the gaps between the lines may not be thoroughly searched.

5. Zone search

   The zone search is a good option for scenes that do not readily lend themselves to the other search patterns. Two commonly encountered situations in which zone searches are ideal are large areas and vehicle interiors. When breaking a large scene down for zone searching, each zone can be searched using one of the common types of search already discussed. Coordination between investigators is important to ensure that no zone is missed or not thoroughly searched. Vehicles in particular lend themselves to this type of search as they are easily visualized as zones made from the different seating areas and the trunk.

Conducting the Search

Prior to commencing any search, investigators must consider what information they may possess about the possible events that have taken place. With this information, and any developed from the initial walk through, decisions can be taken about which areas will be priorities and the specific types of evidence that may be of higher importance, e.g., fingerprints. As the scene unfolds, the evidence located might both add to the information and change priorities that had previously been established.

Searches should progress logically from the least to the most intrusive activities. Initial searching should be restricted to visual searching exposed areas only as this is the least destructive activity. The visual search must encompass all levels, including the ceiling, where important bloodstain patterns and other evidence may be located. For example, if blunt force injury is suspected, cast off blood spatter is often found on walls and ceilings due to the weapon being swung. Visual searching is significantly enhanced by the use of alternate light sources which can highlight valuable evidence that would be missed when using only visible wavelengths of light. During the visual search, no furniture, etc., should be opened or moved, and the evidence located should be documented and collected before moving to the next level of searching.

The next level of searching is that in which objects may be lifted, moved or opened to search areas that were not visible or accessible during the initial search. Prior to any object being moved, investigators must ensure that its original condition has been documented, measured and photographed, and any evidence that could be lost has been collected. Evidence revealed as objects are moved is documented and collected as before. At any stage, it is appropriate to evaluate whether the initial search pattern in use is still the most effective or whether another pattern should be used.

Upon completion of this stage, more destructive techniques may now be introduced. These include chemical screening tests for biological fluids or drugs and fingerprint enhancement techniques. Thorough documentation of visible stains or markings should take place prior to screening tests or enhancements being used. Investigators must be aware of whether the reagents used are known to damage DNA that might be recovered from both biological fluids and epithelial cells on surfaces or in fingerprints. While most enhancement techniques have been determined to be safe to use when evidence will subsequently undergo DNA analysis, there are some that can damage DNA, including prolonged exposure to UV light.

Finally, once investigators are satisfied that they have thoroughly searched and recovered the physical evidence from throughout the scene, the final, and most destructive, stage of the crime scene search begins. This involves physically destroying parts of the scene such as cutting or removing carpets, walls and other items if it is believed that critical evidence, such as a bullet, may be located within or under them. Also at this stage, portions of items believed to be carriers of evidence, such as door frames, may be cut out to be collected and sent for further testing. If bloodstain pattern analysis is to take place, all documentation of stains, including using lasers or strings, should be complete before removing any structural material to avoid damaging patterns. In the case of exterior scenes, this phase of the search may involve cutting projectiles out of a tree, excavation to look for dead animals or dismantling enclosures or fighting pits. If available, ground penetrating radar can be used to identify potential areas for excavation. While most agencies do not have this equipment, many agencies or academic institutions that do are willing to assist.

Alternate Light Source Techniques

The use of alternate light sources (ALS) during all stages of crime scene searching can reveal evidence that is very small or has little contrast with the surface upon which it is lying, e.g., semen stains, gunshot residue or trace evidence. ALS works by using nonvisible wavelengths of electromagnetic radiation, such as infrared (IR) or ultraviolet (UV), to cause materials to fluorescence or luminesce. Users wearing colored goggles specific to the

Table 5.1 Excitation Wavelengths and Barrier Filters for Different Evidence Types

	Excitation Light and Wavelength				
	UV 260–400 nm	Violet 400–450 nm	Blue 450–490 nm	Green 490–560 nm	IR 700–900 nm
Barrier filter	No filter	Yellow	Orange	Red	
Evidence					
Hair/fibers	X	X	X	X	
Gunshot residue			X		X
Bruises/bitemarks	X	X	X	X	X
Body fluids	X		X		
Blood		X			X
Bone/tooth fragments			X		
Questioned documents (charred documents and ink comparison)					X

wavelength in use can then see those items more readily. Fibers, and other trace materials, in particular may become clearly visible using UV wavelengths of light while very difficult to see with visible light, especially if in the coat of an animal. Some biological fluids will also fluoresce under UV light and the coats of sexually assaulted animals may be searched for semen using ALS. Other items of evidence that benefit from using ALS are gunshot residues, blood on dark surfaces and bone and tooth fragments. Table 5.1 shows the appropriate goggles to use, and types of evidence found for different ALS.

There are numerous vendors of ALS which can be purchased in many different configurations and wavelengths. The configurations includes flashlight styles, broad beam, high intensity, head-mounted or even drone-mounted ALS among others (Figure 5.2). LED technology has eliminated the prior need for heavy laser equipment and power sources and has also made alternate lights more affordable. With budget limitations, UV and IR are useful ALS for most common types of evidence.

Vehicle Searches

In some animal cruelty cases, e.g., sexual assault, abandonment or theft, a vehicle must be searched for physical evidence. Zone searching is a very efficient

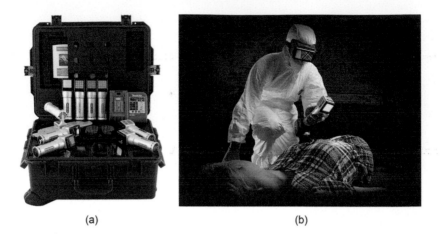

(a)   (b)

Figure 5.2 (a) Crime Lite alternate light source kit. (b) Crime Lite in use showing barrier goggles. (Both photos courtesy of Foster+Freeman Ltd.)

way of processing vehicles as they are easily divided into separate areas, such as passenger compartment (and into further zones within that), trunks and cargo areas. Figure 5.3 shows how a vehicle may be divided into zones for the purposes of a search. Vehicles have many interior compartments, some of which are not obvious, and additional hiding areas are easily created. These must all be considered and must not be overlooked during the search. If possible, vehicles should be moved into a secure, indoor location to facilitate searching and ready access to investigators, though they can be searched at a scene if necessary.

If moving is necessary, vehicles should be on a flatbed truck rather than towed or driven, which could result not only in important evidence under or on the vehicle being lost or contaminated, but also affect the mileage and other data that can be recovered from the vehicle computers. To maintain

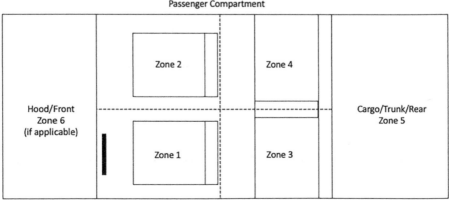

Figure 5.3 Division of a vehicle into zones.

the chain of custody, the flatbed truck should be accompanied on the journey and kept in view at all times. No one should enter the vehicle for any reason prior to the search, and the door, trunk and hood can be sealed with tamper-proof evidence tape to ensure the integrity. Seals should be placed in areas away from those that an individual might touch and leave DNA or fingerprint evidence.

Prior to moving the vehicle, the surrounding area should be carefully searched for evidence such as trace materials or impressions. If the vehicle is on a dirt surface, a control sample of the soil should be taken prior to moving in case of a later comparison to a suspect's footwear or soil recovered from the undercarriage of the vehicle.

Final Thoughts

Context must be considered in the search for evidence to avoid collecting disproportionately large amounts of evidence that do not provide probative linkage information. If an incident takes place at the location where both suspect and animal victim live, finding animal hair or the suspect's fingerprints is often of little importance unless these are found in unusual locations which are associated with the suspected activities. For example, if blunt force injuries to a dog are consistent with an impact against a hard surface, then investigators should consider collecting hairs found on such surfaces, especially when they are unusual locations, e.g., on a wall above the height of the animal, or appear to have been deposited with force rather than a passive transfer.

When searching for evidence and while the scene is still secured, investigators should not overlook the need to collect reference samples for comparison during forensic examinations. This might include items such as rolls of duct tape, garbage bags, ropes/cords, lubricants, carpet and other textiles for comparison to evidence recovered from the victim.

Crime scene searches must not be rushed, and investigators should take their time to do the search thoroughly. Once the scene is released, doubts can be raised as to the integrity of any evidence recovered at a later date.

Bibliography

Edmond G, et al. Contextual bias and cross-contamination in the forensic sciences: The corrosive implications for investigations, plea bargains, trials and appeals. *Law, Probability and Risk.* 2015;14: 1–25.

Gardner RM, Krouskup DR. 2018. *Practical Crime Scene Processing and Investigation,* 3rd Edition. Boca Raton, FL: CRC Press.

Landscape Study of Alternate Light Sources. Forensic technology center of excellence. 2018. https://forensiccoe.org/private/5dd5a78c1ff38.

National Forensic Science Technology Center (NFSTC). Crime scene investigation: A guide for law enforcement. 2013. https://www.nist.gov/system/files/documents/ forensics/Crime-Scene-Investigation.pdf.

Spex Forensics. Forensic light source applications: Wavelengths and uses. Horiba. https://www.horiba.com/fileadmin/uploads/Scientific/Documents/Forensics/ fls.pdf.

Collection and Packaging of Evidence

6

VIRGINIA M. MAXWELL

Introduction

Upon completion of the search and documentation, evidence must be correctly collected and packaged, which initiates the chain of custody for each item. Good collection and packaging of evidence are essential to prevent loss, contamination or degradation of evidence between the crime scene and the laboratory. Issues can arise through poor collection technique and packaging choices, mishandling or inappropriate storage conditions. All of these can be avoided by following accepted crime scene and evidence-handling procedures.

Crime Scene Kits and Equipment

Agencies or investigators who regularly respond to crime scenes usually have a comprehensive crime scene kit at their disposal, sometimes even a crime scene van or other vehicles. Kits are stocked with evidence collection and packaging items suitable for a range of different types of evidence. A wide variety of crime scene kits are available for purchase through specialized vendors, (see references) or they can be assembled by the investigator. Investigators often supplement commercially prepared kits with additional tools and packaging based on personal preference. If the crime scene work is more sporadic, investment in a full-scene kit may be unrealistic but assembling and maintaining a basic scene kit appropriate for small-scale scenes is worthwhile as many important items do not degrade with time and cannot always be easily obtained on short notice. A basic kit can be assembled at relatively low cost. A comprehensive listing of items for use at crime scenes, as well as some suggested vendors, is shown in Appendix A. This list contains many specialty items which are unnecessary for most scenes, e.g., excavation tools are important in dog fighting but less so in other types of cruelty, but other basic items would be necessary at every type of scene.

Items in a crime scene kit may be categorized according to purpose, such as collection, packaging, documentation, screening, etc. Many, such as containers and tools, can be obtained at common retailers, though some must be ordered from specialist vendors. When ordering items with expiration dates,

DOI: 10.4324/9781003090762-6

such as screening tests, quantities needed should be carefully assessed as these items cannot be used after those dates thus overordering can be expensive and wasteful. Expiration dates and batch numbers must be recorded in crime scene notes. Maintaining an adequate supply of personal protective equipment in every kit must not be overlooked; these items must be changed regularly during scene processing and a large-scale scene can take several days to complete. Further, double-gloving is recommended when handling some materials, such as suspected LSD.

Types of Evidence and Collection Techniques

Investigators may be confronted with many types of evidence; thus a variety of different collection and packaging methods must be available at every scene. At times, the decision may be taken to seize an item that is a carrier of evidence, such as fingerprints on a weapon, to allow processing to take place in a controlled laboratory environment. When this is not feasible, a variety of collection methods for evidence will be employed, including swabbing, scraping, cutting, picking, lifting, casting and vacuuming. Though vacuuming requires a specialized evidence vacuum, tools for the other techniques are easily obtained. When assembling these tools, the issue of contamination must be considered. If disposable items are not used, and in some cases, they do not work as well as non-disposable tools, e.g., picking fibers with forceps, then a mechanism by which tools may be sanitized at the scene must be included in the kit. If a tool is used to process multiple items without thorough cleaning, there will be a risk carryover of material from one to the next, and with highly sensitive DNA analyses, this is not acceptable and can compromise an entire case. Scalpels, forceps and other tools are readily sanitized with a 10% bleach or alcohol wipes which can be in a scene kit for this purpose. However, disposable tools are preferable when they are available and suitable for the evidence. Swabs used for either screening tests or sample collection must be sterile and packaged to avoid contamination prior to use.

Collecting and Packaging Carriers of Evidence

Almost anything can be physical evidence and provide important linkages in case investigations. Items as diverse as cocoa powder and fingerprints can be used to link individuals to locations. At the scene, evidence may be easily visible and removed from a surface, while in other cases, it may not be easily seen, and some form of enhancement or casting is necessary. In these situations, investigators have the option of attempting to recover the evidence at the scene using whatever method they have available to them there or to sieve, or sift the "surface" for processing to take place in a controlled environment with more resources available. The decision to seize a carrier of evidence is taken on a case-by-case basis and depends on several factors including ease of removal of carrier, weather (if outdoor scene), resources for processing at scene, time available, light available, personnel present, laboratory procedures or capabilities and other case-specific reasons.

When carriers of evidence are seized, then packaging must be such as to protect the area of interest, so the evidence is not damaged or lost. Fingerprints are easily smudged or smeared through rubbing so the carrier should be immobilized and contact of the area of interest with the packaging should be prevented (Figure 6.1).

Other evidence such as particulate and trace evidence can be dislodged and transferred to other parts of an item, and fragile items can be broken if not packaged carefully.

Numerous different sizes of boxes can be purchased at common retailers and boxes fabricated for specific types of evidence, such as guns, can be purchased through specialty vendors. Zip ties can be used to secure items though they should be carefully placed so that they do not damage evidence. It is prudent to wipe zip ties with alcohol or 10% bleach before use to remove any possible contamination due to prior handling. Bags, either paper or plastic, can also be used though it is hard to immobilize items in bags if that is necessary. Gauze and cotton wool are good choices to cushion fragile items assuming that no easily damaged evidence such as latent prints are on the outer surface of the item (Figure 6.2).

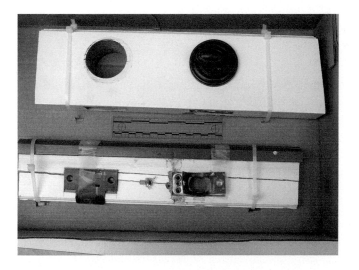

Figure 6.1 Correct securing of an item to protect other evidence that may be located on it.

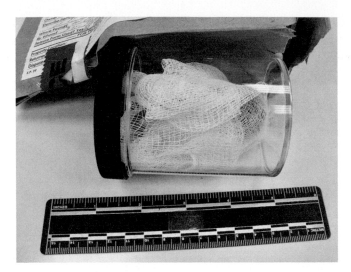

Figure 6.2 Using gauze to protect fragile evidence before placement in an outer container.

Evidence-Collection Techniques

When it is not necessary or practical to collect an item in its entirety, potential evidence can be removed in several different ways at the scene.

Cutting

When feasible, removing a piece of larger items works well. This might be used to obtain material that has soaked into a porous surface, e.g., blood, or material sitting on a surface of an immovable object, e.g., fingerprints. Examples might include carpets or rugs, flooring, sofa cushions, bedding, mattresses and structural materials such as door frames or wallboard. While removal of sections is usually straightforward, attention must be paid to avoid contamination or damage to any evidence on the cut section. Cutting implements used must either be disposable or carefully sanitized using alcohol or bleach prior to each use.

Swabbing

Swabbing is a common technique for recovering biological evidence. It may be used to obtain a small sample for screening tests and also to collect a sample for laboratory analysis. Swabs must be sterile and are usually moistened with sterile phosphate buffered saline (PBS) or distilled water before being gently rubbed on the sample. Care must be taken to avoid the spread of the sample on the substrate during collection and to avoid getting excessive extraneous surface material on the swab.

After use, swabs should be air-dried in a location away from possible contamination prior to packaging; contamination from airborne material should be considered. Boxes and tubes specifically designed to hold swabs are available. Swabs may also be used to pick up nonbiological liquid evidence, such as lubricants, when they are found at scenes.

Scraping

Samples of dry material, such as paint, mud or blood crusts, can be effectively removed from surfaces by scraping them off. It is best achieved using a sterile single-edged razor blade scraped in a direction away from the investigator. A piece of clean white paper or another suitable receptacle is directly below to collect the sample as it falls. While many samples are easily removed, paint samples can require considerable effort when trying to remove all layers of paint from a surface, particularly automotive paint. Caution should be exercised to prevent injury, and plastic holders for blades are available at many retailers and their use is recommended, though they must be sanitized between uses. Blades should be safely discarded after each use, or if significant sample material is adhering to the blade, they can also be collected and packaged.

Picking

Trace materials can be removed from surfaces in different ways; however, picking them off using forceps is an ideal technique as it allows investigators to accurately document the precise location of the materials which can assist when reconstructing the sequence of events. Picking is the recommended primary method for removing evidence such as hairs, fibers, paint chips, glass fragments and other visible trace materials. Disposable forceps may be used to minimize the possibility of contamination; however, in reality, they often lack the fine points that are most effective for many of these samples. Fine point metal forceps may be purchased from specialty sources but must be thoroughly sanitized between uses. Individually packaged alcohol wipes work well for this purpose as they are easily carried into the scene with no chance of spilling liquid onto evidence, and the forceps can be dipped into the open packets and wiped. Keeping a crime scene kit stocked with multiple forceps allows for the use of different forceps in different areas. Picked evidence is usually placed into labeled druggist folds as the primary packaging and then placed into plastic or paper bags (Figure 6.3). In general, each fold should be in a different bag to ensure no cross-contamination, although when several folds all contain evidence picked from the same location, they may be placed into the same outer container.

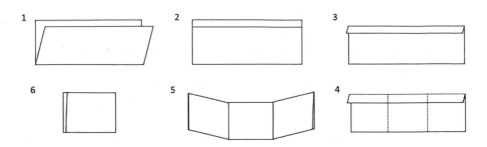

Figure 6.3 Making a druggist fold.

Lifting

Lifting techniques can encompass the removal of two-dimensional pattern evidence and trace evidence. Pattern evidence lifts are primarily associated with fingerprints; however, some footwear and tire evidence can be captured this way when the patterns are 2-dimensional dust and dirt patterns, rather than 3-dimensional impressions. Lifting is achieved with the use of either lifting tape or specialized gel lifters which may be purchased in different sizes or in large pieces that can be cut to size. Lifters consist of an adhesive material on plastic that is attached to its own backing and may be purchased with different color backings, usually black or white, to achieve a high level of contrast between the pattern and backing. Fingerprints are usually lifted after enhancement by physical methods such as powders. Specialized electrostatic lifting technique may be used to lift footwear patterns in dust if available (Figure 6.4); if not, a gel lifter may be used. Examination-quality photographs of all pattern evidence should be taken prior to lifting.

Tape lifting is used at scenes to remove trace materials from items such as bedding, sofas, chairs and car seats. This works well using a zone approach in which a piece of tape is used for a specific small area before a fresh piece of tape is taken for the next designated area. Tape is then stuck to pieces of acetate or page protectors and clearly labeled with the area from which it came. While tapes such as packing tape may be used, specialty tapes with lower adhesive coefficients may be purchased for evidence collection purposes. Lint rollers are also useful for lifting trace evidence from larger areas but whether contamination of the roll can be prevented should be considered.

Casting

While lifting is appropriate for two-dimensional patterns, casting is used for three-dimensional pattern evidence such as toolmarks, footwear impressions and tire tracks. The casting material will vary depending on both the type of pattern and the surface. Tool marks, which require a microscopic level of detail to compare individualizing striations, are best cast with silicone-based

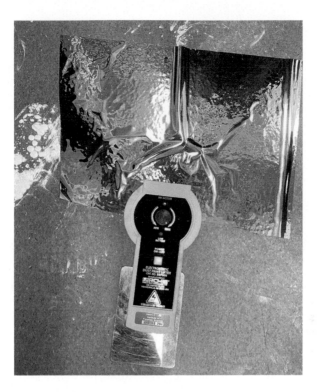

Figure 6.4 Lifting a footwear imprint in dust using an electrostatic technique.

materials such as Mikrosil (Figure 6.5). In many cases, the item holding the tool mark can be submitted in its entirety, but when this is not possible then casting can take place at the scene. Mikrosil and similar materials are prepared from two components mixed immediately before use and produce a robust, rubbery reproduction of a tool mark.

Footwear and tire tracks require less fine detail and are usually cast with Plaster of Paris or dental stone (Figure 6.6). Dental stone is preferred to Plaster of Paris as it has greater strength and a finer texture that captures more detail. Casts are made by placing molds around the area of interest, and larger casts may be reinforced with wire or wood sticks added to the cast as it is poured. Casting materials should not be poured directly onto the impression but should be poured over another item such as a spoon to prevent the loss of important detail. If impressions are in snow, the exothermic setting process can be detrimental to the impression, and snow print wax may be carefully sprayed onto the impression prior to casting to protect it from this issue.

Vacuuming
When highly efficient collection of particulate and fibrous materials is required, specialized evidence collection vacuums are a good choice. These

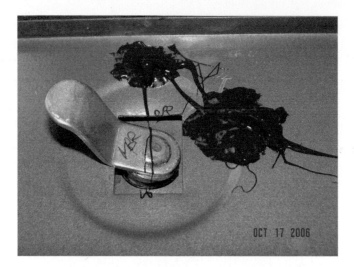

OCT 17 2006

Figure 6.5 Use of Mikrosil to cast toolmark impressions on surfaces.

are compact powerful vacuums with single-use disposable filters through which air is pulled thus trapping any materials drawn up with the air. Though a very efficient technique, this can be a disadvantage as material that was left long before the incident is collected along with more recent deposits. When an investigator uses forceps and picks trace evidence, they can see whether this is lying on the surface or is under other more recent deposits. This temporal information is lost when using a vacuum. Thus, it is often preferable to use a more precise technique like picking first, with vacuuming as a final step.

Wet vacuums have been developed for efficient recovery of cellular material from surfaces for later DNA analysis. It can be deployed at the crime scene on immovable surfaces as well as rocks and stones, and porous surfaces such as soft furnishings and textiles.

While these vacuums may be available for use at larger agencies, they can be a costly item when their use might be more limited.

Appendix B provides a summary of appropriate collection techniques for most common types of evidence that might be found in animal cruelty cases and further information can also be found in the dedicated chapters. Physical evidence can take many forms and individual cases may have unique types of evidence that provide key linkages in the investigation. Investigators must keep an open mind about sources of physical evidence, and in situations where the evidence does not fall into one of the major areas, they should consider the similarities and potential pitfalls in collection when determining the most appropriate collection techniques and packaging. Most forensic laboratories are willing to provide advice to investigators when needed.

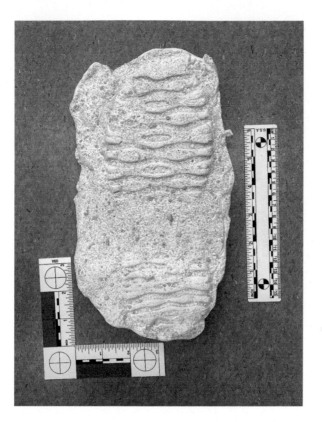

Figure 6.6 Cast of a footwear impression using dental stone.

Packaging Carriers of Evidence

Many types of packaging are available for use with evidence, including boxes, bags, jars, tins, envelopes and paper. The choice of packaging will be dependent upon several factors, primarily the type of evidence but also whether it is wet or dry, the size and whether the packing is to be the primary or secondary container.

Bags

Evidence bags are available in numerous sizes made from paper or plastic and can be used for many types of items. Specific evidence bags may be purchased with tamper-evident seals and preprinted with important labeling information. Plastic bags are commonly used to hold evidence but there are some situations in which they should not be considered the best packing materials; for example, wet biological material should never be packaged in plastic as it leads to degradation of the evidence and hinders the ability to recover a usable DNA profile. Special plastic evidence bags have been developed that allow biological evidence to "breathe", decreasing the likelihood of degradation. When trace evidence, such as fibers, is placed directly into plastic bags, there is a risk of static electricity affecting the successful placement or retrieval of the evidence. If the trace material is first placed into a druggist fold, plastic bags do make excellent outer packages.

Paper bags are good choices for items with biological material as they allow the item to dry and "breathe", thus minimizing bacterial degradation of the evidence; they are also good general choices for many types of evidence. If trace materials are thought to be present on an item, paper bags are more securely closed by folding over the top at least once, preventing loss of trace materials and other evidence through small gaps. Once folded, they can be stapled to secure them before the application of tamper-evident tape.

Boxes

Boxes are useful for larger or heavy items and make good containers to transport castings due to their rigidity. Boxes specifically made for certain types of evidence, such as swabs or different types of firearms, may be purchased from specialty vendors. In many cases, standard cardboard boxes are sufficient. Boxes should not be reused for other evidence. As discussed previously, items may need to be secured within the box to protect important evidence that might be on the item. All boxes should have lids that can be secured onto the box using tamper-evident tape.

Cans

Clean, unused paint cans are useful containers as they have a tight seal which is ideal for accelerant evidence and other volatile evidence such as towels used to absorb airborne substances at hoarding scenes. If they, or glass jars, are to be used for accelerant evidence, there must be no plastic component to them, such as a lining, as this can contaminate the accelerants preventing any useful analysis. If small items, such as bullets, are to be packaged in ointment tins, they should be wrapped in gauze or cotton wool to protect the markings from damage due to movement within the tin or jar. Tamper-evident tape should be placed over the lid and the tin in such a way that the tin cannot be opened without tearing the tape.

Envelopes

Envelopes are used for document evidence and other flat items such as druggist folds. Envelopes should not be used as the primary packaging for any particulate and trace materials as gaps are present which can lead to loss of evidence. Tamper-evident tape should be used to seal the envelope flap.

Paper

If the item is too large for a standard package, then careful packaging in brown paper is the accepted method. The paper should be thick enough that it does not tear when the item is wrapped. The paper should be fastened with tamper-evident tape.

Labeling Evidence

Regardless of the type of packaging used, all evidence must be clearly labeled with important information that allows it to be uniquely identified and maintain the chain of custody. Specialized evidence packaging is preprinted with labeling that needs the investigator to fill in the required information, and preprinted evidence labels can be purchased to attach to any packaging. If labels are not available, the investigator can simply write the necessary information onto the package.

All packages should be clearly marked with, at a minimum, the following information:

Agency
Case number
Date and time seized
Location
Investigator
Package contents

Some preprinted labels have spaces for information regarding the incident under investigation, general remarks and also for initiating chain of custody. Packages must be sealed with a tamper-evident seal, either one that is part of the packaging or tape added after closing. While staples and other fastenings can be used, the tamper-evident tape should be the final seal and applied such that the contents cannot be accessed without breaking the seal. Finally, the investigator should initial and date the seal.

Contamination Issues

A recurring theme throughout this book is that of contamination of evidence. Contamination must be avoided at every stage crime scene processing and evidence collection and packaging. Even the suspicion of contamination can tarnish the integrity of the evidence and may ultimately cause it to have little bearing in the case, no matter how important or compelling that evidence is.

Contamination can occur at many stages in scene processing and beyond. Not only must investigators be mindful of contaminating evidence through sloppy processing or collection techniques, but they must consider cross-contamination of evidence by choosing to package multiple items together. In most situations, each item of evidence should be packaged separately to avoid evidence from one item being transferred to another. Evidence transfer can prove problematic when the location of evidence recovered during later analysis does not make sense. For example, if seizing clothing worn by the perpetrator, packaging all items together can cause transfer of evidence from an outer garment to an inner one or from the outside of a jacket to the inside of a shirt.

With the sensitivity of current methods of DNA analysis, contamination evidence by biological material is of significant concern. As few as ten cells will provide sufficient DNA to obtain a full profile. All personnel at crime scenes must therefore take every precaution to prevent contamination with cellular material at the scene and fully sanitize all tools prior to arriving at the scene and between sample handling. Gloves must be changed often, and investigators should avoid touching their skin with gloved hands. Items that are routinely used and handled with ungloved hands should not be used while gloved to avoid transfer of cells from the item to the gloves and then onto evidence.

Final Thoughts

No matter how good an investigator, veterinarian or scientist, nor whether a laboratory has the best equipment in the world, if evidence is incorrectly collected and packaged, it may be compromised through contamination or degradation and cannot be used in an investigation. Every investigator should be aware of the correct collection and packaging for each type of evidence and should have the appropriate tools and equipment with them when processing a crime scene. It is possible to assemble a comprehensive kit at a reasonable cost, and this kit should be inventoried and restocked after each scene.

Bibliography

Physical Evidence Handbook. 9th Edition. Wisconsin Department of Justice Crime Laboratory Bureau. 2017. https://www.doj.state.wi.us/sites/default/files/dles/clab-forms/2021_physical-evidence-handbook-2017.pdf

Physical Evidence Manual. Oregon State Police. Version 10, 2018. https://digital.osl.state.or.us/islandora/object/osl%3A510583

Trace Evidence Collection and Packaging. Minnesota Department of Public Safety. 2016. https://dps.mn.gov/divisions/bca/bca-divisions/forensic-science/Documents/Trace%20collect-pack-handout%20final%202016.pdf.

Special Considerations for Crime Scene Investigation and Evidence Processing of Animal Abuse*

7

AMANDA FITCH

Introduction

When an animal is seen being treated cruelly or living in inadequate conditions, it can be very easy for responders to the scene to go into "rescue mode" and want to immediately remove the animal(s) from the harmful environment. It must be remembered, however, that in order to prevent further injustices, violations of cruelty laws must be treated as the crimes that they are. In recent years, laws pertaining to animal cruelty have evolved significantly to include both misdemeanor and felony-level offenses. Because these convictions can carry significant sentences, judges and juries want to see the same standard of evidence handling and processing that would be applied to human cases. In order to meet this need, the handling of criminal animal cases has begun to evolve beyond animal rescue to include crime scene processing techniques and protocols, as well as forensic testing.

Regardless of the type of crime or species of the purported victim, it is important to remember that the purpose and goal of processing every crime scene are the same – to locate, document, collect and preserve physical evidence. Therefore, the same steps recommended for processing a human crime scene – assessment, observation, documentation, search, collection and analysis (Gardner & Krouskup, 2018) – should also be utilized for an animal scene. Due to the unique aspects of an animal scene, however, it may be necessary to make some adjustments to this procedure. Most important, however, it must be emphasized that animal scenes require a balance between animal welfare and crime scene and evidence integrity.

DOI: 10.4324/9781003090762-7

Assessment

Although the assessment step begins prior to arrival at the scene, it will continue throughout the entirety of the crime scene investigation. The information received prior to scene arrival will affect many aspects of the response – this is especially true of animal scenes. Like any other type of crime scene, however, it is quite possible for information received prior to arrival to be inaccurate. For example, you think you are responding to a dogfighting scene known to have a few chickens on site, but when you arrive, there are over 100 fighting birds and only a few dogs. Important information to know before scene arrival includes:

- How is the property accessed? Is there space for multiple and/or large vehicles?
- How large is the scene property? Is it a standard residential house and yard or large acreage?
- What is the suspected crime type?
- What species are reported and how many?
- Are animals alive and/or deceased? Are there burials reported?
- How are the animals housed? Kennels, tie-outs or free-roaming?
- Where are the animals housed – indoors or outside?
- Are there any victims on scene – living or deceased?
- Are there any unusual circumstances or dangers that must be addressed, such as disease or aggressive animals?

The size and layout of the property are relevant for two reasons. As such, aerial photographs, property maps or even topography maps should be consulted before scene arrival if possible (Figure 7.1). First, you will need to know whether the vehicles you require on scene (both for personnel and animal transportation) will fit and be capable of accessing the property. Second, the actual size of the property as well as the number and species of animals and how they are housed will be factors in determining personnel needs. Fifty dogs in kennels inside a typical house will require fewer responders. The animals will be close together for processing and it likely won't be as difficult, or as timely, to photograph the property and to create a diagram of the house showing the spatial relation of the animals within it. Additionally, the space inside the house may be limited due to the number of animals, making fewer responders necessary for ease of movement. Alternately, 50 horses roaming free in multiple pastures across multiple acres will require more people to perform the animal processing in a timely manner, and it may require more than one individual to complete scene and evidence documentation due to the expansive property size.

Knowing the suspected crime type, as well as the number and species of animals, will help you to determine the types and amount of equipment

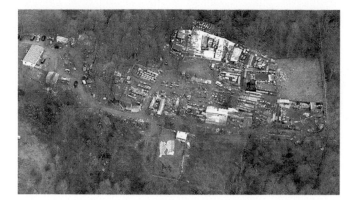

Figure 7.1 Aerial photograph used to plan a large-scale scene response. Information that was not learned until scene arrival was that the road leading from the house into the yard was at a very steep grade. This combined with extreme winter weather conditions made it necessary to alter the removal plan as large vehicles were not able to safely negotiate the steep, icy road. The consultation of a topography map would have illustrated this issue prior to scene arrival.

which will be needed. For example, if the scene is reported as a "puppy mill", you will know to expect various ages of animals as well as pregnant mothers. Identification markers (e.g., collars) of various sizes will be needed as well as the ability to safely transport single and cohoused animals. In this type of scene, the animals are generally housed in pens or kennels. In comparison, bolt cutters are a tool that should be considered when going to a dogfighting scene as they are frequently tethered with heavy metal chains.

Overall Documentation

Once a crime scene has been secured, it is standard for an initial, observational walk-though to be performed prior to the initiation of overall documentation. On an animal scene, however, it is recommended that overall entry photographs and video are taken first. The initial walk-though on an animal scene may include multiple people – investigators, crime scene analysts, veterinarians, members of the removal team, etc. Having these many people enter the scene before it has been properly documented is not recommended. It is also suggested that the overall documentation process includes videography. Remember that your evidence consists largely of live, moving beings. Video allows for the documentation of the animals' normal behavior prior to their normal environment being disrupted. It is also recommended that the individual(s) who performs the overall documentation be cognizant of the animals they are documenting. If an animal appears to be in distress or in need of medical treatment, the veterinarian or vet tech on scene should be contacted immediately and directed to the location of the animal. Prior to an animal being removed for urgent care, it must be photographically documented in place (this process is covered in more detail in the *Search and Collection* section). If a second photographer is not available, it may be necessary for the photographer who is performing the overall documentation to briefly stop and photograph the animal. Once the overall entry documentation has concluded, the other processing steps may proceed as normal.

Observation

During the observation step, it will be important to consider the safety conditions as they are affected by the presence of live and deceased animals. In addition to the normal safety concerns at a crime scene, animal scenes may include inadequate air quality, the danger of animal bites and scratches, and the possibility of zoonotic diseases. Ammonia is a naturally occurring gas, produced by the decay of animal waste. The odor of ammonia is detectable by the human sense of smell at a concentration of 1–5 ppm (parts per million) (Parod, 2014). The National Institute for Occupational Safety and Health (NIOSH) recommends an upper exposure limit of 50 ppm; however, levels over 350 ppm have been documented on animal scenes where there was no air flow and extremely poor sanitation conditions (Figure 7.2a and b).

Live animals can cause both noncontact and contact injuries. While tripping over a chain may not be avoidable, bites and scratches can be. Anyone who is responsible for handling animals should have the appropriate training not only to protect themselves but also to prevent injury to the animals. Likewise, a veterinarian or veterinary technician should be consulted regarding potential zoonotic disease concerns so that the appropriate PPE (personal protective equipment) can be utilized. Another potential safety hazard to be aware of is the presence of sharps. It is not uncommon to find syringes

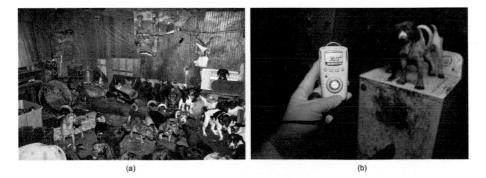

(a)   (b)

Figure 7.2 (a) Large-scale neglect scene where 99 canines were living in a trailer. (b) Ammonia reading of 369 ppm from scene in (a).

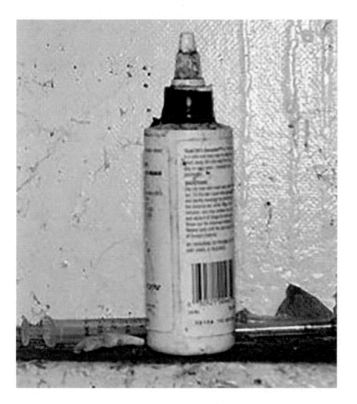

Figure 7.3 Syringe and dog canine tooth found in room with a dogfighting pit.

(Figure 7.3) on an animal scene as they can be used to administer vaccinations or other substances such as (in the case of dogfighting and cockfighting) anabolic steroids.

Documentation

As with human crimes, documentation of the scene and evidence is of significant importance. All of the standard documentary methods (See Chapters 2-6) should be utilized and are equally as important for an animal scene.

Notes should contain information on the environmental conditions, including the air quality, ambient temperature and physical living environment. Information pertaining to the environmental conditions can be of great importance to the veterinarian who will be examining the animal(s), as some of the medical conditions may be attributed to the living environment. As discussed above, poor air quality due to ammonia can be an issue. It's preferable that ammonia levels be documented as soon as possible so that the true levels are not diluted from ventilation. If a room is closed off upon scene arrival and has a strong odor of ammonia, the door should be kept closed as much as possible until a reading can be taken. There are a variety of methods for quantifying ammonia levels; however, a digital monitor is recommended as it is the only method which will result in an exact ppm reading. When considering the purchase of a digital ammonia monitor, consider whether it will be necessary to calibrate the monitor with compressed gas, the maximum level the unit will register and whether the measurements are stored on the unit. Many units are designed specifically for human safety purposes and will not register above 50 or 100 ppm. If the unit does not record readings for future data download, it is recommended that photographs are taken of the digital display. Once the level is documented, the room should be ventilated before work continues, or respirators should be utilized by persons entering the environment.

In addition to the air quality, there are other environmental conditions that should be documented. The ambient temperature should be recorded whether animals are held inside or outside. It may be necessary to take temperature readings more than once as conditions change, such as ventilation of a room or the time of day resulting in a change from sun to shade. It may also be of benefit to take the temperature of the interior of housing structures (e.g., a doghouse). Even though an animal may have shelter from the sun, it may be that the temperature within the shelter is higher than the outdoor ambient temperature. It is also important to note any physical dangers within the living environment. This could include chemicals such as rodenticides, sharp metal or nails used to construct housing (Figure 7.4) or toxic plants.

The photographic documentation of an animal scene can be problematic. It is not uncommon for individuals responding to an animal scene to unconsciously alter the conditions of the scene as they attempt to immediately improve the circumstances of the animal (e.g., filling water bowls or spraying waste from the floor). While it is not within the context of the overall photographs to capture such detail as the contents of food and water bowls or the

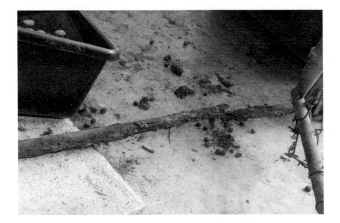

Figure 7.4 Rusted and jagged metal of kennel.

presence of vomitus on a kennel floor, it is highly recommended that the time be taken to ensure other responders know to not alter any conditions without confirming that they have already been documented. Allowing water bowls to be filled prior to documentation could affect the examination results of the veterinarian, as an animal will have had the opportunity to rehydrate, or the question of whether sufficient food and water was available may be contested.

Another particular issue with the overall photo documentation of animal scenes is the size of the property. Scenes may span tens of acres or be confined to small structures. In both situations, it can be difficult to photographically relay the true environment because items of interest are either spread too far apart and require multiple photographs to show a connection, or a space is very confined and only allows for a narrow slice of the scene in each photograph, which will also require multiple photographs in order to get an actual "overall" perspective. If available, a 360° camera can be used to cover these types of areas. Alternatively, a fish-eye (ultrawide angle) lens (which is not typically recommended for forensic work due to the peripheral distortion of the images) can be used on very large or confined scenes to expand the area that is captured in the photograph (Figure 7.5a and b). If a fish-eye lens is going to be used, however, it is recommended that images of the same areas are also taken with a standard lens to ensure the same information is documented without distortion. Another option for creating broad view images, of either large or confined areas, is photo-stitching software. This type of software can be used to create a panoramic photograph using images taken with a standard camera (Figure 7.6a and b).

When creating a scene diagram for an animal scene, it's important to remember why the sketch is being created. Generally, sketches are created to assist in the recreation of a crime scene, and measurements are taken to allow items of evidence to be placed back in the exact same location and position from which they were initially collected. On animal scenes, the specific locations from which items were collected are not necessarily relevant; however, elements of the living environment are. Take, for example, a dogfighting

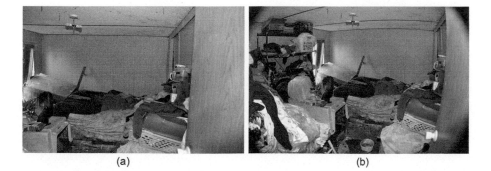

(a)   (b)

Figure 7.5 (a) Regular lens photo of bedroom. (b) Fish-eye lens photo of bedroom.

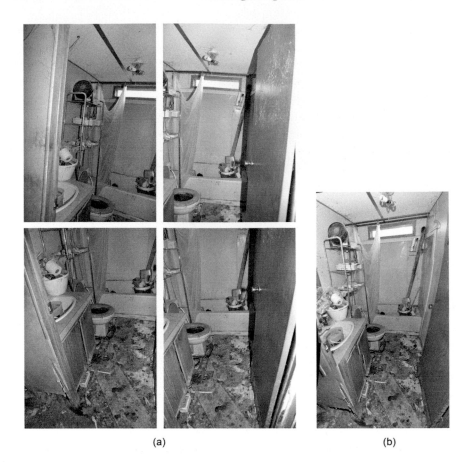

(a)   (b)

Figure 7.6 (a) Unstitched bathroom photographs. (b) Stitched bathroom image.

scene where there is a constructed fighting pit with a break stick laying within its walls. The general location from where the break stick is recovered should be documented; however, it is likely not necessary to know its exact distance from the pit wall and which direction the bite end was facing. Of more importance are the measurements of the pit itself. Obviously, there may be situations where the exact positioning of an item of evidence will be relevant; however, this will most likely be related to scenes of nonaccidental injury.

One of the most important types of evidence found on an animal scene is the animals themselves. Therefore, like any other item of evidence, the location(s) of the animals on the property need to be documented. Depending on the positioning of kennels or crates, it may be necessary to create not only a bird's eye but also a horizontal view if the enclosures are stacked.

A diagram, in addition to the photographs, will illustrate how the animals were confined and their spatial relationship to one another. Diagrams can also help to clarify and "declutter" photographs of scenes that are very confined or busy (e.g., "hoarding" scenes). In addition to the assigned Animal ID number, sketches should include measurements of the accessible living space (whether it is an enclosure or larger open area). The dimensions of enclosures and chain spaces should be documented but also anything that would prevent the animal from accessing the entire space. For example, if there are excess feces in a kennel that limits the floor space where the animal can walk or lie comfortably, then measurements of the nonaccessible area should also be taken. If accessibility of food and/or water may be an issue (e.g., different sized animals housed together), it will be necessary to measure the height of the receptacles and the level of food/water in them. Additional measurements may apply to various other circumstances, such as the length of a tether, or the height of a perch or jump board in the enclosure of a fighting bird.

Sketching large acreages can be not only physically difficult but also time-consuming. If aerial photographs or property maps were available for planning, these can also be used for sketching the overall property. They can be used to divide the property into more manageable zones, and as one walks through the property, measurements can be added to the photo/map and corrections can be made to areas that are different in life. It is also helpful to use the appropriate equipment and methods for large properties. Unless a total station or laser mapping scanner is available, a measuring wheel and/or a range finder is recommended for measuring long distances. It can also be helpful to consider all possible sketching methods. There may be situations where the standard X, Y coordinates or triangulation methods are not ideal due to a lack of straight measuring planes and stationary reference points. In these situations, a baseline can be created by placing a stake in a convenient location, documenting its GPS coordinate and using it as the reference point. A baseline can then be run in a cardinal or other designated direction from the stake. The polar coordinates method can also be useful when documenting items located irregularly across an open area, such as the chain spaces of a dog yard or scattered skeletal remains.

Search and Collection

The search methods utilized on an animal scene will be the same as those on a human scene. Keeping with the recommended protocol, all items of evidence should be photographed prior to collection. Similarly, the packaging of items should follow generally accepted packaging guidelines for whichever evidence type they most resemble. Whether evidence processing occurs on scene or post removal in a controlled environment will be determined by the type of processing conducted and whether the item is going to be collected. For example, some law enforcement agencies not to have the space to hold multiple treadmills from a dogfighting scene. Therefore, the presumptive testing and collection of suspected blood samples may need to occur on scene.

The types of evidence collected will vary depending on the type of animal scene; however, there are some items that are commonly found regardless of the crime type. These include medications and live animals. Any medications or supplements should be thoroughly photographed to include the name, manufacturer, ingredients and directions for administration (Figure 7.7). If the substance is prescribed, all of the prescription information should also be recorded.

As stated previously, live animals should be documented like any other type of evidence. An overall photograph should be taken of the animal(s) in the environment in which it is initially found (e.g., still in their kennel or tethered). Then, identification photos should be taken (Figure 7.8). It's recommended that a white board (or something similar) is used to show the case number, date, location, photographer and Animal ID number and be held next to the animal's head for a "mugshot". Any characteristics that are particularly identifiable, as well as any existing injuries, should also be documented. After the animal has been removed from its enclosure, additional photographs can be taken to illustrate the living environment (Figure 7.9). These should include the contents of food and water bowls, excessive or lack of waste, indications of illness (feces or vomit), items of comfort or enrichment, general cleanliness and any other areas or items of interest (e.g., the end of a nail which may have caused injury). If any of the conditions appear to be the result of the animal being removed (e.g., lack of water due to being spilled), this should be noted, and the information should be shared with the Forensic Veterinarian.

Scenes related to intentional, targeted abuse of an animal may rely heavily on physical evidence from the scene and forensic testing. It is important to consult with a Forensic Veterinarian as quickly as possible so that they might be able to provide information on whether a weapon was used and what type.

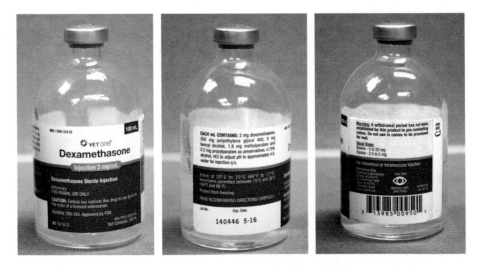

Figure 7.7 Photographs showing the complete information on a medication bottle.

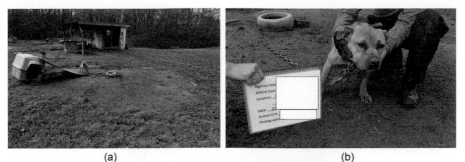

(a)   (b)

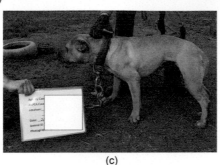

(c)

Figure 7.8 Live animal intake photo series. (a) Overall of animal in its living environment. (b) Identification photo of animal's face and a case board. (c) Identification photo of animal's side and a case board.

In cases of blunt or sharp force trauma, bloody or broken items should be considered as well as any item that is consistent with the animal's reported injuries (Figure 7.10). In cases of sexual abuse, videos and/or literature with bestiality-related content may be found. It is also recommended that the animal's bedding and recent feces are collected so they can be examined for the presence of semen.

Due to the nature of hoarding and puppy mill scenes, the majority of evidence may fall into the category of environmental documentation, rather than tangible physical evidence. Most frequently, collected items will consist of medications and paperwork. In addition to OTC and prescription medications, home-remedy recipes may sometimes be found. These are important to document as it could be an indication that the owner was aware of a medical condition but did not seek standard medical treatment for it. Paperwork may consist of veterinary records or documents related to a rescue or breeding business, such as employee records, breeding schedules and registrations, sales records, 501c3 status and tax returns. Business records may be of importance as it is not uncommon for money-related crimes to be associated with these types of animal cases. Since the general link between these two types of scenes is neglect of the animals, the absence of evidence (e.g., no veterinary records or stock of animal food) may also be considered relevant.

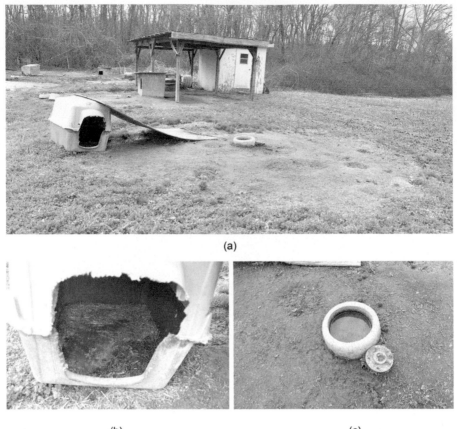

Figure 7.9 Live animal postremoval series. (a) Overall of the living environment. (b) Interior of the doghouse. (c) Interior of water bowl.

Dogfighting and cockfighting scenes will also generally have the same types of evidence. These include training devices (such as treadmills) (Figure 7.11a and b), transport carriers, medical kits, anabolic steroids, fighting pits, blood and documentation. Many items found on fighting scenes, including training devices and carriers, are not specific to organized fighting or illegal to own. The same is true for many items contained in a medical kit; however, the presence of such items may be part of cumulative evidence that supports the crime. The presence of blood on any of these items may also add to that support. Any unlabeled substances (Figure 7.12), or those suspected of being either anabolic steroids or pentobarbital, should be submitted for chemical identification. Whether labeled or unlabeled, both of these substances are controlled and the possession of them is on its own a crime.

Although fighting pits for dogs and birds may look slightly different (e.g., some cockfighting pits may be round instead of square) (Figure 7.13a

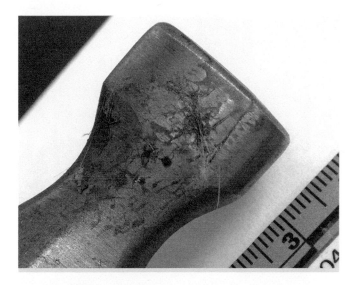

Figure 7.10 Hammer head with blood and fur adhering.

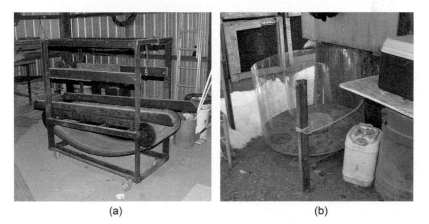

(a)   (b)

Figures 7.11 (a) Treadmill (slatmill) used to condition fighting dogs. (b) Circular rooster treadmill.

and b), their purpose is the same and therefore they are generally processed in the same manner. Fighting pits should be constructed (or reconstructed) including any flooring, so that photographs and measurements can be taken. Measurements should include the length, width and height of the structure, as well as the locations of any markings, such as scratch lines. The presence of suspected blood should be photographically documented as well as the presence of teeth and/or toenails in the carpet (specific to dogfighting).

Other items that may be found specific to dogfighting are heavy chains, break sticks and battery cables. Once the dog is removed from a chain, the chain should be cut as close to its tethering point as possible, and its weight

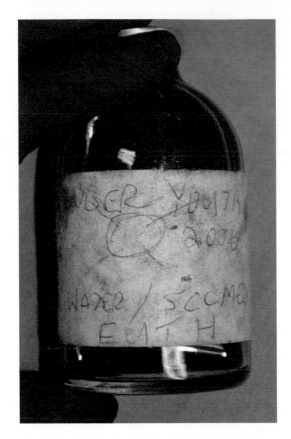

Figure 7.12 Unknown liquid in a bottle with handwritten label.

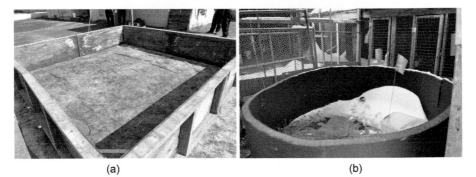

(a)   (b)

Figure 7.13 (a) Dogfighting pit. (b) Cockfighting pit.

documented. This information should be given to the Forensic Veterinarian to compare against the weight of the dog. Break sticks used to separate two fighting dogs should be examined for the presence of blood as well as to trace fur which could have skin cells adhering that can be submitted for DNA testing (Figure 7.14). The construction and material of the break stick should also be considered for latent print processing. The handle portion of these items

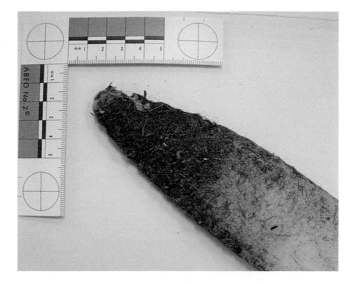

Figure 7.14 Break stick with blood and fur adhering.

is frequently wrapped with tape, which can be processed for the presence of fingerprints on both its nonadhesive and adhesive sides. Battery cables are known to sometimes be used to cull a dog. If these are found on scene, the clips should be examined for the presence of fur or blood (Figure 7.15). Specific to cockfighting, gaffs and knives should be examined for the presence of blood or feathers (Figure 7.16).

Samples of suspected blood can be submitted for DNA speciation or individuation testing. There are two field tests that can be utilized prior to sample collection to help prevent the expense of submitting nonblood samples. Kastle–Meyer test is a presumptive test that will result in a pinkish-purple color change when the components of the test are in contact with hemoglobin. Although a negative result is generally considered a proof of the absence of detectable quantities of blood, false positives are known to

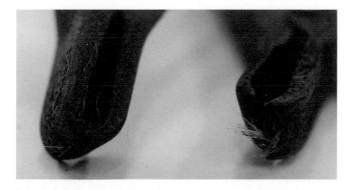

Figure 7.15 Battery charging cables with fur in the clips.

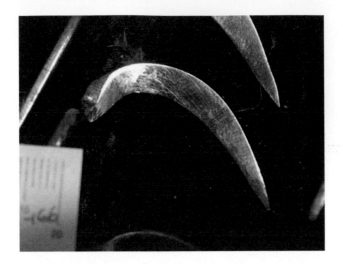

Figure 7.16 Cockfighting knives with blood and a feather adhering.

occur in the presence of some chemicals and vegetable enzymes. The second test utilized is Hexagon OBTI. This test is considered confirmatory for blood, BUT presumptive for human blood as false positives are possible in the presence of nonhuman primates and some Mustelidae (weasels and badgers). The Hexagon OBTI should be performed following a positive phenolphthalein test. Because the suspected blood is hypothetically nonhuman, a negative OBTI reaction could be the result of the testing of nonhuman blood or of a nonblood substance.

Deceased remains can be associated with any type of animal crime scene and may be found in a range of locations including lying on the surface, inside a garbage can, on a burn pile or in a single or mass burial. If deceased remains are fresh or in the beginning stages of decomposition, they should be submitted to a Forensic Veterinarian or Veterinary Pathologist for necropsy. If the remains are in an advanced stage of decay or completely skeletonized, they should be submitted to a Forensic Osteologist or Anthropologist for analysis. Depending on the postmortem interval and the recovery location, the collection of entomological and botanical evidence should also be considered. Environmental concerns should also be documented when dealing with deceased remains. Not only should the remains not be in close proximity to living animals, but they may also be of a public health concern due to contamination of the water table or air quality.

Analysis

As mentioned earlier, based on the evidence type and material, there are various forensic disciplines that can be utilized in animal cruelty cases. In fact, basically, any forensic test that could be used on a human crime scene can also be used for animal cruelty cases. The biggest hurdle, however, is finding a laboratory that will analyze the evidence. It is not uncommon for law enforcement-directed crime labs to have restrictions on accepting evidence related to animal cruelty cases. In some jurisdictions, cruelty toward an animal is considered a property crime, and despite whatever levels of pain and suffering may have been inflicted on the animal, the crime(s) are considered lesser than those of violence toward a human. Therefore, there is reluctance to add the evidence to an already backlogged system and allow the analysis of it to take time away from human-based crimes. The alternative to a jurisdictional laboratory is either a private lab or university lab. University labs that offer analytical services are generally found attached to veterinary colleges or forensic science programs. Unfortunately, many of these labs lack forensic accreditation and the analysts may have no experience (or interest) in testifying to their reported findings. Alternatively, private laboratories can be found which specialize in a variety of forensic testing, such as trace evidence, drug chemistry, and ballistics. Many of the private laboratories have forensic accreditation and do offer expert witness testimony as a service, but both of these matters should be confirmed before submitting evidence to them. While not abundant, laboratories that will perform common analyses such as trace collection, DNA comparisons and drug chemistry analyses can be found. As a relatively new field, it may be even more difficult to find a laboratory or expert to perform a veterinary osteological analysis.

The first part to skeletal analysis is determining who or what the remains belonged to by determining components of a biological profile, including species, sex and age. The skull provides the best information for determining species as all of its characteristics are formed for a specific function. For example, large canines and molars with sharp cusps are used for tearing meat (i.e., a carnivore) and an animal with eyes oriented laterally for a wider range of vision will be a prey animal. Once the general class and order of an animal are determined, the comparison of specific anatomical features becomes important. This is because the closer two animals are in the taxonomic hierarchy, the more similar they will look. Achieving a basic familiarity of those animal crania most frequently encountered on animal scenes, as well as those indigenous to your region, is recommended. Unfortunately, the determination of specific breeds within a species is generally not possible. For the domestic dog, the most basic level of identification that can be determined is based on the shape of the cranium – brachycephalic, mesocephalic and dolichocephalic (flat faced, medium lenghth snout, long snout) – which will give an idea of the size and cranial shape of the dog you are dealing with but not the specific breed.

The sex and age of skeletal remains can also be difficult to determine. For many species, the sex of an animal is displayed in ways that are not visible when looking at skeletal remains (e.g., brightly colored feathers). Within the class Mammalia, many males possess a baculum or *os penis*. If this bone is present, then the animal can readily be identified as a male. However, if the bone is not present, it may be because the animal is a female, or it may be that the animal is a male but the baculum was not collected with the rest of the remains. Similarly, it is much easier to determine the age of younger individuals than it is for older ones. Age is determined by the stages of dental eruption and fusion of the secondary growth plates. After all adult teeth have fully erupted and all of the secondary growth plates have completely fused, age is based on degradation, including the wearing of teeth and the formation of osteoarthritic lesions. Due to individual chewing habits and variations in general lifestyle, however, assessing age through degenerative changes can be unreliable.

The second part of a skeletal analysis is the assessment of anomalies which may be related to the cause of death. The assessment of pathologies and trauma is much less abstract than determining biological factors. This is because, regardless of species, bones are formed by the same chemical and structural components. Therefore, they also react to disease and stress in the same manner – dental disease has the same characteristics in a dog as it does in a human, osteosarcoma on a horse femur looks very similar to that of a cow femur and a healing cranial fracture of a cat appears similar to that of a dog. With the analysis of skeletal remains, it is possible not only to discern natural disease processes from trauma, but also to distinguish between antemortem and perimortem trauma, and postmortem damage. Being able to differentiate these various types of abnormalities not only contributes information possibly related to the cause of death but also to the medical history of the individual. Questions are frequently asked regarding the necessity of osteological analysis. Why is this process necessary when bodies can be X-rayed or digitally scanned? Unfortunately, there are circumstances where fractures and other anomalies may not be visible by these methods. It may be that the animal was not positioned correctly to allow for clear visibility. It is also possible that the injury consists of a nondisplaced fracture. This type of fracture, where there is no gap in the bone and the broken ends have remained in good alignment, can be difficult to visualize due to the lack of contrast.

The goal of this chapter has been not only to introduce the reader to the idea of different types of animal cruelty but also how some of the unique aspects of animal scenes must be addressed in order to maintain crime scene and evidence integrity as well as the welfare of those animals involved in the scene investigation. While it is recommended that the standardized steps of scene processing are preferred, this chapter also exemplifies specific instances when an alternate process is recommended and why. Most important, the reader is reminded that the purpose of investigating an animal cruelty scene is the same as investigating any other crime. Therefore, animal cruelty scenes should receive the same attention to detail and meticulous care as any other types of investigation.

Note

* All figures in this Chapter used with permission, non-exclusive license, and © American Society for the Prevention of Cruelty to Animals (ASPCA).

Bibliography

Gardner RM, Krouskup DR, *Practical Crime Scene Processing and Investigation*. Boca Raton, FL: CRC Press, 2018.

Parod RJ. Ammonia. In *Encyclopedia of Toxicology*, pp. 206–208. Wexler P, ed. Elsevier, Inc., 2014.

Large-Scale Animal Abuse Cases

8

MARTHA SMITH-BLACKMORE

Preparing for a search of a large-scale crime scene containing live and deceased animals must include careful advance planning. The area to search may be vast, with uneven terrain, including multiple structures and numerous animals, both living and deceased. Bodies of animals may be buried below ground, kept in freezers or other containers. Live animals may be fearful, aggressive, or both. Individuals with species expertise should be consulted with in planning the scene response. It isn't every day that crime scene investigators are responsible for corralling evidence that can run, jump, fly or even swim!

Planning must include provisions for animal transport, veterinary assessment, urgent and ongoing veterinary care, and housing of the animals. Capacity planning must include both space needs and sufficient caregiving for the animals (including animals yet to be born) for a protracted period of time. The National Animal Care and Control Association designates 15 minutes of worker time per animal, per day for feeding and cleaning. This means a population of 40 animals requires 10 hours for just basic care. Appropriate care to ensure an acceptable quality of life for a group of animals requires significant additional staff time. Add in walks, behavior assessment and training, enrichment, grooming and veterinary care, and the staffing needs likely double or triple.

Pre-search preparation may include educating animal handlers, veterinarians and technicians on the basic principles of search and seizure to include chain of custody documentation and other processes. While veterinarians can be tremendously helpful to the animal cruelty investigation, they may not understand the rules of evidence and the need to refrain from public comment or posting about their experience on social media. They may also need instruction on photography, note taking and diagramming of exam findings, as well as summary reporting.

Filing criminal charges and seeking a financial bond to care for the animals may help persuade the owner to relinquish some or all of the animals. Even if the animals are not released as evidence by the court or ownership rights relinquished, a prosecutor or judge may allow movement of the animals from the pound or shelter into foster homes for care during the pendency of the trial. Strategy planning for animal care and outcomes will help facilitate swift resolution of the animal care challenge.

DOI: 10.4324/9781003090762-8

Command Structure

When planning a large-scale animal scene intervention, it is helpful to have teams for each process during the search and seizure: investigative, documentation/evidence collection, animal capture and handling, health assessment and transport teams. Because animal hoarding scenes and illegal breeding operations are in fact human-made disasters, it is helpful to structure teams and reporting structures similar to those outlined in the Federal Emergency Management Agency (FEMA) National Incident Management System (NIMS) Incident Command System (ICS). The ICS command structure is a standardized approach to the command, control, and coordination of an emergency response, providing a common hierarchy within which responders from multiple agencies can be effective. Online ICS training is freely available at the FEMA website, and it is helpful for communities to regularly train using tabletop exercises. An animal hoarding scenario makes an excellent training for interagency response practice.

Helpful forms include memoranda of understanding between a lead agency and assisting agencies detailing who is responsible for what parts of the response, an animal inventory form to record all living and deceased animal taken, chain of custody for multiple animal forms, exam forms for each individual animal, transport logs, evidence cage cards and a service tracking spreadsheet for purposes of future restitution.

Documenting the Scene and Evidence

Search warrants for such scenes should be written to encompass all animals, born and unborn, alive and deceased, above and below ground, contained or free roaming, inside or outside. All animal medications, treatments, supplies, animal and financial records (to include food and water bills, proof of ownership documents, care and boarding contracts and agreements, photographs) written or electronically kept, feed, food bags or containers, any and all implements for the training, control, restraint or confinement of animals should be included.

The search warrant affidavit should designate the search to include unattached property such as trailers, sheds, and cars, vehicles and trailers used to transport animals, and the interior of refrigerators and freezers where deceased animals may be stored and cabinets and drawers where relevant evidence may be stored. An animal hoarding or intensive breeding operation search may include the grounds of the property and exhumation of mass graves.

The first responsibility for all investigators and responders is human safety, followed by the dual and competing activities of documenting evidence and rescuing animals from suffering conditions. It is important to remember that most neglected, hoarded animals or animal fighting victims have been in suffering conditions for months or years, and the delay of veterinary care long enough to document the evidence is time well spent. Having a veterinarian at a large scene can help with the triage of animals in need of immediate intervention.

The Preliminary Search

The preliminary search will provide an overview of the entire scene. This "hands in pockets" walkthrough is an opportunity to triage animals in need of more immediate care and will guide the investigator as to what other equipment or resources may be required. For instance, a scene with large numbers of cats unsocialized to people will require box traps, nets and experienced cat handlers.

A video of the initial walk through can capture the scene before intervention and before investigators cause any changes. It is important to either mute the microphone or avoid unnecessary conversation during the walk through.

Unmanned aerial vehicles (UAVs or drones) may be of utility to provide an overview and orientation to the property prior to search, and to document the property from above. Flying drones over private property should be done only under an approved search warrant to avoid Fourth Amendment violations and potential liability. Additionally, the Federal Aviation Administration (FAA) has strict rules about the heights and locations at which UAVs may be flown. Drones with thermal imaging technology can be employed to identify the heat signature of animals in dense brush or wooded property.

Alphanumeric Numbering System

When there are multiple animal-holding paddocks, buildings and rooms, it is helpful to use an alphanumeric organizational designation system. Each building can be designated with a letter, then each room within the building is numbered. Within each room, every primary enclosure (cage or crate) can be designated with a letter, and each animal within that cage numbered. Using this system, the first animal from Building C, Room 2, Cage A would be designated C2A1. This diagram and numbering system can help to create order out of chaos (Figure 8.1).

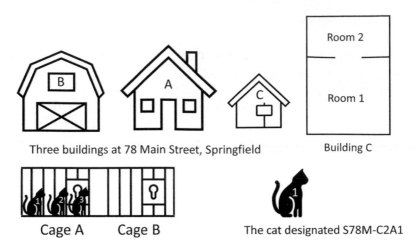

Three buildings at 78 Main Street, Springfield   Building C

Cage A   Cage B   The cat designated S78M-C2A1

Figure 8.1 Example alphanumeric numbering system at 78 Main Street, Springfield, where there is a house (building A), a barn (building B) and a shed (building C). The shed has two rooms, 1 and 2. There are two cages in room 2, A and B. There are three kittens in cage A, kittens 1, 2 and 3. The first kitten removed from that cage would be Springfield 78 Main Street – building C, room 2, cage A, kitten 1, or for short, S78M-C2A1.

Documenting the Animals

Each animal should be photographed as they are within their enclosure, and then photographed out of the enclosure, and the interior of the cage or crate should be photographed after the animal is removed. The preliminary photographs at the scene can be identified with a case card with the alphanumeric location designation present in the photograph. Each animal should be identified with an affixed paper collar or similar system. The alphanumeric designation for the animal can be written on the paper collar or tag as a unique identifier number, see figure 8.1.

The Building/Room/Cage/Animal designations can be used as unique identifying systems for the animals' records throughout the case, perhaps prefaced by a case identifier such as Town Name, street number, first letter of the street name. An animal from 78 Main Street in the town of Springfield might be designated as "S78M-C2A1".

Search techniques described in Chapter 6 should be employed. Different types of large-scale scenes will require specialized equipment and experts. For example, a scene with burial graves, fire pits or exposure of large amounts of bone evidence will benefit from an anthropologist directing the mapping and excavation of the scene or scenes.

Farm Animal Scenes

Farm animals may be hoarded in pens, barns and outbuildings, and will generally be in no condition to be of value at auction or for food production. In chronic, longstanding situations, the manure may accumulate in thickness to the point that fences no longer keep animals contained. Barn or shed-housed animals may have restricted headroom which prevents a normal anatomical position due to the thick fecal base underfoot. Having no animals on a property in producing or salable condition is evidence that the scene is not a farm or agricultural business.

Body condition scoring systems are available for most species of animals kept for agricultural purposes, and they should be employed by a species expert in grading the condition of the animals. Other signs of neglect include overgrown hooves, overgrown teeth, matted wool or fur, pressure sores, rain rot, fly strike and myiasis (the presence of maggots under the wool/fur or in wounds).

The grounds may have hazardous materials that pose dangers to animals and people. There may be exposed rough edges of rusted metal debris, containers leaking toxic chemicals such as pesticides, and standing water harboring infectious disease pathogens. Findings such as these may require specialized equipment and responders. These items should be comprehensively described, photographed and collected as appropriate.

Animal Hoarding and Illegal Breeding Operation Scenes

In animal hoarding cases, it is important to create order out of chaos and to follow all ordinary crime scene documentation practices. Reports should note the amassed debris and filth, describing mixed and matted papers, rotting food, garbage, and human and animal waste, etc. The volume of empty pet food cans, feed bags and feces can be a testament to the chronicity of the hoarding.

Investigators must be prepared to encounter unbreathable air, from ammonia buildup and other bioaerosols. Years of urine and waste can rot floorboards, and scenes with considerable object hoarding may also pose the risk of avalanche or collapse. Planning for safety is an integral part of the investigation and intervention.

Hoarded animals may be kept in enclosures, or they may be free roaming, or both. The house may be uninhabitable due to extreme filth, and the hoarder may live in an accessory dwelling unit, trailer or vehicle on the property, or they may live elsewhere. Sheds, garages, broken down automobiles or buses may also be used to house animals.

Animals should be documented at the scene as described above and tri-aged for the delivery of urgent veterinary care. More detailed exams and pho-tography can happen at the receiving facility due to the amount of time this work takes, the need for equipment at the veterinary clinic, and the need to provide preliminary medical and grooming care.

Deceased animals are of the lowest priority for collection, but like living animals, they should be assigned unique identifier numbers and photographed in situ. It is helpful to assign the deceased animals an alphanumeric designa-tion that makes clear the animal was deceased when found, such as adding a letter -D at the end of the number. A brief exam should detail the condition of the body (fresh, in rigor, early or late decomposition, mummified or skeleton-ized). Regardless of the condition of the body, it is worth collecting and docu-menting, even if a full necropsy is not possible. Once the body is collected, the scene where the body was found should be photographed, and the body should be bagged for eventual postmortem examination as described in Chapter 19.

After all animal evidence has been removed, a comprehensive documen-tation of the scene can focus on the presence or absence of food, water, body fluids and other conditions. This is the time to note and collect any veteri-nary medications or records. Animal hoarders may make some attempts to provide veterinary care for some animals, and this shows knowledge that animals do require veterinary care and may be in a suffering state.

Animal Fighting Scenes

Dog fighters may keep dogs in crates in a house or on the grounds. In urban settings, the animals are likely to be kept in kennels in a basement in order to muffle the sounds of barking dogs, and they may be kept with cloth, wire or leather muzzles on to prevent barking, which is inhumane. In suburban or rural settings, the dogs may be kept in a garage or on tethers, often under tree cover. The shade from trees provides some protection from solar heat, but from the dog fighter's perspective, it obscures the tell-tale dirt circles from aerial observation. Makeshift dog houses may be constructed from 50-gal-lon drums or plywood; airline kennel crates or commercially available dog houses may be used. In general, fighting dogs are friendly to people and aggressive to other dogs, but this cannot be assumed, and caution must be exercised when handling suspected fighting dogs.

If dogs are trained to fight at a scene, there will be equipment used for strength and endurance training. There may be treadmills of various con-struct (from professional gym equipment to homemade "carpet mills"), jenny mill (also known as a cat mill), flirt poles, spring poles, heavy chains, weights or other equipment. A jenny is an apparatus used to exercise a dog or dogs by keeping them separated and chasing one another or a bait. A bait may be a caged chicken, rabbit or other small animal, real or simulated. A flirt pole is a training stick with a cord and bait attached, used to encourage the dog to leap for the just out-of-reach object. A spring pole is an apparatus that a dog is encouraged to jump up and grab, so that they are hanging by biting onto an object. This is usually connected to a heavy-duty spring, giving the dog a sensation of dynamic interaction. This exercise encourages jaw strength and teaches bite, hold and tear behaviors. Long stick-like wedges of wood or other materials may be present to be used as "break sticks" to separate fighting dogs during sparring bouts. There will likely be scales present to weigh dogs as they are pitted against one another in weight classes. All materials potentially used in training should be photographed, measured and, if appropriate, weighed (e.g., heavy chains or weights used in training). If the volume or size of equipment is too large to be collected, a representative sampling should be seized (Figure 8.2).

Dog fighting scenes may have a "pit", the area where the dogs are fought. These are often lined with carpet and walls of sheets of plywood. In less formal operations, pits may be defined by old furniture, mattresses or other materials. If used, these items will likely have abundant blood and saliva evidence. There may be patterns of cast blood from head shaking and tail whips, and there may be transfers of blood and in rub patterns as the dogs push up against the walls of the pit. There may be imprints of blood in the pattern of dog noses or paw prints. There may be evidence of expectorated blood spatter (coughing up blood). The blood and saliva evidence can be photographed and collected for individual profiles to compare against suspected dog fighting victims.

The dog fighter may keep veterinary medications and surgical equipment to crop ears, dock tails and treat fighting wounds. The presence of these materials is evidence of planning for injuries. There may be other drugs or

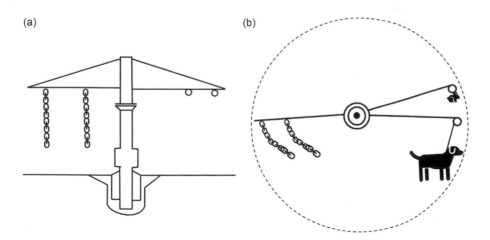

Figure 8.2 A jenny mill side view (a) and top view (b) may be constructed out of a vehicle axle embedded in concrete with arms welded to it to tether the dog and lure. On the opposite, the arm is weighted with chains to balance the mill. When dogs are trained on the mill, they will wear a circular path in the ground.

substances intended to enhance a dog's performance or aggression such as testosterone, amphetamines or cocaine. There may be vitamins and electrolytes for preparation or recovery from training or a fight. There may be buckets or tubs and sponges used to wash the dogs down before fights, as is the custom in dog fighting.

Dog fighters may keep electronic or paper copies of breeding records and fighting histories. There may be stands that a female dog can be strapped to for purposes of forced breeding. These stands are aptly and unfortunately called "rape stands".

Fighting birds ("cocks") may be kept in barns, in enclosures or outdoors, tethered to "a-frame"-type shelters. For both dogs and fighting birds, tethering at a distance where the animals cannot quite make contact increases frustration and therefore aggression; noting tethering distances and the length of restraints is important evidence.

Fighting cocks have long nails on their feet known as "spurs". In cockfighting, blades known as "gaffs" are secured to trimmed spurs to increase the lethality of strikes. In training matches, chicken-sized boxing gloves or "muffs" will be secured. Cock fighters will use cords or leather straps to secure the gaffs or muffs to the birds.

Animal fighters may have equipment used for killing animals, especially the losers of a fight. Animals may be drowned, hung, shot, suffer blunt head trauma or be electrocuted. There may be implements used for drowning such as barrels or tubs full of water, clubs or other implements used to strike the animals on the head, electrical extension cords with one end cut off and exposed wires.

Animal fighters are often known to have large amounts of cash, illicit drugs and weapons on scene. The planning for a search of a suspected animal fighting scene must include appropriate safety planning. Animal fights are a clandestine activity, but there may be provisions for spectators, refreshments and wagering.

After the Seizure

The animals' conditions must be photographed and assessed as described in Chapter 17, The Clinical Exam, or Chapter 19, the Postmortem Exam. Each animal must have their own medical record, and each of the various conditions found in individuals of the entire group of animals can be noted and aggregated on a spreadsheet. The spreadsheet can list the animals down the first column, and conditions noted across the top. This facilitates summary reporting on how many animals suffered from various conditions.

Veterinarians should be notified of any pharmaceutical or drugs of abuse found at the scene. Knowledge of these materials can guide testing of animals for their presence in the animals.

Tracking ongoing care delivered to the animals will provide a record of what was done and prove that the animals did not have any reason for being in a poor condition, other than because of how they had been kept. These documents can also be used to put a financial value on the care given to the animals during their rehabilitation for civil redress or for bond and forfeiture procedures.

Veterinarians involved in the seizure and ongoing care of the animals can serve as both fact and expert witness in these cases. It may be helpful for the initial progress of the case to have the veterinarians provide reports or affidavits of the general condition or the scene, of the group of animals, to include an opinion on the cause of injury or condition and the degree and duration of suffering.

It is also important to note the number of person-hours needed to adequately care for the animals, and the volume of food and water supplied. A forensic financial analysis may be helpful to demonstrate that the hoarder, breeder or animal fighter was not spending the amount of money necessary to provide minimal care to the animals.

Final Thoughts

Large-scale investigations require appropriate planning for resources for the documentation of voluminous evidence and the care of large numbers of animals. Additionally, safety for the investigators is paramount. Perpetrators of animal fighting may also be involved in drug, weapons and financial crimes. Scenes where a large number of animals are found pose a risk of physical injury from the poorly maintained environment or from animals. No single item is necessarily evidence of hoarding, illegal breeding or animal fighting, but the totality of evidence can be quite compelling. A consulting subject matter expert may be needed to opine on the nature of activities indicated by the entirety of evidence.

Animal Abuse Involving Large Animals

9

MARTHA SMITH-BLACKMORE

Generally speaking, "large animals" include cattle, horses, donkeys and other equids, pigs, sheep, goats and other small ruminants, llamas, alpacas and other camelids. Under the law, however, the definition of agricultural animals varies, as do their legal protections. In many states, farmed animals are exempted from the animal cruelty law, and they may be specifically referenced by species, or the activities such as food or fiber production, or animals used in "entertainment" activities such as rodeo can be excluded from protections. Some species of animals such as rabbits may be considered companion animals, food or fiber production animals or wildlife, depending on context.

Livestock clauses in animal cruelty law do not mean that a person cannot be prosecuted for animal cruelty against farmed animal species, as most laws stipulate activities are allowed "when the treatment is in accordance with accepted agricultural animal husbandry practices". So it is imperative that the investigator understand the stipulations of accepted agricultural animal husbandry practices in their state and the applicable laws. Increasingly, states are phasing out extreme methods of farm animal confinement by statute; however, these are generally civil statutes, enforced by fines or similar penalties.

Horses may be treated as livestock, depending on how they are defined under local law. Even horses that are pets may be subject to the legal interpretation of livestock, but police horses may have special protections that exceed the ordinary animal cruelty law. For these reasons, it is recommended that the investigator has familiarity with the definition of "animal" and the local cruelty statute, and with which agency is responsible for investigation and enforcement (e.g., the Department of Agriculture or the Department of Natural Resources).

Animal cruelty may be committed by long-time farmers who have become complacent in animal care, unable to physically keep up with animal care, suffering from mental incapacitation conditions such as dementia, or they may be unaware of, or uncaring about changes in animal cruelty laws. People may obtain farm animals or horses with an uneducated but romanticized vision of self-reliance or organic farming. These types of offenders may commit animal cruelty through neglect of appropriate nutrition, veterinary care or other appropriate animal husbandry practices. It is appropriate to provide guidance on how to improve conditions and plan a recheck visit. If recommendations have not been implemented, it may be time to consider animal cruelty charges.

DOI: 10.4324/9781003090762-9

Animal cruelty crimes to large animals include neglect (a failure to provide adequate food, water, shelter, grooming or veterinary care), abuse (non-accidental injury) or sexual abuse. The particulars of those types of cases are covered in other chapters.

Because of the complexities around large animal abuse cases, it is recommended that the investigator inform the appropriate responsible authority before planning an intervention. In many cases, the Department of Agriculture representatives will already be aware of the situation and collaboration with law enforcement may be the correct next step to ensure good animal welfare.

Biosecurity

When multiple species of animals are housed close together, and particularly when they lack adequate veterinary care and are stressed, there is a risk of inter-species infectious disease transmission. Some of these diseases pose a threat of zoonotic transmission (diseases that spread from animals to people) or a threat to larger agricultural concerns. Spread of infectious disease is exacerbated in close confines, filth and when animals are expressing symptoms, such as diarrhea. Investigators and other responders should be informed and equipped with appropriate protective equipment. There may be regulations related to decontamination of equipment, boots and vehicles between visits to various farm properties.

Preparation

Few municipal animal-impound facilities are equipped to take in farm animal species, so if animal impoundment is anticipated, plans must be made for where the animals are going to go for care during the pendency of any legal processes. Specific equipment and adequate personnel will be needed if downed animals (unable to get to their feet) are present, such as sleds, lifts and slings. Adequate and appropriate transport trailers must be arranged.

Well-equipped farms have paddocks, pens and chutes with good fencing to enable animal movement and sorting. This is not likely to be the case in circumstances of large animal neglect, and teams of people may be needed to move animals with boards and flags. Everyone responding to a farm animal scene must be informed about safety, including the behaviors and risks of working with various species of animals.

In addition to threats such as infectious disease and injury from animals, dilapidated farm scenes may have other risks such as rusted metal, dangerous equipment, noxious fumes and stray voltage. Barns, outbuildings, silos and haystacks may be unstable and at risk of collapse (Figure 9.1).

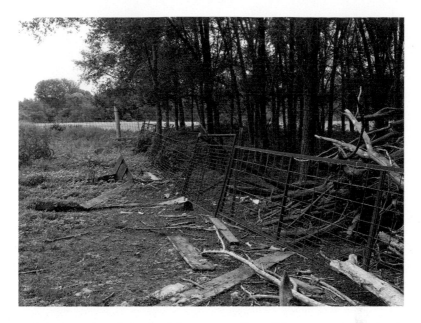

Figure 9.1 Rusted and sharp debris at neglected farm scenes pose a hazard to animals and responders. (Photo courtesy of Companion Animal Protection Society (CAPS).)

Scene Walk-Through and Sketching

The scene should be assessed with an initial walk-through, and the investigator should consider video recording the initial evaluation. Animals may initially present as depressed, but because they are prey animals, instincts and adrenaline may cause them to appear livelier later when there is more activity on scene.

The investigator should be sure to include all aspects of the property, pens, paddocks, fields, barns and buildings in their review. There should be clean, relatively dry (not deep muck) ground for animals to stand on. The presence or absence of shade structures (to include trees) or shelters from the weather should be noted. All feeders and food, water troughs and waterers should be captured and demonstrated to be in working condition (or not). Troughs and buckets should be of an appropriate size for the animal drinking out of it, especially when water levels are low. Water must be clean and potable. Any ponds or streams accessible to animals must be noted as well. Any veterinary treatment medications or equipment should be noted.

It is not normal for farm animals to die on the farm, and if they do die at a properly managed farm, the body will be buried in a deep grave or sent for rendering. The presence of carcasses or bone piles is a clear sign of a poorly run animal operation and the likelihood of significant animal suffering (Figure 9.2).

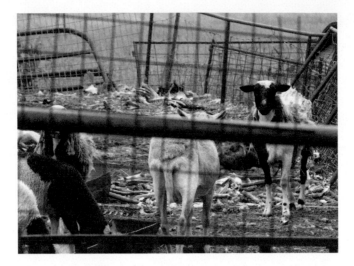

Figure 9.2 Deceased animals in paddocks with live animals pose health risks to people and animals, contaminates groundwater and is evidence of neglect. (Photo courtesy of CAPS.)

The animals should be videotaped without causing them undue stress. Normal and abnormal ambulation (walking) and other behaviors should be captured. Take the time to focus on individual animals so that their body contours and respiratory effort can be captured. Lameness (limping or failure to use a limb) can be secondary to acute injury or chronic conditions and should be recorded. While it may be "normal" or acceptable for a dog or cat to carry a leg while healing from an injury, this is a sign of unacceptable suffering in livestock. The visual of animals struggling to stand can be compelling testimony (Figure 9.3).

Triage

A large animal veterinarian should be on scene to evaluate animals before they are seized and transported. Livestock in borderline condition or juvenile animals are vulnerable to collapse with stress of handling or transportation. Some animals, especially horses, may require sedation for safe transportation. Other animals may be too incapacitated to tolerate transportation and may need to be euthanized on site.

Each animal should have a unique identifier number. If ear tags, notches or leg bands are present, those should be recorded. Animals should be evaluated by a veterinarian, and each photographed from each side, and at an oblique angle to highlight body condition. Photographs must also demonstrate significant findings such as wounds, overly long hooves or other conditions of note.

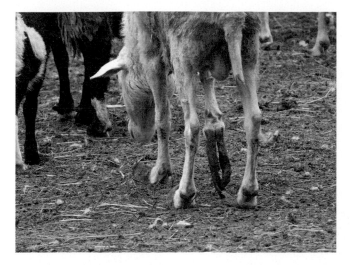

Figure 9.3 Overly long hooves are painful, prevent animals from ambulating normally and can interfere with an animal's ability to access food and water. (Photo courtesy of CAPS.)

Each animal should have its own physical exam record and should be body condition scored according to an accepted scoring system for that species and breed of animal. Some animals may appear shockingly thin to the uneducated observer, but it may be a normal phase of conditioning for that type of animal, depending on the breeding cycle or other factors. It is important to note that animals with heavy hair coats or wool cannot body-condition scored without touching them. Some animals can be too thin, even in the presence of adequate feed due to competition for resources, dental impairment or other conditions. A thinner than normal body condition may be acceptable, provided the animal is under the care of a veterinarian, and measures are being taken to ensure the animal's quality of life. All veterinary records should be gathered and reviewed by a veterinarian.

Postmortem Examination

Deceased animals should be necropsied. As with small animals, the necropsy should be documented with photography and ideally performed in a laboratory setting. However, with large animals, there may be constraints that prevent transport and lab necropsy. Some states require deceased farm animals to be transported in leak-proof conveyance. When anthrax is suspected, the necropsy must be performed in the field, and there should be a tractor available to bury the animal after necropsy (Figure 9.4).

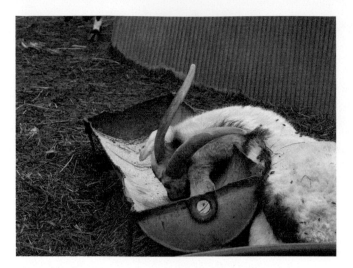

Figure 9.4 Photography of the deceased animal in place, accompanied by a post-mortem exam that supports death from dehydration or malnutrition is an appropriately complete approach to documenting the animal's death from neglect (failure to provide adequate food and water). (Photograph courtesy of CAPS.)

Nutrition and Water

The local agricultural extension office may be able to assist with the analysis of feedstuffs being used for the farm animals, whether hay, silage or grain. Some farms feed leftover waste such as expired bakery products or spent barley and hops from a brewery. These items can be part of a responsible diet if balanced appropriately, but animals fed only these products are subject to malnutrition. A veterinarian or the Department of Agriculture can assist with sending feed to a forage testing laboratory to evaluate feed for quality and for water quality testing.

Water must be available and potable. Water is not potable if it is murky or discolored. Even the most pure water is of no value, if it is frozen and therefore undrinkable. Livestock water requirements vary by species and size, but their water needs will be measured in gallons per water, along the lines of 1–3 gallons per 100 pounds of body weight per animal, per day. In hot or humid weather, water needs will be increased (Figure 9.5).

The amount of feed provided and the linear feet of trough access to feed and water sources are important measures. A trough in the middle of a barn

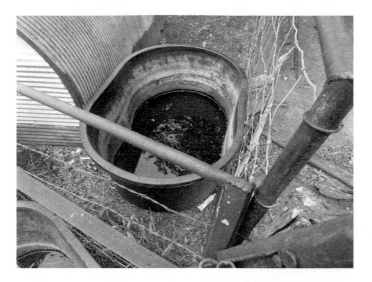

Figure 9.5 Water is not "available" if the animal cannot physically access it, or if the water is contaminated with filth or algae. (Photograph courtesy of CAPS.)

or yard will have access on two sides, so the available linear feed access is double that of a trough of the same size that is against a wall or fence. In animal yards that have a too-high stocking density, a pecking order will develop that will cause more dominant animals to prevent access to food and water by less dominant animals.

Air Quality, Bedding, and Footing

Animals kept in enclosed spaces must have appropriate ventilation, air exchanges and removal of manure. Wet or sloppy surfaces can predispose animals to injury, foot infections, abscesses and skin infections. High ammonia levels can lead to respiratory infections. Fecal samples can be collected to be assessed for fecal parasite counts. External parasites such as fleas, ticks, mites, lice and flies can also plague farm animals, transmit disease and can cause loss of condition (Figure 9.6).

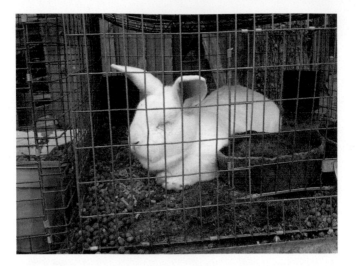

Figure 9.6 Thick accumulations of urine and feces in primary enclosures where animals cannot escape their own filth leads to painful foot, skin, perineal and eye infections. (Photograph courtesy of CAPS.)

Final Thoughts

Agricultural animals and horses may or may not be covered under the local animal cruelty statute, and there may be a mandate that a particular department performs an investigation. Farm animal investigations require preparation for safely and humanely handling large numbers of animals, potentially in poor condition. Preparation for case interventions must include species specialists, the appropriate equipment and a plan for where the animals will go for care. Agricultural authorities must be consulted before moving animals as there may be regulations in place to prevent the potential movement of infectious diseases.

Bibliography

Animal Legal and Historical Center. Farm animal issues. Michigan State University. https://www.animallaw.info/policy/farm-animal-issues.

Cavender A. 2020. Processing forensic cases involving agricultural animal species. Byrd JH, Norris P, Bradley-Siemens N (eds.). *Veterinary Forensic Medicine and Forensic Sciences*, 1st Edition, pp. 327–389. Boca Raton, FL: CRC Press and Taylor & Francis.

HFHA. The hub for biosecurity to protect the herd or flock. https://www.healthyagriculture.org/.

Tremblay R. Overview of management and nutrition in animals. Merck Veterinary Manual. 2014. https://www.merckvetmanual.com/management-and-nutrition/management-and-nutrition-introduction/overview-of-management-and-nutrition.

Releasing the Scene

10

VIRGINIA M. MAXWELL

Introduction

When all crime scene processing activities are complete, the scene is formally released. Upon release, perimeter security is withdrawn and no further entry or exit logs are maintained; therefore, there is no longer control over access and interaction with the scene and the integrity of any remaining materials cannot be guaranteed. If, at a later time, it emerges that a sample needs to be collected, the lack of security means that no chain of custody can meaningfully be initiated, and a subsequent search warrant may be required. Thus, releasing the scene is a critical step and one that should not be rushed.

Hold a Team Meeting

As scene processing draws to a close, the lead investigator should meet with the crime scene investigators and other specialized personnel who are involved, such as veterinarians and animal control officers. This meeting can take place within the secure area established outside the main crime scene or at another location; however, it should always take place away from any media present or other onlookers.

At the meeting, the team should consider the following:

1. What information was initially available and what information may have been developed during, or as a result of, the crime scene processing.
2. What evidence was located and seized? Has this addressed all information and subsequent questions or theories that have arisen?
3. What are the scene findings based on observations and evidence located?
4. What forensic analysis is required and therefore what evidence seized also requires that a control sample or a substrate control, e.g., carpet sample, be collected from the scene? Have all relevant control samples been obtained?
5. What items collected require a known DNA sample, fingerprints or hairs? Will elimination fingerprints be needed? Have warrants been obtained for these samples?

DOI: 10.4324/9781003090762-10

6. Have all relevant notes, measurements, sketches and photographs been obtained?
7. Have all pieces of investigative equipment, chemicals, etc., been retrieved from the scene?

Final Walk-Through

When the team meeting has addressed all questions to the satisfaction of the lead investigator and the scene processing is considered to be complete, the lead investigator should complete one final walk-through of the entire scene to ensure that all evidence collected, all equipment, chemicals, and processing kits, etc., have been retrieved, and no hazardous materials or conditions are being left. All areas of the scene must be inspected and general photo or video documentation of the final condition of the scene should be obtained. Once the investigator is satisfied that the crime scene processing is complete and all evidence accounted for, the scene can be released in accordance with the requirements of the specific jurisdiction.

Case Files

While some cases have a single crime scene to consider, others may have multiple scenes. For example, an animal may be killed in the suspect's house (primary crime scene), but the body is then transported in the suspect's vehicle (secondary crime scene) before being dumped in a remote location (secondary crime scene). Crime scene processing protocols will apply for each of these scenes, and reports, documentation and other documents will be generated. When each scene is complete, the lead investigator must ensure that they obtain copies of all materials generated to be maintained in a central case file along with all other investigative materials for the case. This case file should, at a minimum, contain the following crime scene-related materials:

1. Initial reports from the first responding individual, whether police officer or animal control officer.
2. Any search warrants or consent forms related to the crime scene or to the possession of any animals.
3. Any medical or veterinary reports related to human and animal victims.
4. Any documentation related to the transportation of live animals from the scene.
5. Documentation from the initial walk-through.

6. All crime scene documentation including note, photographs, video and sketches.
7. All documentation related to evidence located and seized, e.g., chain of custody.
8. Any documentation related to the release of the crime scene(s).
9. Any laboratory reports related to evidence seized and tested, though there may be considerable delay between the crime scene investigation and forensic analysis and reports.

Final Thoughts

Though releasing the scene seems such a simple step, it is irreversible therefore should never be rushed and must be undertaken in the same methodical manner as scene processing. The lead investigator should seek input from their entire team, including personnel such as veterinarians, to ensure that all scenarios and related evidence have been considered, and all important photographs and videos have been obtained. All areas of the scene should be considered, including all structures, and above and below ground.

Biological Evidence 11

VIRGINIA M. MAXWELL

Introduction

Biological evidence, and subsequent DNA analysis, can be significant in a wide range of animal cruelty crimes. However, in the investigation of animal cruelty, the analysis is complicated by the need to be able to examine both human and animal biological materials. While forensic laboratories are equipped to identify whether a biological sample is human or animal and to then analyze human DNA, few accept animal samples for DNA analysis due to differences in the analytical procedure and lack of validation for these animal-specific procedures. Significant advances in DNA analysis since its introduction to forensic science in the 1980s have made this the gold standard method of forensic testing. Through its ability to individualize samples and link them to specific individuals, to the introduction of the Combined DNA Indexing System (CODIS) database, DNA has revolutionized criminal investigations. Indeed, the likelihood of recidivism of animal abusers and the proven linkage between abuse of animals and interpersonal violence means DNA evidence can provide a critical linkage in their apprehension. While we consider animals primarily in the role of the victim in animal abuse cases, we must consider that there are also situations in which the biological material of an animal is used to identify an attacker, such as in dog-fighting or predation.

Forensically, the most common biological sample analyzed is blood, though semen is of importance in any case that has a sexual element involving a male. Saliva may be encountered in cases in which there are bite marks and, therefore, will likely be more common in animal than human cases. At the crime scene, reddish-brown stains are screened for blood, though it is common to conduct screening tests for other body fluids, along with species testing, in the laboratory. Advances in crime scene technology have produced simple self-contained field tests for most body fluids, though these may not be available in every agency, and some are human-specific. The principle behind screening tests for biological fluids is a color change catalyzed by some components of the body fluid in question. There is a need for caution when using screening tests for two reasons; first, these are catalytic reactions which means that the reaction, and the color change, will still occur in the absence

DOI: 10.4324/9781003090762-11

of the body fluid, just at a slower rate. Therefore, the results of a color test must be recorded within approximately 30 seconds of the test; they should never be left for several minutes before observation. Second, the tests are not absolutely specific and are subject to false positives. The common sources of false-positive results are well-established and available. For example, the phenolphthalein test for blood will indicate positive in the presence of vegetable peroxidase enzymes. As many of the sources of false-positive reactions to the different tests are visually dissimilar to the body fluid of interest, visual examination is an important first step before testing any stains. Investigators using field testing for biological fluids should ensure that they are familiar with any sources of false positives or cross-reactivity between species. The results of screening tests are used to indicate a particular body fluid may be present but should not be interpreted as definitive identification.

Beyond the use of specific body fluids as biological evidence, epithelial cells present on swabbing of items are now routinely used as a means of developing human DNA profiles in criminal cases. These cells are recovered from items such as clothing, firearms grips and other rough surfaces that have sloughed-off epithelial cells through contact and rubbing. Preliminary research indicates that animal coats are also capable of retaining sufficient human epithelial cells for DNA analysis.

Regardless of the source of the biological material, the goal is linkage to a specific source, human or animal. The sensitivity of modern analytical procedures for DNA analysis is such that less than a dozen cells are sufficient to obtain a full DNA profile. Robust procedures must be in place to ensure that contamination of samples cannot take place, including contamination from investigators or sloppy collection procedures allowing cross-contamination between items.

Sources of DNA

Human

Deoxyribonucleic acid or DNA contains the genetic material necessary for the functioning of all living things. Through ongoing research, different small sections of DNA were found to be highly variable and suitable for use to link biological materials to their donor. When considering nuclear DNA, these sections are referred to as short tandem repeats (STRs) which may be used to individualize the donor of the biological material with the exception of monozygotic siblings, such as identical twins. Specific locations on genes are referred to as loci, and at this time, STRs from 20 loci are tested. These loci have been chosen from among all chromosomes and were selected based on the variability of types within the population, and many countries use the same 20 STR loci. STRs that are specific to the Y chromosome have been identified and may be used in certain cases. These are referred to as y-STRs but are not as individualizing as regular STRs as they are inherited paternally, thus all relatives in the paternal line with a Y chromosome will share the same y-STR profile. Nonetheless, they allow a male profile to be analyzed separately out of a mixed sample. Further, when multiple males may be involved in a case, they allow investigators to estimate the minimum number of male donors to the profile and include or exclude male suspects. When nuclear DNA is not available in a case, such as when only hair shafts are available, or the samples are highly degraded, mitochondrial DNA may be used as an alternative way to link individuals to biological samples. Mitochondrial DNA (mtDNA) is located within the mitochondria of cells, but it is present in a much shorter loop, only 16,500 base pairs long, and does not contain the STRs of nuclear DNA. Instead, the base sequences of two regions of mtDNA, hypervariable region 1 (HV1) and hypervariable region 2 (HV2) are used. Like y-STRS, mtDNA does not provide the same individualizing power as nuclear DNA; however, in contrast to y-STRS, mtDNA is inherited maternally via the X chromosome regardless of the sex of the offspring.

Animals

Animals also have both mitochondrial DNA and nuclear DNA, and both types can be analyzed. However, the analysis of animal DNA for forensic purposes is by no means as routine as it has become for human DNA. First, human DNA is exactly what it says it is; it comes from humans, a single species. While certain species are more common than others in animal cruelty cases, it has to be considered that animal DNA could come from a multitude of different species with differing number of chromosomes and useful STR markers. While identification of the species is a relatively straightforward task, analyzing the DNA brings forward some critical issues. The STR markers used for human DNA analysis are well-defined, have been extensively tested and statistics are widely available. This is not the case for animal DNA; in fact, when animal DNA is encountered, the specific markers that provide the required variability for a high level of association may not have been established for the species in question. Once developed, the markers must be extensively tested, and statistical occurrences developed for each through the construction of databases containing numerous animals from the same species. This is not an easy and quick process, even finding sufficient samples of a species to establish statistical significance can be an almost insurmountable hurdle in some cases. Finally, there is a high likelihood of a legal challenge at trial if DNA results from an as-yet untested species is introduced. However, in many cases, it may be sufficient to simply identify the species from which a sample originated if there is no doubt as to the specific animal involved.

CODIS and CanineCODIS

CODIS was established by the FBI in the 1990s and was initially populated by the nuclear DNA samples from convicted sex offenders. Later, the offender database was expanded to include all convicted felons beyond just those convicted of sex crimes. CODIS provides a database of known DNA samples which could be used as a reference for comparison to DNA samples from criminal cases in which no suspect had been developed. Should no match, or "hit" be obtained, the unknown evidentiary sample remains in a separate database, regularly run against the offender database which continually expands as new offender samples are collected and entered into the database. A third database within CODIS contains samples developed for the identification of missing persons. CODIS is administered and controlled by the FBI, and samples entered into the database must meet certain standards with regard to quality.

Like CODIS, CanineCODIS is a DNA indexing system that can be used in animal cruelty casework though it is limited to dog-fighting cases. Initially populated from the genetic profiles of dogs seized during a large-scale dog-fighting investigation in Missouri, it has continued to expand through the submission of new samples from dogs seized during dog-fighting investigations as well as unknown samples seized from dog-fighting scenes, such as blood in the fighting ring. CanineCODIS allows investigators to determine relationships between dogs and to expand dog-fighting investigations into the breeding and training of fighting dogs. Though all analysis takes place at UC Davis, it is a joint initiative by the Humane Society of Missouri, the ASPCA, the Louisiana SPCA and the UC Davis Veterinary Genetics Laboratory.

Field Testing, Collection and Packaging of Blood and Body Fluids

Many items at crime scenes can be collected as possible sources of DNA. An investigation is best served through thoughtful collection of items rather than indiscriminate gathering of large numbers of items, especially as obtaining DNA profiles no longer requires a visible stain. Considering which objects are foreign to the crime scene or possible activities within the scene can narrow down which samples are likely to be probative. Table 11.1 shows a range of items to consider when collecting evidence, though each case will have other items to consider.

Blood

Blood is present in a wide range of crimes and may originate from both victim and perpetrator. In animal cruelty, it can be found in nonaccidental injuries, sexual assaults, animal fighting and even in neglect/hoarding cases where the

Table 11.1   Items from Which DNA can be Recovered in Animal Cruelty Cases

Item	DNA Location
Cigarette butt	Surface
Leash or collar	Surface – fabric areas are best
Ligature or rope	Surface
Dog crate	Surface
Tape	Both sides – cells stick to adhesive
Bite marks	Swab nonbloody area for saliva
Feces	Epithelial cells from sources will be present
Used condom	Exterior (victim) and interior (perpetrator)
Fighting/training paraphernalia	Surface or soaked into porous material
Documents/envelopes	Stamp/envelope adhesive
Guns	Grip
Nonfirearms weapons, e.g., bats, knives	Handle (aggressor), tip (victim)
Gas cans	Handle
Clothing	Areas in contact with skin, e.g., collar, cuffs
Hats	Bills and bands
Plastic bags	Knots
Firearms	Grip, possibly magazine
Zip ties	Rough areas

living environment includes dangers such as broken glass, wire, etc. It should also be considered in cases where cannibalism or predation is suspected.

At the crime scene, stains thought to be blood can be screened using a variety of reagents. Common screening tests include Kastel-Meyer, o-Tolidine or Leucomalachite Green, but there are several others in common use, often in convenient stick or laminar flow forms (Figure 11.1). A screening test includes blood as a possible source of the stain but false positives do occur. Determinations regarding the result of the test must be made within approximately 30 seconds, with a positive screening test usually sufficient to make a determination to collect a sample for further examination but should never be considered as definitive identification of blood. A negative result excludes blood as being the source of a stain.

Some field tests can provide confirmatory information that human hemoglobin is present in a stain, thus confirming that human blood is at least a component of the stain, though it does not mean that the stain cannot be a mixture of human and animal origin, or indeed contain more than one type of body fluid (Figure 11.2). The number of these tests is increasing, and a variety may be found on vendor websites. RSID (Rapid Stain Identification) series were some of the earlier field confirmatory test kits and these are available for blood, semen, saliva and urine. It is worth reiterating that the common field confirmatory test kits are confirmatory for human samples and will likely not react with animal samples; therefore, selection of the screening and confirmatory tests when

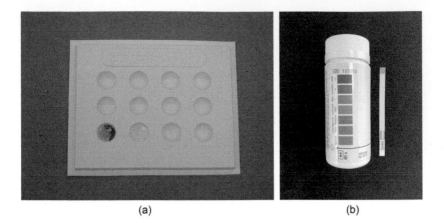

(a)   (b)

Figure 11.1 (a) Well plate showing a positive reaction to Kastel-Meyer reagent as indicated by the pink coloration. (b) Container of Hemastix which may be used for screening blood-like stains.

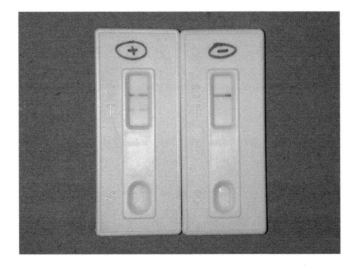

Figure 11.2 HemaTrace cards showing positive and negative results for the presence of human hemoglobin.

searching for animal body fluids should be done with care. Regardless, investigators using field tests for biological fluids should ensure that they are familiar with possible sources of false positives or cross-reactivity between species.

With all tests, it is important to be vigilant of expiration dates and any tests or reagents past the expiration date, even by only 1 day, must be discarded. Depending on the test, it may be necessary for the investigator to have a positive blood control sample to verify the efficacy of any test prior to its use on evidence. Batch numbers and expiration dates of all reagents and tests used should be included in scene documentation.

Chemical enhancement of bloodstains is recommended if they are very dilute or an attempt to clean them has been made. Several reagents are available for use at the scene, such as Luminol or Blue Star, which react with blood to produce luminescence. These reagents are highly sensitive, work with old samples and do not interfere with DNA analysis. Luminescence is temporary and photographic documentation is essential. The area of luminescence may be marked in some way to assist with further testing or recovery. Any area in which these chemicals will be used must be made virtually dark in order to view the luminescence.

When patterns in blood are noted, chemical enhancement can be used to visualize further detail, especially in areas where the blood is faint. O-tolidine is the most commonly used reagent but this must be used with care as it is considered to be a carcinogen. The reagent should be gently sprayed onto any areas of interest avoiding overspraying the area which may result in reagent and blood running down a surface. It is better to gently mist a few times rather than flood the area.

Before sampling bloodstains, the investigator should consider any specific pattern as this might be significant in crime scene reconstruction or may indicate that there are two or more possible sources of blood. This is important to recognize and to sample appropriately as it may provide a critical linkage of a perpetrator to a suspect at a time both were bleeding. If fingerprints or other pattern evidence in blood are noted, they should be carefully documented with evidentiary quality photographs. Note that the blood must be carefully sampled to identify the source.

Depending on the substrate, a stain may be swabbed off or simply cut out, while crusts can be scraped off into a druggist fold. Dry stains may be packaged and sealed, but wet stains must be dried prior to sealing to prevent degradation of the biological material. When blood is in snow, the sample can simply be scooped into a sterile container with care taken to maximize the amount of blood and take as little additional snow as possible (Figure 11.3). All items used for collection must be sterile and cross-contamination between samples must be avoided.

Semen

At the crime scene, semen might be found on bedding, soft furnishing, towels and rags. It may also be found on the coat of any animal victims. Semen generally dries to crusty white or off-white stains that fluoresce under UV lighting (See Figure 22.6). As fluorescent areas are located during ALS examination, they can be marked for later screening tests or removal. Screening tests are sensitive and require very little sample; however, screening tests for

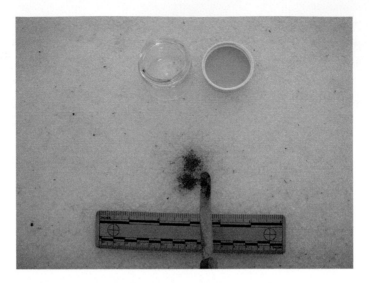

Figure 11.3 Collection setup for blood located in snow.

semen are not usually conducted at the crime scene. Stains on readily seized items can be left in place for lab testing, whereas those on immovable objects should be either cut out or swabbed depending on the substrate. Swabbing is performed via a sterile swab, moistened with saline, which should then be air-dried before packaging and sealing.

Saliva

Saliva is more common in animal cruelty cases than human cases due to bites being both a defensive and aggressive response of animals. Note that animals can be both aggressor and victim in animal cases, and saliva might be used to show that a particular animal attacked another versus being a victim defending themselves against a human act. For example, in a sexual assault case, the animal might bite their assaulter. Saliva in bite marks may also be used to determine the species of the biter when predation or scavenging might be a consideration.

Saliva can be found both in bite marks on bodies and on other items. Like semen, saliva will fluoresce with UV light, and while screening tests do exist for saliva, field tests for saliva are not generally used. In general, it is best to submit the entire item for analysis, but if this is not possible, bite marks can be gently swabbed with a moistened sterile swab to collect saliva. Excessive rubbing should be avoided so as to prevent superfluous epithelial cells being collected along with the saliva. Areas with commingled blood should be avoided if possible. If the bite mark is on the body of a dead animal, the skin can be excised with the bite mark intact and should be refrigerated.

Other Body Fluids

Urine, fecal material and vomit are also useful sources of DNA evidence in specific circumstances. For example, fecal material on a perpetrator's shoe can be linked to an animal through cells sloughed from the animal's intestines. While context is important, these sources of DNA are significant if no prior linkage exists between the animal and human.

No field tests for these body fluids are in common usage so cuttings or swabbings should be sent to a laboratory for screening prior to DNA analysis. Fecal material can be collected in a suitable container and frozen prior to examination.

Touch DNA

Sensitive analytical procedures now allow identification of individuals from items they have touched not just through the deposition of blood or other body fluids (Table 11.1). Sufficient epithelial cells slough off individuals through contact with other items such as clothing or rough surfaces. This leads to the possibility of linking individuals to items and locations through the recovery of epithelial cells by swabbing with a moistened sterile swab. While it becomes tempting to swab indiscriminately, it must be used judiciously to provide any real meaning in a case. For example, swabbing the door handle at the suspect's home is meaningless; however, swabbing the zip ties used to hold closed an abandoned crate containing a neglected dog or the collar of a dog that has been hanged is far more meaningful. Further, investigators must consider the likelihood of numerous people touching the same item. When cells from more than one person are inadvertently recovered, the analytical result is a mixture of DNA profiles which cannot be unequivocally resolved. Rather than individualizing a stain to a source, when mixtures are present, the source can only be considered as a possible donor to the mixture, decreasing the statistical significance of the result. Thus, when considering utilizing swabbings of an item to link them to an individual, it is worth the time to think about what areas are likely to be touched by only the person of interest and whenever possible to use items that would be touched only by the person of interest.

Control Samples

With the exception of no-suspect cases in which the CODIS database is to be utilized, all crime scene samples are compared to a known sample taken from the suspected source. The generally accepted known sample for DNA analysis is a buccal swab. This is a sterile serrated swab that is gently rubbed against the inside of the cheek for approximately 10 seconds to remove and retain nucleated epithelial cells. The swabs should be carefully air-dried before being returned to their package and sealed. If a buccal swab is not possible, blood may also be used and should be collected in a purple-top (EDTA) tube and refrigerated. The subject, human or animal, should not be allowed to eat or drink for 20 minutes prior to the collection of a buccal sample.

Bloodstain Pattern Analysis

Interpretation of bloodstain patterns at a crime scene for reconstruction is a discipline requiring considerable specialized training and certification. Nonetheless, every crime scene investigator should be able to recognize and document bloodstain patterns at the scene. With high-quality documentation, the patterns can be interpreted by a specialist at a later date; the better the documentation, the narrower the variables in the interpretation. Bloodstain patterns analysis (BPA) yields information about the events at different locations within a scene, and can show movement of both victim and perpetrator, whether a prolonged and sustained attack took place, and even the minimum number of heartbeats that occurred after an artery is breached. An expert can assess the approximate time frame of a sustained attack, provide an opinion of the attempts of the victim to escape or estimate the minimum length of time the victim appeared to be conscious during an event.

While a detailed discussion of bloodstain pattern interpretation is beyond the scope of this book, this chapter will provide the general recognition characteristics of commonly encountered patterns. Of note is that most experiments leading to the current body of knowledge in this discipline have not considered the coat, thicker skin and differing musculature of many animals. While the patterns of blood impacting a surface will be the same regardless of species, the injuries that are the source of the blood may not form as readily as in human bodies.

As blood is a viscous liquid, patterns are created by different events following the principles of fluid dynamics, including gravity, viscosity and surface tension. The fundamental laws of physics also apply to the creation of patterns from the events that occur at the scene. Not only are fluid dynamics important in pattern formation, but two other variables must be considered; the surface upon which the blood lands and the angle at which it impacts the surface. Blood drops that impact a rough surface will look considerably different to a similar drop impacting a smooth surface at the same angle and velocity. Though it may be considered counterintuitive, blood drops that impact smooth surfaces produce numerous satellites while a rough surface tends to cause far fewer, if any, satellites.

When blood impacts a surface at 90° (perpendicular) the drops, or main drop on a smooth surface, will be round in appearance. As the angle of impact changes and the surface is no longer perpendicular, drops will elongate further and the surface deviates from 90°. As the angle deviates further from the perpendicular, a satellite is developed in front of the main stain, thus

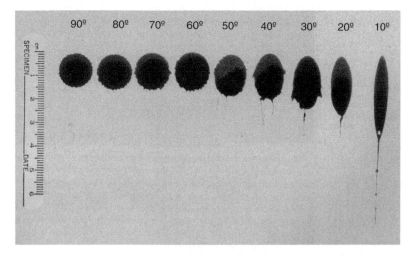

Figure 11.4 Effect of the angle of impact on the shape of the bloodstain produced. (Photo courtesy of Dr. Peter Valentin, University of New Haven.)

enabling determination of direction of impact on the surface (Figure 11.4). The angle of impact may be calculated by measuring the width and length of the main body of the bloodstain to calculate the inverse sine of the angle.

$$\text{Angle of Impact} = \text{Arcsine}\left(\frac{\text{width}}{\text{length}}\right)$$

With an understanding of the complexities of pattern formation, investigators can use the dimensions of drops and simple geometry to calculate the directionality and angle of impact, establishing the approximate location of the blood source.

Spatter Patterns

Spatter patterns are created when blood impacts a surface with some velocity created by the force of an object against the source of the blood or the movement of a bloody object. This might be a projectile entering or exiting a body, a blunt object being used on a body or the movement of a bloody object through the air. These stains may be classified by the velocity of the contact with the blood source, or by the mechanism by which the blood is thrown off against a surface.

High Velocity

High-velocity blood spatter is produced in limited circumstances and requires considerable force for its production. It is usually seen in shooting cases as the velocity of the projectile into or out of a body is sufficient to generate this

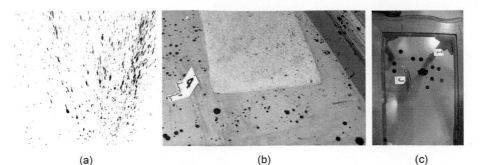

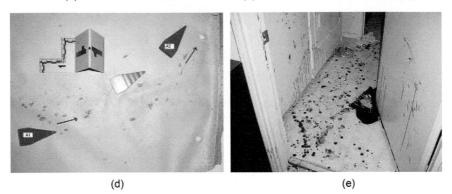

Figure 11.5 Appearance of common impact bloodstain patterns. (a) High velocity. (b) Medium velocity. (c) Low velocity/drip. (d) Cast off. (e) Arterial spurting. (Photos courtesy of Dr. Peter Valentin, University of New Haven.)

pattern. High-velocity patterns are characterized by an aerosol-like appearance with very small blood droplets, less than 1mm in size (Figure 11.5a). This may be seen with both forward and back spatter from the entrance and exit wounds of a bullet, respectively. There are few other common situations in which this pattern might be seen.

Medium Velocity

Medium-velocity patterns present blood drops with sizes of 1–4mm. Common situations would be the use of a blunt object to strike the source of the blood (Figure 11.5b), human or animal. Medium-velocity patterns are ideal for the measurement to determine directionality and angle of impact, thus providing substantial information about the events of the crime.

Low Velocity

Low-velocity patterns, in which blood drops are 4–8mm in diameter, are produced with low-force events such as dripping from an existing wound or a nosebleed (Figure 11.5c).

Cast-Off

Cast-off patterns occur when a bloody weapon moves through the air, as it is being raised to strike another time, and centrifugal forces cause blood to leave the end of the object impacting other surfaces. They are recognizable as medium-velocity patterns occurring in a linear configuration (Figure 11.5d). They may be present on vertical surfaces or ceilings depending on the relative positions of victim and suspect as well as the specific weapon used. The width of each linear pattern and appearance of the blood drops can in some cases indicate what type of weapons was used. For example, a narrower weapon, such as a metal bar, versus a broad weapon, such as a piece of wood. Investigators can also count the number of patterns to estimate the minimum number of times the victim was struck, keeping in mind that the first strike would not produce a cast-off pattern. The skin and coat of an animal can complicate this interpretation of the pattern.

Arterial Spurting

As the name suggests, arterial spurts occur when an artery is cut open usually in a sharp force injury. The high pressure of the blood in an artery leads to arterial blood spurting out of the wound onto an adjacent surface. Each time the heart beats, a new spurt will be produced; however, as the victim weakens, the spurts will diminish until the blood pressure becomes too low to produce further spurting (Figure 11.5e). Arterial spurts may be used to show the movement of a victim and also to estimate the number of heartbeats, and therefore approximate elapsed time, for the duration of the pattern.

Transfer Patterns

Transfer patterns are contact patterns produced when a clean object comes into contact with a bloody surface, or a bloody object contacts a clean surface.

Wipes

A wipe pattern is produced when an object moves through the blood that is on a the surface. Based on the appearance of the pattern, it may be possible to determine the identity of the object (Figure 11.6a).

Swipes

A swipe pattern is produced when a bloody object is moved along a clean surface. As with a wipe, the appearance of the swipe can give an indication as to what the object created the mark (Figure 11.6b).

Pattern Transfer

When a bloody object is placed on a surface or wrapped in something, the object may be identifiable based on the pattern. An example might be a

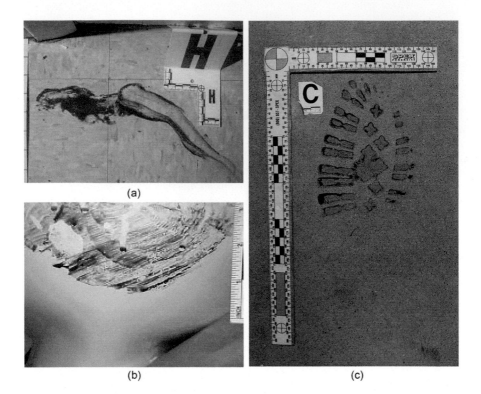

Figure 11.6 Common bloodstain patterns produced by transfer. (a) Wipe. (b) Swipe. (c) Pattern transfer. (Photos courtesy of Dr. Peter Valentin, University of New Haven.)

knife. Fingerprints, canine nose prints or footprints in blood are of course also a pattern transfer; though in their case, they can be used to identify the individual who left the pattern (Figure 11.6c shows a sneaker pattern in blood).

Other Bloodstain Patterns

Pools

Pools are formed when blood runs from a source into low or level points on surfaces and remain undisturbed (Figure 11.7a).

Flows

Blood flows can provide valuable information in determining whether items or bodies have been moved. Blood will always passively flow downward; thus flows that are not consistent with gravity indicate that the victim or object has been moved (Figure 11.7b).

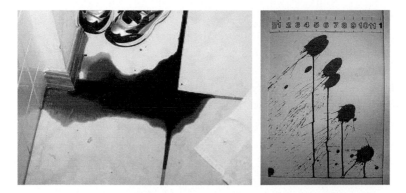

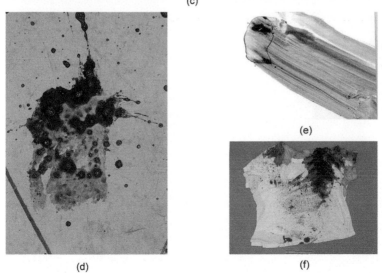

Figure 11.7 Other bloodstain patterns that may be found at a crime scene. (a) Pool. (b) Flow. (c) Drip trail. (d) Aspirated. (e) Skeletonization. (f) Void. (Photos courtesy of Dr. Peter Valentin, University of New Haven.)

Drips and Drip Trails

Drip patterns are produced by blood falling from a source simply under gravitational force. A drip trail is caused by movement of the blood source. This might be an injured person or animal, or it might be a bloody item being held as the person moved. If drip trails are to be used for reconstruction, the source, or sources, of the blood must be identified (Figure 11.7c).

Aspirated Blood

This blood pattern is characterized by air bubbles in the blood. It is created when blood is forced out through the nose or mouth or from certain types of wounds. When forced through the mouth, the blood may also be lighter in color due to dilution with saliva. Under certain conditions, a mist-like appearance of aspirated blood can be mistaken for high-velocity spatter, but the presence of air bubbles is the distinguishing feature (Figure 11.7d).

Skeletonization

Blood drops and pools dry from the periphery in. If a drop of blood is wiped before it is fully dry, a ring consistent with the original size of the drop may be left. The thickness of the ring can be used to estimate the time between deposition and wipe; however, as atmospheric conditions such as humidity can affect drying time, this must be considered an estimate only (Figure 11.7e).

Voids

Voids are noticeable gaps in a bloodstain pattern produced when an intermediary object was located between the source of the blood and the surface upon which the blood would otherwise land. Voids can provide an indication of the location of an assailant (whose clothing would then have the "missing" blood on it), whether doors were open or closed at the time of bloodshed, or whether some object at the scene was ultimately moved (Figure 11.7f).

Documentation of Bloodstain Patterns

Bloodstain patterns at the scene must be thoroughly documented to provide sufficient information for interpretation by a certified analyst at a later date if necessary. Documentation will be through a combination of photographs, sketches and accurate measurements of both dimensions and angles. Photographs must have scales and, in some cases, protractors present, and the use of a tripod to ensure perpendicular photography is recommended.

A combination of distance-, medium- and close-range photography is necessary to ensure that both the entire pattern and individual drops are recorded. As the source of the blood must be identified through DNA analysis (or simple species testing), a sample must be taken and the drop(s) used for this purpose should be noted. Major stains and patterns should also be recorded in the general scene documentation.

When documenting the entire pattern, scales may be used in one of two ways; either a grid of known dimensions can be placed on the pattern or a border of rulers is placed around the entire pattern, with smaller scales used next to each drop for closeup documentation. Disposable adhesive paper scales, rulers and evidence markers are available and are advisable to prevent contamination.

The change in shape of blood drops with angle if impact can be used to determine the approximate area of convergence, which is the point on a two-dimensional plane from which the blood drops originated. By considering straight lines through the elongated drops, a point at which they all converge can be readily established. Caution must be exercised when bloodstains originate from repeated events and interpretation becomes complex.

The area of origin uses a three-dimensional approach that determines not only the approximate height of the origin (if looking at a wall) but also the position in relation to the surface. The most common method of establishing the area of origin is by the use of strings and a protractor to position each in relation to a specific blood drop through calculation of the angle of impact. A tripod, or other stand, is used to support the strings.

Comprehensive documentation should occur throughout any determination of area of convergence or area of origin. Regardless, bloodstain pattern analysis and interpretation are extremely complex, especially when there are multiple bleeding events, and the assistance of a certified bloodstain pattern analyst is highly recommended.

Final Thoughts

Biological evidence can provide critical DNA linkages in animal cruelty cases. The sensitivity of current DNA analytical procedures requires that investigators must take every precaution to avoid contamination of samples. Further collection and packaging of biological samples must ensure that degradation is avoided.

Bloodstain pattern analysis is a valuable tool in the reconstruction of a crime scene; however, the interpretation requires significant training and experience. Through careful and complete documentation of any patterns at the scene, those individuals with this expertise can be involved at a later stage in the investigation if they are not available at the time of scene processing.

Bibliography

Bloodstain pattern analysis. *Wisconsin Department of Justice Crime Laboratory Bureau Physical Evidence Handbook*. 9th Edition. 2017. https://www.doj.state.wi.us/sites/default/files/dles/clab-forms/2021_physical-evidence-handbook-2017.pdf.

DNA evidence and standards. *Wisconsin Department of Justice Crime Laboratory Bureau Physical Evidence Handbook*. 9th Edition. 2017. https://www.doj.state.wi.us/sites/default/files/dles/clab-forms/2021_physical-evidence-handbook-2017.pdf.

NIST. *The Biological Evidence Preservation Handbook: Best Practices for Evidence Handlers*. 2013. https://nvlpubs.nist.gov/nistpubs/ir/2013/NIST.IR.7928.pdf.

Wolson TL. Documentation of bloodstain patterns. *Journal of Forensic Identification* 1995;45(4):396–408.

Trace and Chemical Evidence

12

VIRGINIA M. MAXWELL

Introduction

Trace evidence is usually considered as small, even microscopic, pieces of evidence, but the size is actually not the determining factor, and it includes most types of nonbiological materials evidence. Often considered to be simply circumstantial evidence, it can provide important linkages and should always be considered and collected. When circumstances dictate that fingerprint or DNA evidence may be of little value, trace materials can provide critical investigative information; when probative DNA or fingerprints are present, trace evidence can be used in the reconstruction of the events that took place. Trace evidence is rarely individualizing; however, depending on the material in question, e.g., soil, the likelihood of two similar samples having a common origin is very high. Individualization occurs when a physical match of pieces of trace evidence is possible; larger pieces of glass are particularly suited for this due to their brittle nature; however, tapes, paint, wood, plastics, metal and fabric can also be physically matched in some cases. A true physical match is considered to be absolute as it shows that the pieces were once a single item (Figure 12.1).

Some types of trace evidence provide investigative leads through specific manufacturing characteristics or the use of databases. These include

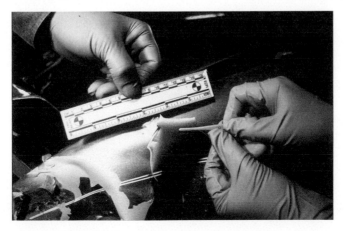

Figure 12.1 Automotive paint chip being physically fit to the location on the vehicle from which it originated.

DOI: 10.4324/9781003090762-12

pressure-sensitive tapes, cordage and automotive paint. Consultation with industry specialists can assist with many types of trace evidence.

Any object can carry trace evidence, though the specific facts of a case will dictate which objects will be of greatest value and which types of trace evidence will provide the important linkages. The greatest success in using trace materials as physical evidence comes from keeping an open mind as to the possible sources of the evidence and where it may be deposited. With the need to find all possible linkages, the search for trace evidence should encompass not just the scene but also the victim, suspect and any potential weapons.

Types of Trace Evidence

Trace evidence is a large category when many types of material are considered, though some are more common and found at many scenes. This includes hairs (both human and animal), fibers, paint, glass, soil, pressure pressure-sensitive tapes, plastics (such as garbage bags and zip ties) and ropes/cordage. These materials may not come from items that were touched deliberately but transfer through incidental contact such as walking across a carpeted floor, fiber transfer from wrapping of an animal as it was transported to a dump site, fibers from the vehicle's trunk on the animal, or mud from the dump site splattered onto the side of a vehicle or on the soles of a pair of sneakers.

In its entirety, trace evidence can comprise almost anything and the following list gives examples of the scope of this area; however, it should not be considered as complete listing and many other materials can be considered depending on the specific circumstances surrounding each case:

Hairs	Paint	Construction Materials
Fibers	Inks/dyes	Pollen
Ropes/cordage	Tapes	Wood
Soil	Plastic	Garbage bags
Glass	Paper	Zip ties
Metal	Lubricants	

It should also be noted that specific identification of some items listed, e.g., pollen and wood, might necessitate the expertise of people other than crime laboratory scientists.

Individualization, Identification, and Physical Match

Before discussing different types of trace evidence, the concept of individualization and identification must be clearly understood. When evidence is individualized, it is linked unequivocally to a source to the exclusion of all others, for example, we generally consider DNA evidence and fingerprints to be individualizing. Identification, however, links something to a source but not to the exclusion of other similar sources. To understand this, we can consider a silver paint chip identified as being consistent with a 2017 Honda Civic. While this paint chip can certainly come from a Honda Civic driven by a suspect, we cannot exclude other cars with exactly the same paint system. While this seems problematic, investigative information developed will exclude virtually all 2017 Honda Civics as they were not in the vicinity at the time of the crime. Despite this, we cannot unequivocally say that the paint chip came from one specific vehicle to the exclusion of all others.

There is a specific circumstance with materials evidence where the individualization of trace evidence is realistic. This is when a physical match can be made; two items can be shown to fit together three-dimensionally. This can occur with types of evidence that break or tear randomly, such as glass, tape, paint, fabrics and rigid plastics. As the likelihood of two items randomly breaking in exactly the same way is virtually zero, when a physical match occurs, it is considered to individualize a piece of evidence to a source.

Hairs

Hairs, both human and animal, can be used to provide linkages through transfer between parties or deposition at a location. Microscopic animal hair comparisons are not generally performed by regular forensic laboratories; however, the species can easily be determined. While human hairs can be compared microscopically, microscopic human hair comparisons are rarely accepted in court without additional DNA testing being undertaken; nuclear DNA, if tissue is present on the root, or mtDNA, if only the shaft is present. Microscopic human hair comparisons can never associate a hair with a specific person; only DNA testing can provide a higher level of association.

Hairs undergo a defined growth cycle which has three stages: anagen, catagen and telogen. During the anagen, or actively growing, phase, hairs are firmly attached to the follicle as they grow and do not passively fall from the follicle; they must be forcibly removed taking tissue attached to the root with them. Although it is not possible to determine how a hair was forcibly removed, the presence of numerous forcibly removed hairs is of note as it suggests some kind of violent event. Hairs in the catagen and telogen phases are no longer growing and cannot be used to determine if they were forcibly removed.

A phenomenon called postmortem banding, characterized by a dark band near the root, occurs in hairs during the decomposition of a body.

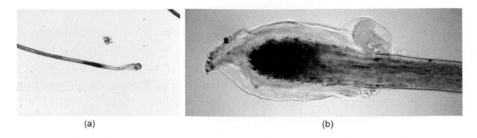

(a)   (b)

Figure 12.2 (a) Postmortem banding in a hair. (b) Hair root with a tissue tag.

Animal hairs that exhibit postmortem banding found on suspects, items such as blankets or tarps, or in vehicles, indicate contact with a deceased animal (Figure 12.2a).

Hair evidence is collected by picking with forceps and should be packaged in a labeled druggist fold before being placed in some sort of outer packaging such as an envelope or evidence bag. Hairs do not need to be refrigerated for storage.

If microscopic human hair comparisons are required, usually as a precursor to DNA testing, then a known sample of hair from all possible sources must be collected. A suitable known head hair sample consists of 50–100 hairs *pulled with forceps*, never cut, from all over the head. Though they can all be packaged together, hairs should come from the front, back, sides and top of the head to ensure that a representative sample is collected. A suitable pubic hair standard consists of 20–40 hairs, also pulled, from all over the pubic region. It is desirable to collect all known samples in a timely manner; many labs actually require that this be within 1 year of the incident. If the unknown hairs have tissue attached to the root, then DNA analysis of the tissue must be considered (Figure 12.2b).

Fibers

With their presence all around us, textile fibers are common trace evidence and, depending on the type and color of the fiber, can provide important associations. Fibers may be classified as natural or manufactured depending on their origin. Natural fibers, as the name suggests, occur as fibers in nature, examples being wool, cotton, hemp, sisal, linen, silk and jute. Manufactured fibers can be subclassified into two classifications, synthetic and regenerated. Synthetic fibers are fabricated polymers spun into fibers; these include nylon, polyester and acrylic. Regenerated fibers are made from natural polymers but, unlike natural fibers, regenerated fibers have been dissolved and spun into fibers rather than occurring in their final configuration in nature. Examples of regenerated fibers include acetate, triacetate, rayon, Tencel and Lyocell.

Manufactured fibers can show variation in the microscopic appearance and cross-sectional shape from one type to another, even manufacturer to manufacturer within a single fiber type. Color is also an important discriminating factor in fibers; thus, between cross-sectional shape and color, there can be a great variety in fibers making them valuable trace evidence. One important caveat is that white and blue cotton are in such widespread use that they are generally considered to be of little evidential value unless extenuating circumstances exist.

Fibers can be collected in several ways, but investigators must be vigilant to possible sources of contamination, particularly their own clothes or dirty crime scene tools. Fibers are easily transferred and are not always easily seen. Collecting potential carriers of fibers evidence should be considered as well as searching for fibers in the coat of an animal if the nature of the cruelty suggests that close contact with the suspect occurred. The location of the fibers can provide important reconstruction information.

Many fibers will fluoresce when exposed to UV light; thus ALS is an important tool in locating them at the scene, veterinary examination or necropsy. When photographing in UV light, a filter of the same wavelength as the goggles worn by the investigators should be placed in front of the camera lens. If significant distributions of fibers are seen, photographic documentation, with detailed diagrams, is important for reconstruction.

At the scene, fibers may be collected by picking, tape-lifting or using a trace vacuum. More than one technique can be used, though it is recommended that initial collection is by picking as the specific location can be documented. Once picking is complete, tape-lifting or vacuuming can be used to collect any remaining trace materials. When tape-lifting, a zone approach works well, and each lift should be clearly labeled as to the area of origin.

Picked fibers are placed into labeled druggist folds and then into an exterior container. Tape lifts can be placed sticky side down on acetate page protectors or some other similar objects before being placed into an exterior container.

Cordage

The term cordage includes rope, string, twine and other similar items. While cordage will ultimately require a fiber examination, the construction of these items is an important feature. As physical evidence, they are common in situations where the victim is restrained or killed by strangulation or hanging. The act of tying cordage can result result in epithelial cells from the perpetrator being deposited on the cordage. If the cordage is removed, but later seized from the suspect, hairs and other biological material may be recovered. If cordage remains on the animal, any knots should be left intact for examination as they can provide investigative information, and human hairs, trace materials and epithelial cells may be recovered from the knot. When removed from the victim, the cordage should be cut, and the cut ends clearly marked. Paper bags are suitable packaging for cordage.

Soil

Soil can place people or objects at locations or, when layers of soil are present, show the route taken by a person or vehicle. Soil can be compared to known samples but can also be used to identify a location based on its mineral composition and other components. The potential uses of soil evidence are numerous and the extensive variation in soil composition, both horizontally and with depth, makes it valuable associative evidence. Soil has three main components: minerals, organic matter and other inclusions such as pollen or anthropogenic materials. Minerals make up about 40% of the composition of soil and come primarily from the bedrock assuming no topsoil has been added. Organic materials are both vegetative and animal/insect in origin and are indicative of the flora and fauna at the location of the soil. Finally, the inclusions can be an important part of a comparison or in identifying a location whether through natural material or indicators of human activity.

Correct collection of soil evidence is critical to the success of the analysis. Inadvertently collecting extraneous material along with the soil sample can lead to a false exclusion due to apparent differences in compositions of known and questioned samples. For example, if a chunk of soil is collected from a vehicle floor mat along with loose sand that has been deposited over the course of a winter season, then the quartz component will appear to be much larger than it actually is which will lead to a flawed forensic examination.

To minimize extraneous materials, carriers of soils, such as footwear or automotive floor mats, should be collected; though if chunks of soil are clearly visible, they can be collected and placed into a leak-proof container such as an ointment tin or plastic tube. Large items, such as shovels or picks that are difficult to package, should have the head with soil attached carefully wrapped to prevent the loss of soil samples. Soil from the undercarriage of a vehicle may be removed and placed into a sealed container. Wet soil should not be placed into sealed plastic to prevent degradation of the organic component. Paper will allow samples to breathe as they dry.

Known samples of soil should be collected from as close as possible to the location in question, keeping in mind that composition can change rapidly with vertical and horizontal distance. Tools used for collection should be carefully cleaned between samples to prevent contamination of one sample by the next.

Both known and questioned soil samples must be packaged to prevent the loss of any of the soil samples as this could ultimately impact the ability to link them.

Pressure-Sensitive Tape

Pressure-sensitive tapes include common categories such as duct tape, electrical tape, packing tape, etc. In animal cruelty cases, it is often used to immobilize victims or to prevent them from making noise or biting their assailant. It may be used to seal containers in which animals are placed such as boxes and garbage bags. Not only is tape valuable associative evidence when compared to a roll recovered from a suspect, but it can also be individualized through the physical matching of tape ends and hold other important types of evidence such as fingerprints, DNA and trace materials. Many types of tapes are manufactured to different specifications depending on their likely end use. Thus, investigative leads may still be developed by examination of a piece of tape in the absence of a possible source.

Tape recovered from an animal or object should be kept as flat as possible. When the adhesive sides of tape stick to each other, they can be difficult to separate without distortion or losing fingerprint and DNA evidence located on the adhesive. If multiple pieces are layered, such as wrapped around an animal's muzzle, the tape should be cut at one location (which should be initialed) and then removed and packaged. No attempt should be made to separate the layers. Once the tape is removed, it can be placed inside a sheet protector or stuck to a piece of acetate prior to packaging. It should never be stuck to paper or card or placed in packaging with the adhesive side exposed.

Paint

Paint has widespread use on surfaces for both aesthetic and protective reasons and is therefore found as evidence on many different types of cases. Forensically, the most common types of paint are automotive and architectural but, depending on the case, other types such as tool paint and spray paint can provide important linkages. Automotive paint might be found if an animal was struck, either accidentally or deliberately, by a fast-moving vehicle, and while make, model and year of the vehicle can be determined via an automotive paint database, the driver's intent cannot be ascertained this way.

Architectural paint is used on structures, whether walls, window or door frames, and other parts of buildings. It is primarily used as evidence when found on tools used in forced entries but can also be important if painted wood is used as a weapon. Further, in the issue of pica, it can link some nonfood items eaten back to a source, such as in neglect and abandonment cases. Other types of paints can provide linkages if painted objects are used as weapons in blunt force injury cases or chopping and cutting cases.

Paint is usually applied in layers; thus, collection of known paint samples must take this into account. Paint chips located at a scene or on an animal can be collected with forceps and placed into a druggist fold and an outer container. Paint chips should never be placed loose into an envelope as these do not seal completely and the paint chips can leak out of the envelope. It is also best to avoid plastic bags as primary packaging, as static electricity can then make retrieval of paint chips, and any other trace evidence, difficult (Figure 12.3).

When collecting known paint samples, investigators must obtain all layers of the paint. This is best achieved using a clean single-edged razor blade and pushing it down to the substrate beneath the paint. Samples should be taken from close to the area of interest but not actually in any damage. Known samples are also placed into a druggist fold and then into an outer container. If the precise location of interest is unknown, then multiple samples may

Figure 12.3 Paint chips leaking out of improperly sealed plastic bags.

be taken when the possibility of differences in the paint exists. Each known sample should be collected using fresh blades and placed into separate packages that clearly state where the sample was taken. When differences in paint exist, being able to pinpoint where the contact between victim and object occurred can be important.

Easily transported items can be seized as potential carriers of paint evidence rather than attempting to collect the sample at the scene.

Glass

Glass is a stable, widely used material. It is found in eyeglasses, doors and windows, household and scientific goods and containers such as bottles, all with differences in composition and glass quality. Chemical analysis of glass can never provide more than an association; however, glass can be recycled many times creating compositional variations within a specific use category allowing meaningful comparisons to be made. From a case perspective, glass is generally used in forced entry cases, motor vehicle cases and where a glass item such as bottle is used as a weapon. Where a glass object is used as a weapon, glass may be recovered from wounds and compared to the suspected source. Due to mass production, glass examination produces inclusion and exclusion with regard to the known sample, but the brittle amorphous nature of glass is ideal for physical matches if the glass pieces are large enough (Figure 12.4).

Questioned glass fragments may be found on clothing, embedded in footwear soles, in wounds and in the coat of animals. If they are visible, then they may be picked using forceps and placed in containers. Envelopes should never be the primary container due to the possibility of leakage, but tins and plastic tubes are ideal. If glass is suspected but not clearly visible, then potential carriers of evidence may be collected but should be packaged to prevent the loss of glass fragments. Tape-lifting glass fragments is not recommended as adhesive residues left on the fragments can be detrimental to a lab analysis.

When collecting a known sample of glass, a representative sample should be taken. Glass is not always homogeneous in nature and samples from several different areas should be included but can be packaged together in a leak-proof container.

Miscellaneous Trace Evidence

Plastics and Polymers

Though polymers are present in major trace categories such as paint and tape, plastic itself is found as garbage bags and zip ties. Animals may be placed into

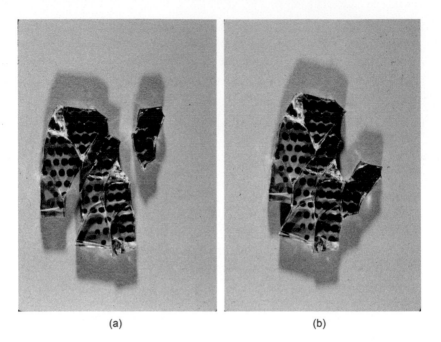

(a)   (b)

Figure 12.4 (a and b) Pieces of automotive glass physically fit back to each other.

garbage bags, dead or alive, and zip ties may be used to immobilize a living animal or to seal containers such as bags and crates.

While plastic is generally class evidence, and a questioned sample must be compared to a known sample, there are instances where individualization is possible, either because of a match between two pieces or alignment of manufacturing striations on garbage bags that are sequential in a roll.

When collecting plastic bags, the possibility of identifiable fingerprints must be considered, and the position and orientation of those prints can be important in establishing how they were deposited. While most zip ties are not large enough to have sufficient ridge detail for fingerprint comparisons, some of their surface is rough and can slough off human epithelial cells from which a DNA profile may be obtained.

When physical match, fingerprints or DNA are not options, plastic items can be compared to known samples to determine if they are consistent with each other and could therefore have a common origin.

Pollen

Pollen is both robust and morphologically distinctive. Through collaboration with an expert, it is possible to identify the specific flora from which the pollen originated, and even identify areas where less common flora are found. Further, not only do pollen "fingerprints" exist due to the location-specific variety in plants, but these "fingerprints" are also seasonally specific. Pollen can be deposited on bodies or their coverings, the clothing of individuals and vehicles, or their undercarriages, used for transportation. Pollen has even been used to link a gas can to the location of two partially burned bodies. The structure of both animal hair and pollen grains assists in the retention of pollen on the coat of an animal once deposited, and further deposition can result in layers that can provide temporal information.

The existence of pollen "fingerprints" allows investigators to link people and objects to other locations and is of value when pollen is found that is not part of the individual's usual surroundings. Pollen can be recovered well using tape-lifting. The location of the pollen on an individual's clothing or on an animal can be important and so tape lifts should be of specific areas not just one general lift and should be carefully labeled as to their origin. For example, each side of a deceased animal should be collected separately, as we might expect to find differences in pollen species if the animal was dead at the time it was left at the location versus an animal living at that location that subsequently died there.

Accelerants and Other Chemicals

Burns can be caused in different ways, including by thermal and chemical means. Thermal burns may be caused by igniting a flammable liquid poured over the animal. Chemical burns are caused by contact with corrosive chemicals, such as bleach or drain cleaner, which may be poured over the animal. In either case, the agent used must be identified. Flammable liquids are volatile and will evaporate if samples are not collected quickly.

If an animal was standing on a porous surface such as carpet, wood or even dirt at the time the flammable liquid or corrosive chemical was poured, a sample of that porous material can be collected for analysis. The animal's coat may also be tested for residues if sufficient hair can be recovered from the area of damage, alternatively a collar may also retain residue. If flammable liquids are suspected, samples should be placed into clean unused paint cans and quickly sealed to prevent vapor escaping. They should never be packaged in plastic or in a glass or metal container that has a plastic-lined lid as the plastic will contaminate the evidence. Conversely, corrosive chemicals might react with a metal can and should be packaged in inert plastic or glass containers.

Gunshot Residue

Discharge of a weapon produces firearms discharge residues, referred to as gunshot residue (GSR). GSR consists of burned and unburned gunpowder along with primer residue and metal abraded from the ammunition and barrel. GSR is propelled down the barrel and exits the muzzle toward the target, as well as coming out of any openings on the gun such as the cylinder gap or ejection port. GSR also tends to come back onto the shooter. GSR exiting toward the target only travels 2–3′ before gravity causes it to fall onto any available surface. If a target is within that distance, the residues can land on the target in patterns that can give an indication of the muzzle-to-target distance. It should be noted that an intermediate surface will prevent the residue hitting the intended target. The coat of an animal is not an ideal surface to establish muzzle-to-target distance using conventional lead and nitrate/nitrite residue testing; however, IR light and photography can reveal sooting, which can distinguish between close-range and distance shots.

Gunshot residue can be collected from a suspected shooter's hands using a purchased kit, though this must take place within a few hours of the shooting as the nature of GSR is such that little, if any, will remain on the hands of a living person after 4–5 hours. The subject should not be allowed to use the bathroom or wash their hands before testing as handwashing will remove the GSR. It should be noted that GSR can be transferred onto hands from any surface in which it is present, and care should be taken to ensure that the subject does not come into contact with any such surface.

The same type of kit can be used to sample a surface, such as the coat of an animal, for the presence of GSR. As this will remove any surface GSR, it should not take place until after any IR photography used for a potential distance determination, and the animal should not be washed for necropsy until after any samples are taken.

Distance Determination

Distance determinations, or muzzle-to-target distance estimations, in human shootings use chemical enhancements of lead and nitrate/nitrite residues on clothing. As this is not possible in an animal cruelty case, specialized IR photography can record the presence of any sooting around a wound which would indicate a close-range shot, assuming no intermediate surface, but that is the likely extent of any possible distance determination.

It should be noted that GSR is a very fine particulate residue and does not permanently adhere to a surface. Thus, extreme care should be taken to avoid any transfer or wiping of this residue when handling the victim. This is to avoid both distortion of the pattern on the body but also to avoid contamination of other surfaces through intermediate transfer via an investigator.

Final Thoughts

Trace and chemical evidence is a large and diverse category. While some types of evidence, such as fibers, are very common evidence, some cases may produce more unusual materials to provide linkages and investigators should keep an open mind to this possibility. Although individualization is not common, the linkages provided by trace evidence are valuable and can provide important investigative information.

Chemical evidence such as accelerants and gunshot residue cannot be associated to a specific source but, like trace evidence, provide information that can be integral to an investigation. Gunshot residue found in the coat of an animal shows that the shooting was within a few feet which could contradict a suspect statement, especially when combined with a bullet trajectory.

The main issues with these categories of evidence lie in careless collection at the scene or lack of understanding of their use leading to trace and chemical evidence simply being ignored.

Bibliography

American Society of Trace Evidence Examiners. Scientific working group for materials analysis. https://www.asteetrace.org/swgmat.

American Society of Trace Evidence Examiners. Trace 101. Introduction to Trace Evidence. https://www.asteetrace.org/trace101.

Santa Barbara County. Sheriff's Office. Forensic Unit. Collection of trace evidence at crime scenes. https://www.sbsheriff.org/wp-content/uploads/2019/12/SOP-CSI-004-12-Trace-Evidence-Collection.pdf.

Pattern Evidence

13

VIRGINIA M. MAXWELL

Introduction

Pattern evidence encompasses a range of evidence types including firearms, fingerprints, imprints/impressions and questioned documents. All have the possibility of individualization; thus good documentation and careful collection and packaging are important. Examination-quality photographic documentation can be used for comparison purposes should there be any issues with the collection, such as casting, enhancement or lifting, at the scene.

The individualizing characteristics have a different origin in each type of evidence, but each has the potential to definitively show that a person or vehicle was at a particular location, authored a document, or that a particular gun discharged a bullet or cartridge case. These linkages are made through the presence of individualizing markings, though sufficient markings for this level of discrimination are not always present; however, it may still be possible to include or exclude a source in these cases. For example, a bullet may be too damaged to provide sufficient striations for individualization but still exhibit sufficient characteristics to be included as coming from a particular weapon but not to the exclusion of all others.

Firearms

Firearms may initially be characterized by the length (or intended length) of the barrel, as handguns and long guns. The barrels of long guns are sometimes crudely sawn off to shorten the barrel for concealment purposes. Beyond the barrel length, firearms may be further characterized based on their design and the number of rounds that can be discharged with a single-trigger pull. This gives categories of single shot, automatic, semiautomatic, revolver and shotgun, with different mechanisms of action leaving specific markings on ammunition that may be used to link the two together.

With the exception of shotguns, gun barrels are manufactured with a twisted interior pattern consisting of lands (raised) and grooves designed to impart spin on the bullet as it moves down the barrel. The nominal diameter of the barrel is referred to as the caliber of the weapon and is measured in

DOI: 10.4324/9781003090762-13

different units depending on the country of origin of the firearm. In the US, it is measured in hundreds of an inch, the United Kingdom uses thousands of an inch, while the rest of Europe uses millimeters.

In addition to the twist direction and dimensions of lands and grooves, which are called class characteristics and do not individualize, the barrel manufacturing process, and subsequent wear and tear from use, leave microscopic striations which are transferred to the bullet as it passes along the barrel, as shown in Figure 13.1. These striations are considered individualizing as they can link a bullet to a single barrel to the exclusion of all others. Thus, a bullet removed from a body or scene may be linked unequivocally back to a specific gun if the gun is also recovered. Further, the discharge of a firearm causes the base of the cartridge case to hit the breech face of the weapon with sufficient force to transfer the pattern and manufacturing striations onto the cartridge case along with a firing pin impression. These markings also have the potential to be individualizing. One additional source of individualizing markings comes from the mechanisms used to eject cartridge cases and reload live rounds in semiautomatic weapons.

Shotguns are notably different from other firearms as the barrel interior is smooth. Shotgun ammunition consists of numerous balls or pellets which are much smaller in diameter than the barrel and therefore a rifled barrel could not impart spin, and so shotgun pellets do not have individualizing striations. Shotguns do have firing pins and a breech face, and therefore, spent ammunition left at the scene could be linked to a specific shotgun using those markings.

The potential for recovery of cartridge cases at a shooting scene is related to the type of weapon used. As semiautomatic ejects spent rounds after

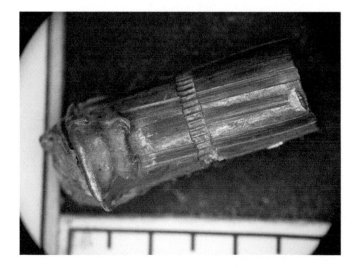

Figure 13.1 Striations on a bullet caused by transfer of markings from the interior of a gun barrel.

discharge, the rounds may be found at the scene, assuming they have not been collected by the shooter. Revolvers function using a rotating cylinder that holds the ammunition. After discharge, the spent cartridge case is rotated out of alignment with the firing pin and the next round moves into place. The spent rounds are not ejected by the weapon after discharge and will not therefore be left at a scene unless the cylinder is deliberately emptied. Most shotguns do not eject spent shells and unless the shooter manually ejects and reloads at the scene; there is unlikely to be any spent ammunition there.

Ammunition

Ammunition generally has four components: a bullet, primer, main charge and a cartridge case. The diameter of the ammunition will be similar to the caliber of the weapon from which it is designed to be fired. Shotgun shells differ in which the bullet is replaced by shot (small metal balls) separated from the main charge by wadding, and these are contained within a plastic shell. The base of the shotgun shell is, however, still metal and contains a primer and main charge.

The bullets used in regular ammunition have several possible configurations. Bullets may be unjacketed (rare), semi-jacketed and fully jacketed, and the tips may be rounded or hollow point. Different materials may be used for the bullet though they are typically metal, such as lead-jacketed in copper or nickel. Discharge of a weapon ignites the primer which in turn ignites the main charge creating a large amount of hot gas, propelling the bullet down the barrel due to the pressure of the gas. The chemical residues from this process create gunshot residue (GSR) though GSR cannot be linked to a specific weapon. The GSR that exits the barrel behind the bullet is particulate and will land on available surfaces, including the shooter's hands and clothes, but when the shooting is within approximately two to three feet, the GSR can also be found on a shooting victim.

Firearms Evidence

The evidence recovered at the crime scene will depend on the weapon and ammunition used. As discussed, revolvers do not eject cartridge cases after discharge, whereas semiautomatic weapons do. However, the absence of cartridge cases should not be considered as conclusive proof that a revolver was used as spent cartridge cases may be collected by a shooter. If an exit wound is apparent on the animal, then the bullet may be found at, or in the vicinity of the scene, though any bullet could travel a significant distance until it is stopped by an obstacle. Establishing the bullet trajectory with the assistance of a veterinarian can provide a viable area in which a bullet may be found. Outside of biological evidence, it is worth keeping in mind that a bullet may retain material from any object it penetrates or ricochets off. While this may not be important in every case, if there is any suggestion of an accidental shooting where the victim was not the intended target, this should be explored (Figure 13.2). If the wounds are consistent with a shotgun, then wadding or fragments of plastic ejected from the barrel with the discharge of the shotgun might be found at the scene or in close close-range shots, in the animal's body.

Shotgun shot disperses with distance, though the actual degree of dispersion is dependent on both the shotgun and the use of a choke on the muzzle. Thus, the presence of shot will depend on the distance involved. The wound size and the extent of shot spread can be indicative of the rough distance involved. If the shot is at a close range, there is also the possibility of the wadding being blown into the wound which, along with shot pellets, can be recovered at necropsy.

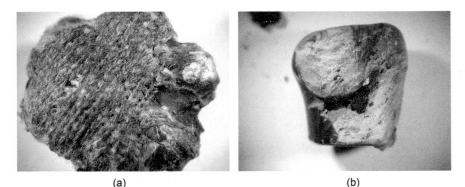

(a)   (b)

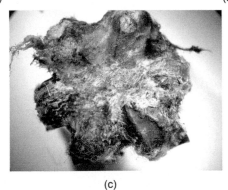

(c)

Figure 13.2 Bullets with foreign material from clothing and contact with other surfaces due to ricochet or impact. (a) Fabric from clothing. (b) Asphalt and paint. (c) Fabric and biological materials.

Firearms Evidence Collection

With the possibility of individualization of firearms evidence, it is of utmost importance that all markings on spent bullets and cartridge cases are protected from the possibility of damage. Spent bullets and cartridge cases should be carefully wrapped in gauze or cotton wool before being packaged in an envelope or other suitable exterior container. They should not be packaged loose and unprotected to ensure that they do not rub against a hard surface potentially damaging their markings. Initials are marked on the evidence with a scribe in a position away from evidentiary markings, e.g., the base of a bullet has no useful markings, nor does the side of a cartridge case. The same precautions should be used for the metal base of a shotgun shell. Any other components of the shell located, such as the wadding, should also be collected.

Firearms should never be held by placing an item, such as a pencil, inside the barrel as preservation of the interior rifling and striations is critical to a successful forensic examination and comparison. The sides of the trigger guard or a textured grip are good areas to hold when seizing a gun (with gloved hands). The serial number of a firearm should be recorded as this is a unique identifier of the weapon. In some cases, serial numbers are obliterated by scratching or sanding but the number can often be restored by a trained analyst. A firearm must ALWAYS be checked and unloaded before packaging, keeping in mind that removal of the magazine from a semiautomatic weapon does not fully unload the weapon as a live round may remain in the chamber. Thus, the chamber must always be checked, and any live round should be removed and packaged separately from the magazine and contents (Figure 13.3). The magazine can be left loaded with any remaining live rounds, but the number of rounds and magazine capacity should be documented. The position of the rounds in a revolver chamber should be noted prior to unloading. Any position that is empty should be marked in case there is the possibility that the shooting was an accidental discharge. A firearm should never be pointed toward anyone even if it is thought to be unloaded.

When collecting a shotgun that has been fitted with a choke, the position of the choke should be documented and left unchanged. The choke affects the scatter of the shot as it exits the barrel which can change the general spread used for a distance determination estimate.

Tool Marks

Tool marks are markings made on surfaces by a moving or stationary tool such as scissors, bolt cutters, pry bars, etc. Tool marks may be impressed as a general shape in cases where the tool does not move along the surface, though these markings usually only lead to class characteristics such as shape and

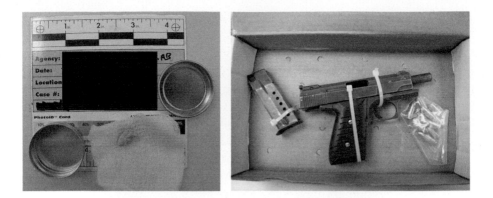

(a)   (b)

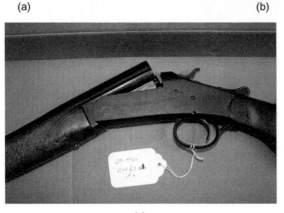

(c)

Figure 13.3 Correct packaging of firearms evidence to preserve individualizing striations and clearly indicate weapons are unloaded. (a) Bullet packaged with gauze. (b) Handgun secured with zip ties with open chamber. (c) Shotgun packaged to show it is unloaded.

size of the tool used. However, when moved across a surface, markings left by the tool can be used for individualization if sufficient detail can be obtained through some recipient surfaces, such as wood, may not be suitable for fine detail. Individualizing marks are a result of the manufacturing process of the tool followed by wear and tear from repeated use. Together they can link a specific tool to a mark. When only class characteristics are left, a specific tool can be included or excluded based on the size and shape of the mark.

Tool marks should be considered in many types of cases based on the incident and use of the tool. Any crime involving a forced entry should be considered as having tool marks evidence at the point of entry, such as a pried door or window, and anytime something is cut, such as with bolt cutters on padlocks and chains. When animals are stabbed or chopped, either as the cause of death or for disposal of the body, markings may be made in bone by the tool used. Though

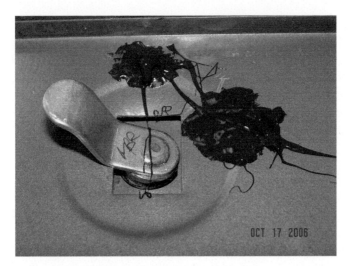

Figure 13.4 Casting a tool mark at the scene using Mikrosil®.

bone has not always proved to be an ideal surface for individualization, it should still be examined as markings can indicate the type and size of tool or weapon.

Evidence containing tool marks can be seized directly for laboratory processing of the tool marks. When the mark is in an immovable object, the relevant area in question should be removed and collected, e.g., part of a door frame. If this is not possible, the tool mark should be cast at the scene using a casting material, such as Mikrosil® or a similar product, to make a permanent cast of the mark and any fine details present (Figure 13.4). Once set, the cast is removed and packaged.

Items seized for comparison purposes should be packaged with care to ensure that the striations are protected from the possibility of damage. The tool should never be placed into the questioned tool marks as this can not only damage the tool mark but can also lead to transfer of trace evidence between the two.

A note of caution with regard to tool marks in bone and in wood. Tool marks that are made when the animal is alive or recently dead will shrink as the bone dries out over time. The hygroscopic nature of wood means tool marks in wood can also change in size; if the wood dries, the tool mark will shrink and vice versa. This is important when wood with tool marks is collected in a humid or damp area and then stored in an air-conditioned location for a period of time. Thus, casting at the scene as well as seizing the item may be considered.

Imprints and Impressions

Impressions are three-dimensional markings made in soft materials such as mud; imprints are two-dimensional and made when an object deposits material in the pattern of the object on that surface such as footprints in blood or grease. Footwear or tire imprint and impression evidence can be used not only to link a person or vehicle to a crime scene, but in some cases, a trail of footwear or paw imprints and impressions will show movement around a scene providing important information for a crime scene reconstruction. If no suspect has been identified, the Shoeprint Image Coding and Retrieval database (SICAR), purchased by some, but not all, crime laboratories, can provide investigative leads through the identification of shoes and tires based on the patterns left at the scene (Figure 13.5).

Beyond footwear and tires, other types of imprints or impressions are patterns left on the bodies of victims which can, in some cases, provide strong linkage for a particular item used as a weapon, e.g., a shoe sole pattern in a stomping case, or the general shape of a weapon.

A critical step in the crime scene collection of any imprint or impression is obtaining examination-quality photo documentation prior to any attempt to cast or lift them (Figure 13.5b). If problems arise in the collection of the evidence, these photographs ensure that a comparison can still take place should a potential source be identified. Other important information that must be documented through careful measurement are stride length for footwear and tire measurements or axle width for tire tracks.

The choice of collection method will depend on the size and type of evidence. Three-dimensional impressions are generally cast while two-dimensional imprints are lifted, though the mode of lifting depends on the medium on which the imprint is found.

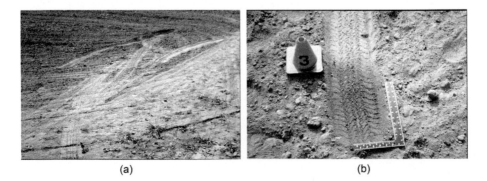

(a)   (b)

Figure 13.5 Tire tracks from a pickup truck at the scene of a shallow grave. (a) Overall photographic documentation. (b) With evidence marker and scales to take evidence-quality photographs before casting is attempted.

Dental stone or plaster of paris is the casting medium used for footwear and tire impressions, though dental stone has a finer texture, capturing greater detail, and is stronger when dry. Casting materials are mixed in Ziploc bags or bowls immediately prior to use. Molds are placed around the impression and the casting medium is poured carefully into the mold to prevent any damage to the fine detail of the impression. The medium is either poured around the perimeter of the impression and allowed to flow into the impression or poured over a spatula held over the impression. Larger casts may be reinforced during the casting process by laying chicken wire or wooden sticks into the cast during pouring. Impressions in snow may be stabilized using snow print wax, a spray, prior to casting, and a fine coating of snow print wax can also be used to provide some contrast when photographing the impression prior to casting. In all cases, investigator initials and case number are scratched into the cast before it is fully set. Once dry, casts should be placed in a sturdy box for transportation. The scale of tire impressions can be challenging for casting. Rather than casting the entire impression, areas with the best detail, or in which individualizing characteristics have been observed, are cast. Prior to this, both the entire impression and the areas of particular interest should be photographed (Figure 13.6).

The choice of collection method for imprints is dependent on the medium of the imprint which can be as diverse as blood, grease, paint or dust. Imprints in blood are enhanced using o-tolidine spray in the same manner as for

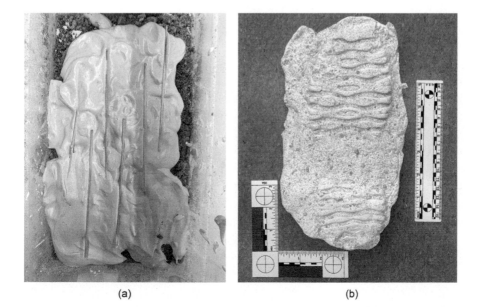

(a)   (b)

Figure 13.6 Casting a footwear impression. (a) Using wooden sticks for reinforcement. (b) The finished cast.

fingerprints in blood. This provides additional detail, particularly at the edges, which may become clearer. If the bloody imprint is on a surface that can simply be removed, such as a piece of cardboard, then that can be seized without enhancement. Examination-quality photographs should be taken before attempting enhancement. If the surface cannot be removed, e.g., a tile floor, then additional examination-quality photographs must be taken following enhancement. All photographs must be taken perpendicular to the imprint and with a scale in the frame. A plumb line, or level, and tripod are recommended as shown in Figure 4.4. Any deviation from perpendicular will create distortion of the pattern rendering the photographs unusable for comparisons.

Imprints in other materials may be recovered at the scene using lifters. As these imprints are fragile, photographs must be taken prior to lifting. Lifters must be placed down onto the imprint without any motion that might result in smudging of the imprint. Tire imprints should be photographed in a sequence if the area of interest is significant as a single photograph is unlikely to adequately capture the imprint in a way that can be used for a comparison. An overall photograph is essential, but the size of the imprint will prevent this from being perpendicular and it cannot be used for comparison purposes.

Fingerprints and Other Friction Ridge Prints

Fingerprints are friction ridge skin found at the tips of the fingers. Friction ridge skin is also found on the palms of hands and the soles of feet. Friction ridges are formed in utero and do not change through the individual's life, except to increase in size, unless the skin is damaged right down to the dermal layer, though the actual ridge pattern itself is not altered, but scars, etc., may be visible. Though fingerprints may be classified by three general ridge patterns: loops, arches and whorls; other friction ridge skin does not have identifiable patterns for similar classification. However, all friction ridge skin has minutiae in the ridge detail that may be used for individualization, definitive identification of the individual who made the print. While the average finger has over 150 minutiae, most crime scene prints have far fewer identifiable minutiae. It is therefore imperative to properly enhance and collect friction ridge evidence to ensure the best chance of recovering sufficient identifiable prints that can be compared to known samples.

Fingerprints (and other friction ridge prints) are classified as being latent, patent or plastic depending on their appearance and the surface on which they were deposited. While patent and plastic prints are clearly visible and require little or no enhancement, latent prints are deposited in colorless sweat and sebaceous material from the pores located on the friction ridges and require either physical or chemical enhancement to be seen. Enhancement techniques work by physical adherence to the print or a chemical reaction with one of the

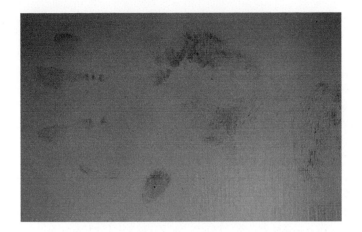

Figure 13.7 A bloody palmprint enhanced at the scene using o-tolidine.

chemical components of the print, such as proteins or metal ions. At the scene, enhancement is usually by powder, which adheres to the residues, followed by lifting. Chemical techniques are used primarily in the laboratory except for bloody fingerprints which are often enhanced at the scene by gently spraying the prints with o-tolidine after taking examination-quality photographs (Figure 13.7). However, it is better to collect carriers of prints whenever possible and limit field enhancement to those surfaces that are not easily removed. With the development of portable devices, it is now possible to undertake superglue fuming at the scene. While not all scenes are ideal for this, the enclosed interiors of cars work well with these devices.

Patent prints are those that are made by friction ridge skin that has some sort of material on it that is deposited in the pattern of the print. This might be blood, paint, ink, dirt, grease or any other similar type of material. These fingerprints rarely require enhancement, though the careful use of blood enhancement reagents can make additional features of a print visible, particularly at the outer edges. Plastic prints are made in some sort of soft medium and are three-dimensional in nature. Media such as putty, paint and even soap can hold a plastic print. They require no enhancement in the field.

In addition to human prints, animals also have sources of skin with ridge detail, for example, the noses of dogs. While they are referred to as individualizing, the lack of common usage and large-scale studies would indicate that using these prints should be done with caution and with the mindset that they are no more than an "inclusion" rather than the individualization associated with human friction ridge skin. If scars and other distinguishing marks are present, then a higher level of association can be considered, but conclusions should not reach the level of individualization.

At the crime scene, the decision to use enhancement techniques, and which to use, is based on the location in which prints are believed to be present and whether the prints are made in blood. Easily seized carriers of prints are rarely processed at the scene. Nonporous surfaces work the best for on-scene processing, mainly by powder dusting but, as mentioned before, superglue can be used if needed and a suitable enclosure can be made. Porous surfaces, such as paper, are usually developed using chemical developers and should be seized and sent for processing at a laboratory.

Fingerprint powders are available in a wide spectrum of different colors, including fluorescent, to obtain maximum contrast between the print and the surface. A variety of fingerprint brushes are available, and most investigators have a personal preference. Magnetic brushes differ from others as they do not have any physical bristles but have a magnet at the tip of the handle which, when used with magnetic powders, forms a "brush" from the powder particles themselves. When the magnet is retracted, any remaining powder is released from the handle. When using powder, gentle circular movements will avoid smearing the print. It is better to start with less powder and build up the print rather than overloading it with too much powder (Figure 13.8).

Once prints are dusted, they should be preserved using fingerprint lifters attached to a backing which may be black or white and chosen for maximum contrast with the print. Prior to any lifting attempt, prints should be carefully photographed before lifting. Lifts can be packaged in envelopes or evidence bags.

Items seized for laboratory processing for latent prints must be handled carefully to prevent smearing of fingerprints during packaging and transportation. Packaging should be chosen to prevent items moving around as this

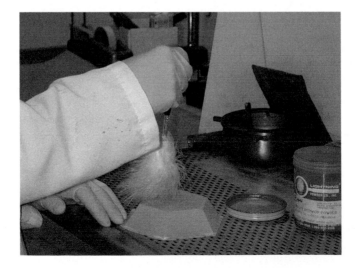

Figure 13.8 The correct technique for dusting a fingerprint using powder. The examiner is using a feather brush and nonmagnetic fingerprint powder.

can also cause prints to be smeared through contact with the outer container. If necessary, zip ties can be used to hold an item in place and should be carefully placed to avoid damage to prints.

As many unrelated latent prints will be found at any crime scene, investigators must ensure that elimination prints are collected from all individuals who have normal access to the scene, e.g., family members. These prints can be collected as inked rolled prints on ten print cards, or through electronic means if available. The Automated Fingerprint Identification System (AFIS) and Integrated Automated Fingerprint Identification System (IAFIS) are tools that can be used to attempt identification of unknown fingerprints. All individuals who are fingerprinted as part of an arrest or through their occupations, e.g., military, teachers, etc. have their prints uploaded into these databases, thus elimination prints do not need to be obtained from people whose fingerprints are already in these databases.

Questioned Documents

Questioned documents include any item marked with characters, alphanumeric or otherwise, for which authorship must be established. In addition to handwriting and signature comparisons, this evidence may also include obliterations, erasures, alterations, indentations, charred documents and ink or paper comparisons. Documents produced by mechanical means, such as typewritten, photocopied, faxed or printed, are also examined though only typewritten documents support individualization. The paper and inks used in documents may be further examined in cases of suspected forgery or document alterations, for example, forging prescriptions or signatures for veterinary medications or pedigree certificates.

Some categories of questioned documents have the possibility of individualization to a source, including handwriting, signatures and typewritten documents. However, when considering handwritten documents, sufficient characters must be present to observe individualizing characteristics; thus, one or two words in uppercase are not good candidates for this, while multiple paragraphs of cursive writing can be individualized. Other categories of documents may lead to inclusions or exclusion, including printers, fax machines and photocopiers. Questioned document evidence should always be considered in cases of neglect, hoarding, animal fighting and breeding mills.

Collection and packaging procedures are similar for most questioned documents. As other types of evidence, such as fingerprints, DNA and trace materials, are likely to be present, all questioned documents should be handled carefully and packaged to avoid compromising other evidence examinations. Most documents can simply be packaged and sealed, without folding, in appropriately sized envelopes or plastic evidence bags. Charred documents are very fragile and should be stabilized between two pieces of card for support before being placed in an outer container. Writing implements can be placed in envelopes or bags.

Critical to the success of any questioned document examination are the exemplars that are obtained for comparisons. These will vary depending on the type of documents in question.

1. Handwriting exemplars

   Exemplars for handwriting comparison may be either requested or non-requested, and there are situations in which each might be the preferred type. Requested handwritings are obtained specifically for comparison to the seized document. The individual should be provided with paper and a writing implement similar to those used for the questioned document. They should be in a comfortable writing position in a well-lit location. The passage selected for the writing sample should contain specific letters and letter combinations that are in the question document, but the passage should not be the same as in that document. The passage should be dictated, and once complete, the sample should be removed and a new paper provided. The same passage should be dictated and that sample removed. This procedure should be repeated multiple times to combat any attempts at disguised writing.

   Non-requested writings are those made by the individual in everyday life. These might include notes, letters, journals, etc., though they must be authenticated before use for comparison. The advantage of these writing samples is that it is possible to obtain older samples of the individual's writing if the questioned document was not created recently.

   Exemplars for signatures should be obtained in a similar manner as requested writing samples using similar writing implement and paper and removing signatures from view.

2. Typewriters

   Though typewriters are no longer common, typewritten documents are still found especially in older cases or in forgeries of older documents. The entire typewriter should be seized for examination in the laboratory, including both the inked and correction ribbons. The typewriter should not be used at the scene as examination of the ribbon can reveal prior letters and numbers typed which can be compared to the questioned document.

3. Printers, photocopiers and fax machines

   These machines do not produce characters in a mechanical way that can lead to individualization; defects from scratches or lack of cleaning can lead to repetitive marks appearing on documents. Smaller machines can be seized directly; however, exemplars must be taken from larger machines at the scene. Multiple sheets of paper should be put through the machines to determine if markings seen on questioned documents are permanent and repeatable.

Final Thoughts

All types of pattern evidence have the possibility of individualization and should be considered during scene processing. The collection of known samples and exemplars for comparison purposes must not be overlooked as examinations and the ability to individualize rely on them. Examination-quality photography is essential before attempting enhancement or collection as comparison to known samples can still take place using photographs. These photographs must always be precisely perpendicular to the pattern and contain a scale, and the equipment needed to achieve this, such as a tripod and plumb line should be readily available at all scenes.

Bibliography

NIST. The Organization of Scientific Area Committees for Forensic Science. Footwear and tire subcommittee. https://www.nist.gov/osac/footwear-tire-subcommittee.

Physical Evidence Bulletin. Documentation of shoe and tire impression evidence. https://oag.ca.gov/sites/all/files/agweb/pdfs/cci/reference/peb_23.pdf.

Physical Evidence Bulletin. Firearms evidence collection procedures. https://oag.ca.gov/sites/all/files/agweb/pdfs/cci/reference/peb_12.pdf.

Scientific Working Group for Forensic Document Examination. https://www.swgdoc.org/index.php/standards/published-standards.

US Department of Justice. *The Fingerprint Sourcebook*. https://www.ojp.gov/pdffiles1/nij/225320.pdf.

Drugs and Controlled Substances

14

VIRGINIA M. MAXWELL

Introduction

Drugs are referred to by several different names, including controlled substances and narcotics. Strictly speaking, narcotics are only one category of drugs when the principle pharmacological effect is used as the classification scheme. However, in law enforcement, many agencies refer to their specialized unit as narcotics. Controlled substance is the nomenclature that arose out of the Comprehensive Controlled Substances Act of 1970 (CSA), a landmark law in the long running efforts to regulate drugs, their distribution and use, which introduced the term "controlled substances" as the accepted way of referring to these materials. With many years of disjointed approaches, the CSA was regarded as the definitive means of classifying drugs, also providing storage and sentencing guidelines, though it must be noted that tobacco and alcohol are excluded from the CSA. Classification by the CSA is into one of five schedules based upon accepted medical use in the United States and the potential for abuse, with Schedule I containing those drugs without currently accepted medical uses and a high potential for abuse, such as heroin. Since 1970, however, there has been a rapid and ever-evolving increase in the number of "designer drugs" produced in clandestine laboratories. They require additional legislation for both the final product and the precursors used in their manufacture. Further, more recent changes in public attitude have led to the decriminalization of marijuana in many states. With confusing nomenclature, for the remainder of this chapter, the term "drugs" will be used to cover this particular category of illicit substance evidence.

With detailed instructions for clandestine laboratory preparations of controlled substances now widely available on the internet and requiring little sophistication to successfully produce, investigators may encounter, not only controlled substances but also the precursors and paraphernalia used in their preparation and use, which must also be recognized and seized. Clandestine laboratories can be very dangerous due to the chemical reactions taking place and the by-products of different steps in the preparation may themselves be highly toxic, e.g., phosphine gas is the by-product of one synthetic pathway for heroin. If the early walk-through of the crime scene indicates a clandestine laboratory is in operation, the investigators should immediately leave the scene

DOI: 10.4324/9781003090762-14

and request assistance from a trained clandestine lab response team. Typical indications might include chemical smells, glassware and empty containers of common precursors in the garbage. Specialized personal protective equipment, including respirators, must be worn for the initial entry and walk-through if a clandestine laboratory is suspected.

Drugs and paraphernalia can be found at any scene and may be unrelated to the animal cruelty under investigation. Regardless, they cannot be ignored for both safety and legal reasons. Animal cruelty crime scenes at which controlled substances are common include animal fighting, hoarding and animal sexual assault. Drugs associated with animal-fighting cases fall into three categories: training and performance enhancement, "veterinary" care and those for human use, either for personal recreational use or on a larger scale, for dealing at the fight. It is common for animal-fighting cases to come to light as a result of investigations into other infractions such as controlled substance offenses. Sedatives may be used in animal sexual assault cases, and hoarding cases might have legal veterinary drugs present but used for additional animals to those for which they were prescribed or veterinary drugs obtained illegally from overseas online pharmacies.

Classification of Drugs

Though the CSA was considered to be the most unambiguous method of classifying drugs, they can also be classified based on several other criteria. For example, if classified by origin, the different classes are natural, synthetic or semisynthetic. A further, and common, classification scheme is that of predominant pharmacological effect. In this scheme, drugs are placed into the following categories: narcotics, stimulants, depressants, hallucinogens and anabolic steroids.

1. Narcotics:
   Drugs placed into this category have a common effect of dulling the senses and relieving pain. This includes opium, its derivatives and semisynthetic substitutes, collectively known as opioids. Examples include heroin, fentanyl, Vicodin®, OxyContin®, codeine and morphine. Drugs in this category can be smoked, injected, snorted or swallowed. The appearances can vary and include tablets, capsules, powders, chunks, liquids and skin patches. The colors of the powders range from white to shades of brown and even black.
2. Stimulants:
   As their name suggests, stimulants speed up the body's systems. This class of drugs may be manufactured illicitly or diverted from legal prescription markets. The most common examples of this category include cocaine, crack cocaine, methamphetamine and synthetic

cathinones ("bath salts") and prescription medications such as Ritalin®, amphetamines (Adderall® or Dexedrine®) and diet aids (Didrex®, Fastin® and Adipex P®, among others). Stimulant drugs may be injected, swallowed, smoked or snorted. They can be found as powders, pills, liquids and rocks.

3. Depressants:

Depressants relieve anxiety and induce sleep by slowing down the body's systems. This category is primarily manufactured legally as prescription medication but is diverted for illicit use. The main drugs in this category are the barbiturates (including phenobarbital, Pentothal®, Secotal® and Nebutal®), benzodiazepines (Xanax®, Halcion®, Valium® and Ativan® among others), methaqualone (Quaaludes®), Ambien®, Lunesta®, Rohypnol® and gamma-hydroxybutyrate (GHB). Rohypnol® and GHB are common drugs used in drug-facilitated sexual assaults. Drugs in this category may be found as pills, injectable liquids and syrups. They are swallowed or injected. Some cases of animal sexual assault may include drugs from this category.

4. Hallucinogens:

This category of drugs is mood and perception altering in their action and may be produced synthetically or come from plants and fungi. Drugs with hallucinogenic responses include marijuana, Ecstasy (MDMA), LSD, Ketamine® (veterinary anesthetic), psilocybin (mushrooms) and peyote buttons (cactus). Hallucinogens are swallowed, smoked, injected and may be found as vegetative materials, tar-like oil (hash), pills and blotter papers (LSD). Ketamine® can be used not only as a veterinary anesthetic, both legally and illegally such as in dog fighting, and it is associated with drug-facilitated sexual assaults.

5. Anabolic Steroids:

Anabolic steroids and synthetically produced versions of the male hormone testosterone. They may be produced legally and illicitly diverted, often from abroad. They include testosterone, oxymetholone, trenbolone, nandrolone, stanozolol and oxandrolone. Steroids may be found as tablets, capsules, liquids for ingestion or injection, patches, implants, gels and creams. They are administered by swallowing, injection, rubbing and subdermal insertion. Steroids may be found as evidence in animal-fighting cases.

Drug Evidence

As seen above, investigators must be aware of the range of ways in which drugs can be found and that even prescription drugs may have been illicitly diverted from their intended use or recipient, while some drugs found may be for use by both humans and on animals. Thus, close attention must be paid to the labeling on prescription medications in regard to the medical/veterinary practitioner and the intended recipient.

Beyond the actual drugs, paraphernalia and precursors can also be found at crime scenes. Paraphernalia encompasses those items used to both make and take drugs. Clandestine lab equipment can be both rudimentary or more sophisticated depending upon the operator and scale of the laboratory. Some laboratories are crude setups in basements using household items, while larger laboratories can be far more sophisticated using scientific equipment and chemicals. The equipment includes that needed to measure ingredients, cook, filter and package the final product. However, any paraphernalia is likely to have important residues which can yield important evidence and information that may be used to link cases together. Items related to taking drugs will vary based on the drug and mode of ingestion but may include bongs, rolling papers, needles, syringes, teaspoons, foil and flame sources.

Precursors, reagents and solvents are the ingredients used in the production of illegal manufacture of illicit drugs in clandestine laboratories. Precursors are classified according to whether they are immediate precursors within one step of the finished drug, or more distant. Examples of precursors include ephedrine and pseudoephedrine (methamphetamine and methcathinone), piperidine (phencyclidine) and acetic anhydride (heroin and methaqualone). Reagents undergo reactions with precursors and include iodine (methamphetamine and amphetamine), hydrochloric acid (cocaine, MDMA, LSD and fentanyl) and potassium permanganate (cocaine). In addition, many different solvents are used for different synthetic pathways including acetone, diethyl ether and toluene. Thus, when drugs are involved, the crime scene search is complicated as many of these materials are legal to purchase and when used as intended, such as pseudoephedrine in cold medications. With this in mind, it is important to document the quantities of these materials found at the crime scene.

Prescription Medications

Some controlled substances found at crime scenes may be legal prescription medications, whether they are prescribed for an animal or a human. However, just because the controlled substance is legally produced for prescribed use by an individual or animal does not mean that the person using it, or the animal being treated with it, is the one for whom the prescription was written. Prescription medication at scenes should not be ignored and the labeling should be carefully documented including the prescribing doctor or veterinarian, as well as the intended recipient and the quantity prescribed and remaining. The amount of prescribed medication left in the container should also be documented. The improper use of veterinary medications is common in hoarding, puppy mill and animal-fighting cases, and these medications should be considered as evidence and seized during scene processing. Prescription medications may be identified using the Merck Index through manufacturer markings on the medication.

Controlled Substances at the Crime Scene

Controlled substances may be found as plants and plant material, pills, powders, liquids, blotter papers and edibles. They may be loose on a surface or packaged in various ways such as plastic bags or foil. Once identified as a potential controlled substance, they must be carefully documented and handled with care to ensure the safety of investigators. Screening tests can provide an indication of whether the material is included as being a controlled substance or excluded. While there are now many controlled substances, the general appearance can guide the investigator as to how to proceed with testing. For example, if the material is a white powder, marijuana can be excluded but testing for cocaine would be important; similarly, if the material is vegetative, controlled substances such as heroin, methamphetamine and cocaine are excluded. With the constant arrival of new designer drugs, investigators can stay current through information found at the Drug Enforcement Agency website and in their published Resource Guide (see Bibliography). When nonprescription pills are found, the markings on them should be carefully documented as they are often indicative of the clandestine laboratory that produced the pills. A common example of this is ecstasy which is usually found as brightly colored pills with some sort of impressed marking on them, such as a butterfly. Not only can these markings be used to link batches together, but through a tool mark examination, they can be linked to specific pill presses if the laboratory is located.

Field Screening Tests

Several types of field tests exist to screen suspected drugs at the scene. These are generally color tests and self-contained versions have been developed specifically for convenient field use. These generally consist of a plastic pouch containing reagent vials. Once a small sample of the questioned material is added to the pouch, the vials are broken, and any color change should be noted. Specific color changes, not any color change, are considered to be a positive screening test for the drug in question.

It is imperative to remember that color tests are only screening in nature and are NEVER considered as definitive identification of a specific drug; definitive identification requires sophisticated laboratory instrumentation. While some instrumentation does exist in field portable format, it is expensive and unlikely to be widely available for regular crime scene use. Thus, when correctly using a chemical screening test at the scene, the results may be considered as (a) positive – the material could be a certain drug, or (b) negative – the material is not a certain drug.

Field tests are very sensitive and require only a small amount of sample; in fact, just a few particles are generally sufficient. However, high sensitivity brings the risk of contamination which will alter the screening test results, potentially giving false positive or negative results. For example, a clean toothpick can be used to place some sample in the testing pouch, but if that toothpick is reused with a second sample, there can still be sufficient residue remaining to affect the results of the second field test. The advantage of high sensitivity is that very little sample is consumed to perform several color tests; as the weight of drug is very important in the judicial process, minimal consumption at the scene will have little impact on the total weight. Most common screening tests for drugs have been developed in a field testing format and are readily available for purchase, such as NarcoPouch® and NIK®. Many more screening tests exist; however, they are not yet available in this format but evidence submitted to a laboratory can be tested. Of significant importance is the availability of testing strips for fentanyl. The potency and widespread occurrence of fentanyl is an important safety issue at any crime scene, and these test strips should always be part of the crime scene kit.

Safety

Outside of the safety issues of clandestine laboratories discussed previously, when suspected drugs or paraphernalia are located during any crime scene search, investigators should proceed with caution and due attention to personal safety. Not only are puncture wounds and cuts from needles or other sharp objects a danger, but some drugs are highly toxic in very small doses, e.g., fentanyl, LSD and others can be absorbed through the skin. Fentanyl in particular is one of the current major dangers at any crime scene in which drugs are located as just a few grains can be fatal. Thus, any unknown white powder should be approached with caution. Not only must the wearing of PPE be mandated for all entering the scene, but investigators should ensure that they do not touch exposed skin or mucus membranes prior to removing gloves and thoroughly washing their hands. Gloves should be changed regularly, and immediately, if they are punctured or torn. As fentanyl is toxic in very low doses, it is worth considering keeping naloxone to hand when the presence of drugs is suspected. Naloxone is available in both nasal spray and injectable formats. Further, investigators should familiarize themselves with the signs of an overdose.

One word of caution with regard to conducting color tests at the scene, most color tests contain strong acids. While the tests are self-contained in pouches, care should still be taken to ensure that the contents do not spill when shaken or after completion of the test. Used tests should be disposed of appropriately.

Collection and Packaging of Drug Evidence

Specific issues in the collection of drug evidence are the preservation of the evidence and safety of personnel. All drug evidence must be carefully collected to ensure that no loss or contamination of the sample can occur, and the safety of all personnel who may handle the packaged evidence is assured. The weight of the drug is an important factor in charging individuals. Careless consumption of excess samples in field tests or sloppy collection and packaging will result in loss of sample and a lower weight recorded at the laboratory. Further, screening tests will be repeated at the laboratory; thus cross-contamination of samples by poor collection techniques may impact those tests.

Drugs or other materials that are already in containers may be kept in those containers as long as some form of tamper-evident outer packaging or seal is used. Care should be taken to avoid damage to existing labeling, including that of pharmacies, on the containers. Loose powders or dried vegetative material may be packaged in plastic or vials, but any item used to transfer the material must be new or thoroughly cleaned before use. Liquids should be packaged in glass to avoid any solvent issues with plastics. All paraphernalia must be packaged so that any residue is preserved for testing with due care and attention being paid to fingerprint or DNA evidence if this is thought to be important. Any needles or other sharp objects must be placed into specific "sharps" packaging or some other rigid outer container.

Final Thoughts

To reiterate the safety concerns of handling drug evidence, personnel must remain vigilant regarding PPE. Drugs may be absorbed through skin and mucous membranes; thus careless touching of exposed areas while working with this evidence, even gloved, can result in exposure to toxic levels of these substances.

Bibliography

Drug Enforcement Administration. DEA announces the seizure of over 379 million deadly doses of fentanyl in 2022. www.dea.gov.

Drugs of Abuse. A DEA resource guide. https://www.dea.gov/sites/default/files/2020-04/Drugs%20of%20Abuse%202020-Web%20Version-508%20compliant-4-24-20_0.pdf.

Guidelines for the Collection and Submission of Forensic Evidence. Delaware Department of Health and Social Services. Office of the Chief Medical Examiner, pp. 39–45. https://projects.nfstc.org/fse/pdfs/evidienceguidelines_101508.pdf.

Digital Evidence

15

VIRGINIA M. MAXWELL

Introduction

Historically, digital evidence was limited to computers, but it has now expanded to be any information stored or transmitted in binary form. While digital evidence was initially seized for electronic crimes ("e-crimes"), such as fraud or child pornography, the explosion in the use of digital devices has led to digital evidence being an important part of many different types of investigation. For example, investigators can not only obtain files saved on a computer but also can now determine a person's location at any given time, as well as their social and business connections among many other things. From the perspective of crime scene investigation, digital evidence is essentially invisible, it is the potential source of evidence that must be recognized and collected. Further, this evidence can be easily destroyed and altered, not just in person but also from a remote location or automatically, via embedded code or other means, triggered by the unwitting actions of crime scene personnel, bringing additional challenges to the collection of the evidence. It is also the nature of today's electronic communication and connections that information can be transmitted globally in a split second, rapidly crossing local, national and international jurisdictions.

Digital Technology

Technology is expanding at a rapid rate, and it is difficult for the average person to maintain consistently up-to-date knowledge of all possible forms of digital evidence. As recently as 10 years ago, most people might have access to a computer and many would also have a cell phone, but that phone would be relatively rudimentary compared to the modern smartphone which is essentially a computer in our hands 24 hours a day. Smartphones now are more than just phones and may contain financial information, written communications, text and phone logs, videos, photographs, social media and numerous other apps and internet searches. Not only do we verbally communicate but we can also transmit photos and videos almost instantly. They can also be used to track our locations, either voluntarily

DOI: 10.4324/9781003090762-15

through applications such as Find My iPhone, family and friend location apps, and via triangulation from cellular towers through subpoena to a service provider.

Digital technology has expanded far beyond computers and phones in recent years. Wearable technologies such as watches and fitness devices are increasingly common. Our homes contain smart speakers and digital assistants from various vendors, smart TVs and even appliances such as refrigerators and washing machines are now connected to the internet. We protect our homes with camera and alarm systems and automate them with numerous available devices such as thermostats, light switches and bulbs, door locks and even water meters. New devices are regularly marketed as being compatible with home automation and digital assistants. All of these items, and more, can be used to identify routine or anomalies in behavior, track movements or obtain video footage of activity at a location and many more things. Investigators should be creative in considering what digital evidence might be present and how it can be used in an investigation, though obtaining information from service suppliers, even with a warrant, is not always easy.

Other items of digital technology that should be considered when animals are involved in cases are microchips and other RFID trackers (for example, on cattle) as well as the emerging popularity of GPS collars used by pet owners to track the location of their companion if separated. Also gaining in popularity are internet devices to watch and interact with animals while away from home.

Digital evidence can be subdivided into two categories, volatile and nonvolatile. Volatile evidence is considered to be nonpersistent and is lost when a device loses power. An example of volatile evidence in the computer's RAM. Nonvolatile evidence does not change. This distinction is of particular importance when digital devices are encountered as evidence.

Computers and Peripherals

Computer forensics has been part of forensic analysis for many years. The widespread ownership and usage of both PCs and laptops have made them increasingly common evidence in a wide range of crimes. Not only can they be searched for illegal material such as child pornography, but they also contain seemingly innocent items that can be important evidence in animal cruelty cases. For example, the records of pet food purchases in a neglect case or e-mails to rescues and shelters for the purposes of obtaining more animals in a hoarding case. With reliance upon electronic communication and digital means to obtain information, trade items and even gamble, computers have the potential to open a Pandora's Box of information for an investigation. Beyond e-mail, internet history and social media, photographs and videos related to animal cruelty acts carried out by the owner of the computer may be stored on the hard drive or associated external storage devices. In addition, photographs and videos downloaded from the internet can give insight into the person and may themselves be illegal or linked to associated criminality. For example, in organized animal fighting, files may contain training and fight records, "pedigree" documents for the fighting dogs themselves or digital images of signatures to create documents, communications related to organizing fights, sales records and gambling records.

Beyond the computer itself, investigators must search for any associated storage devices such as external hard drives, CD/DVDs, memory cards and flash media. They should also recognize that flash media comes in different forms beyond the expected appearance, such as models, pens and even watches. While few computers still used floppy discs, if the computer has slots for those discs, then it is likely that some can be found.

Mobile Devices

Mobile devices, such as smartphones and tablets, are almost considered an essential item in today's world and can yield important evidence. While a high percentage of people own a smartphone, many also have a tablet. Some people also own multiple phones to keep different aspects of their life and activities separate. It is important to ensure that all devices are seized for examination and to establish both ownership of the devices and the person responsible for associated cellular and data plans. Evolving technology has brought increased power, speed and storage capacities to smartphones and tablets thus they are used for many reasons and hold significant personal information, information related to the person's activities, movements and even motivations. Further, information is often synced to cloud storage and among other digital devices.

The general types of information that can be obtained from mobile devices include the following:

1. Communications: Communication data include contacts, call logs, text messages, e-mail and social media accounts. This can help establish communications between an individual and external entities and identify an individual's family members, friends, acquaintances and foes. The data show a network of a person's "close associates", which can assist with investigations such as dog fighting.
2. Applications "Apps" data: Information stored within third-party applications on the mobile devices. This includes social media,

ridesharing, shopping, cloud storage providers and finance-related apps, among many others.

3. Device backups: Mobile devices may be backed up in different ways to including to computers and the cloud. Obtaining access to backups can provide not only the most recent information on a mobile device but may also contain historical data from previous backups and even previous and additional devices. Backups and settings from linked wearable technology, such as Apple watches, are usually stored on the associated mobile device.

4. Location data: Mobile devices can track location through their connections to cell towers, Wi-Fi networks and hotspots, roaming cell networks and proprietary networks. These leave a trail of locations that a person has visited and at what times they were there. Some mobile devices also store analytic information regarding usage and charging.

5. Multimedia files: Mobile devices now have storage capacities that can rival some computers. Thus, thousands of pictures, videos, audio and other files can be stored on them, and distributed via them. As with a computer, these can be used as evidence, and it can also be determined where and when they were downloaded in some cases as location-based data are often embedded in them.

6. Internet history: Internet history, cache and bookmarks are stored on mobile devices. Bookmarks and frequently visited sites may also be shared among linked devices.

Wearable Technology

Apple watches and other wearable technology are purchased for specific purposes such as fitness tracking, but they also store a lot of information that can be obtained and used in investigations. This information includes the following:

1. GPS and activity tracking: Wearable technology is often purchased for the purposes of fitness and workout tracking. Thus, they can record data on the individual's location, speed and routes; they do not even have to be working out for this to be stored. Information about heart rate, blood pressure and other similar data may also be stored. Even if this data are not located on the device itself, it may be downloaded to a linked phone or other device.

2. Calendars, schedulers and other apps: While some wearable devices are limited to activity tracking, more sophisticated ones also monitor

many other aspects of user's life. For example, calendar events, such as appointments and reminders, shopping lists, to-do lists, photos/videos, social media and even search histories, are accessible via some wearable devices. This data may be synced between the device and phones or computers. Further digital assistants, such as Siri, may be accessed from wearable technology.

3. Text messages and phone calls: Recent wearable technology models can connect directly to cellular networks and feature smartphone capabilities. They can receive and send text messages and phone calls directly while noncellular enabled devices have the same capabilities only through Bluetooth connection with a paired phone.

Home Automation

The home automation market has increased in size and scope dramatically over the last 5 years. Most houses now have smart speakers and digital assistants, such as Amazon Echo and Google Home, in one or multiple rooms, as well as lights, cameras, thermostats and home appliances that are all connected to the internet and collecting data on the household's activities. Some devices have enabled microphones waiting to hear "wake words" but are always capturing short surrounding sound bites. Home automation runs through the home Wi-Fi network and can also be controlled via cell phones and other devices, thus leaving a digital trail of activity within a location. Examples of home automation include security systems, interior and exterior cameras, light bulbs and light switches, plugs, sockets, door locks, thermostats, appliances, water meters and more, with new devices continually being brought to market. The digital history of all of these devices is a way to assess the normal activity and identify any anomalies that might be related to a crime.

Cameras

Though home security cameras might be considered part of home automation, the use of video in animal cruelty cases is important and finding sources of video outside that taken at crime scenes and during investigations can be of critical importance in cases. As discussed, in Chapter 4, shooting video of abused animals is important for the assessment of injuries, current and prior, as well as pain and response to people, food and other relevant things. Additional sources of video can be used to determine the progression of injuries or deterioration of the animal's overall condition with time; they can even be used to obtain real-time footage of acts of cruelty taking place. In areas where properties closely abut, neighbors may also have relevant video footage. While some cameras store video on local devices, others upload to cloud storage maintained by the camera manufacturer; however, the video may not be stored indefinitely.

Collection of Digital Evidence

The goal in the collection of digital evidence is to prevent any changes taking place to the device and the loss of any data. While this is very simple for some items, it becomes far more complex when considering computers and other networked devices, as well as those synced through the cloud to other devices. Two things should be at the forefront of every investigator's mind; first that code has been embedded in devices that will wipe them or irrevocably change them if they are carelessly powered up or connected to the internet or cellular network, and second, that information can be changed or removed through cloud syncing. The same home security cameras that can hold important evidence can also be used to forewarn a person of a search of their premises and enable them to remotely wipe or encrypt everything.

Requesting assistance from a digital forensic specialist is strongly advised in cases where it is believed that digital evidence will be of high importance in the investigation. Many police departments either have specialist personnel on staff or access to a state-level facility. Specialists can ensure that computers and peripherals are safely powered down and dismantled in a way that will prevent any changes taking place to the hard drive and preserve any volatile memory before it is lost. While many investigators are very competent with technology, the issues that can arise from incorrectly trying to dismantle a system are numerous and best handled by trained experts.

At the scene, it is of the utmost importance that investigators do not turn on any devices that appear to be turned off or in sleep mode. Destructive processes can be triggered through incorrectly waking devices or trying to guess the password. If devices are awake and the screens are on, then investigators can photograph what is visible on them, as well as any cables and attached devices. The cables, power sources and connections should be clearly labeled, and tamper-evident tape should be placed over any USB or other port to prevent insertion of unauthorized devices.

If possible, put any mobile device into airplane mode (if applicable) and disable any internet connection. Mobile devices can also be placed into Faraday bags. The ability to receive alerts from cameras and other items can allow an individual to remotely wipe their devices if they are aware of a search. Simply put, if the device cannot be reached, it cannot be wiped.

Final Thoughts

Investigators should keep an open mind as to which digital devices and evidence might be of importance in an investigation. Our reliance upon digital devices for every aspect of our lives can yield important information in unlikely places. Even a reminder entered into an innocuous app can ultimately be an important piece of evidence. Investigators must never forget that most devices can now be accessed remotely leading to the loss of critical evidence if internet or cellular access is not disabled. Finally, many people consider themselves to be competent with digital devices, but no investigator should be overconfident and forgo assistance from trained digital forensic specialists. One impulsive step can wipe a computer or activate a program that will destroy evidence.

Bibliography

Judish N. 2009. *Searching and Seizing Computers and Obtaining Electronic Evidence in Criminal Investigations*, 3rd Edition. Office of Legal Education Executive Office for United States Attorneys. https://www.justice.gov/file/442111/download.

Massachusetts Digital Evidence Consortium. Digital evidence guide for first responders. https://www.iacpcybercenter.org/wp-content/uploads/2015/04/digitalevidence-booklet-051215.pdf.

Massachusetts Digital Evidence Consortium. Handling mobile devices. https://www.iacpcybercenter.org/wp-content/uploads/2015/04/Handling-Mobile-Devices.pdf.

Scientific Working Group on Digital Evidence (SWGDE). Best practices for collection of damaged mobile devices. 2016. https://drive.google.com/file/d/1XToRyBB1cGpcEUHaxYjwz67qBBjBVNRt/view.

Scientific Working Group on Digital Evidence (SWGDE). Best practices for digital evidence collection. 2018. https://drive.google.com/file/d/1ScBeRvYikHvu6qtE_Lj3JtbOl94a5FDr/view.

Scientific Working Group on Digital Evidence (SWGDE). Guidelines for video evidence canvassing and collection. 2021. https://drive.google.com/file/d/1PGxsQYECQIqwUj1RrjvVLHVNswOZDJAE/view.

The Forensic Veterinarian at the Crime Scene

16

MARTHA SMITH-BLACKMORE

Potential Roles for the Veterinarian at the Crime Scene

A veterinarian at the scene of a suspected crime can contribute to the investigation and response in several ways that can enhance the investigation through recognition and documentation of evidence that might otherwise be overlooked. Additionally, the veterinarian can triage the animals on scene and sort animals according to their immediate veterinary needs. Depending on the circumstances and resources available, the veterinarian may be able to perform physical exams on scene and record the animal's condition as found at the time of the intervention.

Immediate exams on scene are preferred over transport and examination at an offsite facility, because this prevents any idea of the animal's condition being related to transportation or delay. Delaying an exam allows for time passage and potentially raises the concerns that an animal's condition was acquired after the intervention, or at the holding facility. There are times that only a visual or cursory exam may be performed on scene, and a subsequent full exam with radiographs, laboratory work or other modalities can be performed at a veterinary facility. This, along with thorough photographic documentation of the animal on site, can help refute an allegation that the animal's condition was secondary to transportation or holding at the veterinary facility.

If appropriately trained, and with the right equipment, veterinarians may assist with chemical capture (tranquilizer darting) of rogue feral animals, or sedation of dangerous, aggressive animals or with the administration of pain medications to animals for whom capture, or transport may be painful or overly distressing. Chemical capture requires specialized equipment and delivery systems such as a blow gun and pressurized darts. The use of such equipment carries some risk, and so, the decision to sedate or anesthetize animals must be made in balance with risks to the animals and people involved, depending on circumstances. In some cases, after consulting with a veterinarian, the decision may be made to use box traps, nets or other capture equipment rather than chemical capture.

Beyond the direct animal care role that a veterinarian fulfills, the veterinarian may also assist in identifying important evidence on scene.

DOI: 10.4324/9781003090762-16

A veterinarian can evaluate feed quality, water quality and other items on scene such as medications and wound treatment materials. There may be behavioral marks on the scene such as scratch marks, chew marks or patterns in the dirt or other substrate that the veterinarian may be able to interpret as related to behaviors that are consistent with struggles or suffering.

A veterinarian's familiarity with species-specific behaviors may help with directing where to search or what to look for. A veterinarian can help identify veterinary medications and treatments on scene, the presence of which may indicate an understanding on the part of the caregiver that in some circumstances, the animals need veterinary care.

Preparation

The time to involve a veterinarian in a scene response is before the warrant is written, and ideally, the law enforcement officers have a previously established working relationship with a veterinarian. It is beneficial if the veterinarian has training in veterinary forensics, but that isn't always possible, and investigators can guide veterinarians in capturing the necessary information.

Animal-involved scenes can be chaotic and messy. It is important that there is a structured approach using consistent processes when approaching a dynamic scene. As it pertains to crimes against animals, the crime scene may be an entire property, dwelling, room, kennel or the animal itself. A veterinarian can be of assistance to help in determining whether a crime has apparently been committed and assist with the determination of whether a case is likely to lead to charges.

Before a Scene Intervention

Veterinarians may not be familiar with the process leading up to a search and the steps in a crime scene investigation. The more a veterinarian is educated about the process, the more useful they will be to the investigation. While both intelligent and educated, a veterinarian may have never studied constitutional law, and they may not be familiar with the Fourth Amendment. Terms such as *probable cause* and *affidavit* may be foreign concepts. Just as veterinary medicine has terminology and jargon that are specific to that profession, it is important to be clear about the meaning of words that are being used in cross-professional collaborations, especially when a word has one meaning to the investigator, and a different one to the veterinarian.

Probable Cause

A veterinarian may need to be informed about the concept of "probable cause", which exists when there is a fair probability that a search will result in evidence of a crime being discovered – reason to believe a crime has been committed, based on the officer's training and experience. Consulting with a veterinarian can help to establish probable cause in a suspected animal abuse case. Probable cause is not equal to absolute certainty. That is, a police officer does not have to be certain that criminal activity is taking place to perform a search or make an arrest. It is important for the veterinarian to understand that probable cause can exist even when there is some doubt.

Search Warrant Affidavit

An affidavit is a written statement confirmed by oath or affirmation that is an integral part of the application for a search warrant. A sworn officer writes an affidavit, in the context of their training and experience and outlines the probable cause that a crime has been committed. The affidavit is submitted to a judge for approval before a search can commence. Search warrants should be sufficiently detailed to include all animals and places evidence can be expected to be found such as "all animals, born and unborn, live and deceased, above and below ground; medication in cabinets and refrigerators, digital evidence," and so forth. A veterinarian can help with the affidavit to ensure it is sufficiently detailed. A lack of detail can interfere with the ability to seize evidence.

A judge may issue a search warrant if the affidavit in support of the warrant offers sufficient credible information to establish probable cause. The veterinarian can be quoted as lending credible information to the affidavit. There is a presumption that police officers are reliable sources of information, and affidavits in support of a warrant will often include their observations. When this is the case, the officers' experience and training become relevant factors in assessing the existence of probable cause. Information from victims or witnesses, if included in an affidavit, may be important factors as well. Veterinarians can serve as witnesses in the establishment of probable cause.

Elements of the Law

Veterinarians may not be fully familiar with the applicable animal cruelty statutes and definitions in the state where they work. It can be helpful to review the statutes with a veterinarian and a prosecutor before taking steps to engage in a search. Understanding the definition of "animal", and what species are covered or excluded by local law, and understanding other necessary elements of the law is vital to engaging in proper process.

Before the Search

If not experienced in the execution of a search warrant, the veterinarian must be educated on the principles of proper conduct at the scene, to include roles and responsibilities of each member of the scene investigation team, what resources are available, what measures have been taken to ensure safety, who has authority at the scene, who should be allowed access, who will establish and maintain the perimeter, what the process of identifying, documenting, protecting and securing evidence will be, what entry logs and timelines are and who maintains them, and above all, what measures must be observed to prevent contamination of the scene. Veterinarians may not know that nothing can be touched until after it is photographed, and even then, there may be limitations on who can handle evidence, and with what precautions.

A veterinarian should have a firm understanding of what teams will be present at the crime scene, who is responsible for what activities and what the expected role of the veterinarian will be. Like disaster responses, the crime scene search team may benefit from team structure, particularly when there is a large scene, or a large amount of evidence is anticipated to be encountered. Teams may include a physical evidence team, an animal evidence team, animal handlers, evidence collectors and packagers, scribes or note keepers, photographers and videographers.

Many veterinarians are accustomed to being the lead and sole decision maker in their day-to-day activities in an animal hospital. It is helpful for veterinarians understand incident command structured systems, and to request that involved veterinarians become familiar with the principles of incident command by undertaking the ICS 100 training course online that is freely available at the Federal Emergency Management Administration website, https://emilms.fema.gov/is_0100c/curriculum/1.html. This training is for the coordination of various agencies in disaster response, but it can effectively lay the groundwork for command systems at a crime scene. While an agency may not use the exact Incident Command model as described in the course, it helps the veterinarian to understand the reasons for organizational structure and common processes in planning and executing searches. Familiarity with this type of process will ease communication at the actual event.

Conversely, the veterinarian may have significantly more experience than the investigators with the involved species and may be part of the planning and direction of animal capture. Veterinarians may advise on the inclusion of other animal professionals such as animal control officers, animal handlers or animal trainers.

Scene Walk-Through

Just as investigators take an initial walk-through of a scene before commencing with the documentation and collection of evidence, the veterinarian should also be brought through the scene to gain an overview of the total scene, to understand how many and what types of animals are involved, what the general condition of the group of animals may be, and the scope of resources and care that will be needed. Only after the scene walk-through, individual animal collection and documentation should proceed.

Evidence Identification and Interpretation

The careful examination of animal-involved crime scenes by a veterinarian may help to elucidate the sequence of events and aid in the identification of salient evidence. The variety of evidence can be as varied as the crime scenes themselves. It is important for veterinarians to know the limitations of their roles in evidence documentation and interpretation.

Veterinarians aren't blood spatter experts, for instance, but they may help identify a cast pattern that is consistent with a particular animal behavior, such as a wagging tail. Dogs wag their tails in different positions whether they are highly aroused prior to aggression, when they are happy and in a signal of submissive behavior. Animals struggling to get to their feet may "helicopter", or whirl their tails, leaving sweep marks. It is important to have the veterinarian accompanied by a crime scene analyst throughout the scene to reduce the risk of overstepping bounds.

A veterinarian may not know what they don't know, or what they aren't certified to comment on. For example, a veterinarian might offer to look at evidence under the microscope to determine if there are sperm cells present. While a veterinarian may ostensibly be able to do so, they are not representing a certified crime laboratory, and it is important that the evidence follow ordinary channels, as it would from any other type of crime scene. Additionally, a veterinarian inspecting a portion of evidence might consume scant valuable information.

There may be paper evidence such as receipts for feed or other animal-related expenditures, banking records, animal breeding or pedigree records, fight "champion" records or medical records. These records may also be digital, contained on computers, tablets, cell phones and other devices. Empty food bags or cans, feed sacks, the feed itself, troughs, bowls and their contents may present important information. The veterinarian may be able to review paper and trash evidence, and provide insight into its meaning or value to the investigation.

The presence of large numbers of empty cans may help the veterinarian to make a calculation of the possible minimum duration of a situation. Conversely, a veterinarian can be asked to perform a calculation on how much food a group of animals would require on a daily or weekly basis, helping to provide proof that insufficient feed was purchased, and therefore fed.

A veterinarian may be able to assist in the determination of what was done on scene. For example, accelerants may be used in the torture or disposal of animals and hot liquids may harm animals either accidentally or nonaccidentally. The burn pattern on the animal may hold important information about whether an accelerant was sprayed, poured or splashed. Veterinarians may be able to identify premortem ("antemortem") vs. postmortem injury on scene, or it may require a postmortem exam to make this determination. If there is evidence of the hot liquid or accelerant being distributed in a dynamic manner (as part of a chase as opposed to a spill for example), this would be consistent with nonaccidental injury.

Animal Evidence

Animals cannot articulate their suffering in words, but behavioral expressions of pain may be evident to the veterinarian. Signs of pain in animals include decreased appetite, reduced sleep, alterations in gait and locomotion, alterations in facial expression, abnormal posture, or reluctance to move, aversion to gentle palpation, changes in grooming activity, self-mutilation (including excessive licking or scratching), vocalizing and aggression. A veterinarian can review animals in person to witness behaviors that are consistent with pain expression, and veterinarians can administer pain medications that alleviate pain. It is important that the veterinarian notes the behavior that informed the veterinarian of the pain the animal was suffering in the medical record, and the behavior changes that indicated the administration of pain medication was effective.

While veterinarians can begin the assessment of animals on scene, note that it is difficult for veterinarians, who are trained as caregivers, to resist the immediate alleviation of suffering. They may want to do this by cleaning an animal's eyes and shaving mats, for example. Remind veterinarians that documentation should precede treatment whenever possible. It is a helpful reminder to point out that it took months for animals to get to a particular condition. Fifteen additional minutes spent on documentation before administering treatments won't make that much of a difference in the life of the animal, but it could make a big difference in the outcome of a case.

Final Thoughts

When the veterinarian can't be on scene, be sure to document the scene thoroughly. This includes careful and complete photography of the scene, and animals at the scene, and also documenting the scene after the animals have been removed. Consider videotaping any animals that are vocalizing, appear to be moving abnormally or when first offered a drink of clean water. Make sure, if you are working with a veterinarian that does not have the benefit of being on scene, that they receive all available scene findings, narrative reports and theories. It is important to capture the entire scene so that the evidence is understood in context. The reason a crime scene is processed, and evidence is collected, is to reveal the presence of any link of a suspect to a victim, the suspect to the scene, and/or the victim to the scene, and to objectively document this link. Making these materials available to the veterinarian will assist them in the objective formation of opinion based on the totality of information available.

Information collection continues after intervention, the veterinarian can comment on the animals' response to the provision of adequate food and water, to grooming care and other improvements in all aspects of animal care. The veterinarian must also be informed of the complicated status of animals as evidence – they may simultaneously be property of the owner, seized evidence and patients in need of veterinary care. As property, the animal belongs to the owner unless and until the animal is willingly surrendered by the owner or the legal process determines they cannot own the animal. As evidence, the defense can have their own expert examine the animals.

In general, the animals cannot be altered (spayed or neutered) without a court order, and any offspring are also the property of the owner. Animal welfare must be a priority, and treatment of any suffering conditions must be provided. There will be occasions where humane euthanasia must be performed on an emergency basis because suffering cannot be relieved by any other means, or because an animal poses a severe and certain risk to human safety. In these cases, veterinarians can provide records and reasons for the court to help convey the urgency of the situation.

Bibliography

Fowler M. *Restraint and Handling of Wild and Domestic Animals*. Germany: Wiley. 2011.

Kreeger TJ, Arnemo JM. 2018. *Handbook of Wildlife Chemical Immobilization*. 5th Edition. Minneapolis: University of Minnesota. ISBN: 978-0692118412.

Touroo R, Fitch A. 2018. Crime scene findings and the identification, collection, and preservation of evidence. Brooks J (ed.). *Veterinary Forensic Pathology*, pp. 9–25. Germany: Springer International Publishing.

Physical Examination of Living Victims

17

MARTHA SMITH-BLACKMORE

The Importance of the Physical Examination

The physical exam of the suspected abused animal is important for both the criminal investigation and the welfare of the animal. A physical exam should be conducted with the dual goals of documenting the animal's condition for forensic and treatment planning purposes but also to identify conditions that may be exculpatory. It is important to note that the presence of disease does not exclude criminal responsibility but may further define what was done to the animal (or what was omitted from the necessary provision of adequate care).

The physical examination of an animal is the most basic and important assessment of an animals' health performed by a veterinarian. It includes visual inspection of the animal (both from a distance and closeup using magnifying instruments), physical palpation (touch and feel), auscultation (listening) and even olfaction (smell). During the physical examination, veterinarians are also observing the animal's movements, posture, facial expressions and responses to handling.

The physical exam will also guide the veterinarian to further modalities to be used to document an animals' condition and influence treatment choices. The veterinarian may recommend imaging such as radiographs ("x-rays"), CT scans or ultrasound, laboratory tests such as complete blood counts, chemistry profiles, urinalysis, fecal analysis, toxin screens, infectious disease screens and so on. A veterinarian may be able to feel a broken bone, but without radiographs, they are unlikely to be able to opine on what types of mechanics led to the fracture.

Record Keeping

Veterinarians are taught a specific record-keeping system referred to as the "SOAP".

- "S" stands for "subjective": The veterinarian's initial impressions of the condition of the animal. Oftentimes, this section will contain terms such as Quiet, Alert and Responsive or Vocalizing, Dull and Minimally Responsive.

DOI: 10.4324/9781003090762-17

- "O" stands for "objective": The veterinarian will list findings that can be measured, counted or described in a manner that represents what is discovered on exam. The objective section of the exam is ordinarily described by system: The system headings such as EENT (eyes/ears/nose/throat), CVL (cardiovascular/lungs), GI (gastrointestinal), GU (genitourinary), MSI (musculoskeletal/integumentary, meaning skin, hair or feathers and nails), neuro (neurological system), and PLN (peripheral lymph nodes) is one typical breakdown of systems. Measured assessments such as weight, temperature, blood pressure or oxygen levels would also be listed in this section, along with a body condition score.
- "A" is for "assessment", or the veterinarian's conclusion of what problems are affecting the animal. Veterinarians may list "differentials" or various conditions that would possibly explain the animal's signs (the equivalent to symptoms in people), and the differentials are often listed in order from most likely to least likely.
- "P" is for the "plan" of next steps, whether for more diagnostics or for treatments.

In veterinary records that are likely to also be forensic records, it is important that the veterinarian note behaviors that indicate the animal is in pain, and behavioral responses to the administration of pain medications. These are the types of details that are not ordinarily recorded in clinical veterinary records, but that are very important in the forensic veterinary record. When a veterinarian is asked in court, on the stand, years after the incident, "how did you know the animal was in pain?", it will be far easier to answer that question if they wrote down that the animal was pacing, guarding its abdominal musculature, or whining, that it had dilated pupils or was crouching and withdrawn. Additionally, after the administration of pain medication, the veterinarian should record behaviors which reflect the resolution of pain signs, such as sleeping comfortably, breathing more steadily or cessation of vocalization.

Veterinarians are not trained for the formation or expression of opinion in veterinary medical records. They are meant to be objective, fact-recording documents. The veterinarian may opine in the "A" – assessment section that a constellation of injuries is most consistent with nonaccidental injury, or malnutrition may be one of the differential diagnoses listed for an emaciated animal, but an opinion of animal maltreatment may not be clearly delineated in a typical SOAP. For that reason, it can be helpful to ask the veterinarian to write a summary document, in lay terms, that outlines the findings and the veterinarian's opinion as to whether the condition is directly related to something that a person did or failed to do. It is important to note that the veterinarian may not be able to describe exactly what happened to an animal, but they can be certain that a set of injuries are inconsistent with a report of household injury (i.e., "fell down the stairs") or hit-by-car injury. It can be helpful to assure the veterinarian that they are not responsible for knowing "who-done-it" or even exactly what happened. The most helpful part of a veterinarian's exam may be the expression of an opinion on what is not plausible to have happened.

Veterinarians may require education on the process of evidence packaging and chain of custody process. A physical exam of an animal for court purposes may also be referred to as a veterinary medicolegal examination.

Methodology

The veterinary medicolegal examination is intended to detect and document evidence of criminal animal maltreatment and is performed in the same manner as the general physical exam, with the main differences being attention to detail, and careful documentation. Most veterinarians work the animal over from nose to tail, and from the tip of each limb toward the body and examine the animal with each system in mind (EENT, CVL, GI, GU, MSI, Neuro, PLN, etc.).

The nose should be examined for discharges or abrasions, in cases of hyperthermia, the shape of the nares (nasal openings) noted. The eyes should be inspected carefully with an ophthalmoscope and the ears with an otoscope. In some cases, the only evidence corroborating a report of blunt trauma to the head may be anterior uveitis (inflammation to the front of the eye) or bruising seen deep in the otic (ear) canal. The lips, gums, teeth and tongue should be examined for bruising, lacerations and broken or discolored teeth. The mouth should be opened, jaw joint motion noted and hard palate inspected. Every aspect of the head should be felt for symmetry, swelling, heat or crepitus (crunching sensation).

The neck should be flexed and extended in all anatomically normal ranges of motion, the spine palpated by putting pressure on each individual dorsal spinous process and each rib palpated along its length. The chest should be carefully ausculted for heart and lung sounds, and the abdomen palpated for masses, fluid-wave or other abnormalities.

Every nail should be examined for fraying; each foot and toe pad should be observed for abrasions or lacerations. Every long bone and joint should be palpated for symmetry, swellings, heat, range of motion and response to touch. Subcutaneous emphysema (a "crispy" feeling of air trapped under the skin) should be noted. The color of fur, especially fur that should be white, should be noted. Any marked odors (e.g., accelerants, smoke, filth or infection) should be noted, and patterns of missing fur recorded. Short whiskers and fur should be examined for singes (tapered curled ends), cutting (blunt ends) or breakage (frayed ends). Any bruises, lacerations, abrasions, or other marks should be noted on a body map diagram, measured for size and in relation to anatomic landmarks (triangulated) and photographed, first in an overall perspective, then regionally and finally up close with and without a scale (See Appendix C for example forms). The fur should be parted, and the skin examined for parasites and any other debris present. The tail should be palpated to its tip and lifted so the anus, perineal region and genitalia can be examined.

A "negative" physical exam does not exclude the possibility of animal abuse. In cases where an animal was observed to be struck or otherwise harmed, and yet the veterinarian finds no evidence on physical exam, there are plausible explanations. Dogs and cats have thicker skin than people, and a different capillary distribution, so bruising is often not as visible on the outer surface of the skin. Most animals are quadrupeds (walking on four legs), so they can mask a sore foot or leg more easily by shifting their weight. In many species, especially prey species, hiding signs of injury or illness is an instinct. In these cases, a veterinarian may write a report detailing why physical signs of abuse may not be noted, and that it does not preclude abuse. Reports of an animal trying to get away from an abuser or crying out in pain are evidence that the animal was trying to escape pain or suffering painful sensations.

Important Measurements and Notations

Veterinarians should be sure to weigh animals, take temperatures, perform a body condition score assessment and note these findings in the medical record. If not known, the age should be estimated based on dentition or ocular examination. In some cases, it may only be possible to record an animal's age in a broad category such as pediatric, juvenile, young adult, adult or geriatric. Any collars or tags present should be collected, photographed and preserved as evidence. The animal should be thoroughly scanned for a microchip. The animal should be photographed from both sides, front and rear, from the top and the underside, if possible. If the offense included confinement in a small enclosure, the animal should be measured from nose tip to tail base, from the floor to the top of the head and in lateral recumbency (laying on its side) from the bottom of the feet to the top of the head. It can be helpful to also measure the thickness of the animal at its widest point with radiography calipers. Dogs that have been "over kenneled" will have weak, flat feet, sometimes referred to as "starfish feet." These should be noted and photographed at intake and over time, as the feet will become stronger and more "square" during rehabilitation.

Any material removed from an animal should be preserved as evidence to include collar and tags. If the animal is heavily matted, the shaved fur should be weighed, packaged and preserved. If possible, blood and urine should be collected for laboratory testing before administering pain medication or sedatives, especially in cases where it is suspected that the animal may have been drugged. Starved animals may require a careful re-feeding plan supervised by a veterinarian as feeding too much, too soon can trigger life-threatening diarrhea or electrolyte derangements. Previously starved animals should be examined, weighed, body condition scored and photographed regularly as they regain good condition.

When radiographing animals with known or suspected nonaccidental trauma, full body radiographs should be taken if possible. In cases of "battered pets", there may be signs of old or poorly healed fractures along with fresh injuries. There are a variety of published scientific papers that can help a veterinarian understand if a collection of injuries are consistent with accidental or nonaccidental injuries, and there are a number of books and articles available that can guide the exam of an animal suspected to have been victim of particular types of abuse (e.g., sexual abuse, burns and sharp trauma).

Opinion Formation and Testimony

Veterinarians can be qualified as experts in a court of law based on knowledge, skill, experience, training and education. As experts, therefore, they may give opinions regarding evidence that falls into their area of expertise during testimony. This means that a veterinarian is not only a fact witness but also an expert witness.

The veterinarian's scientific, technical and other specialized knowledge serves to assist the jury or judge to understand the evidence or to determine an issue in dispute. Expert testimony must be based on sufficient facts and data and be the product of the reliable application of principles and methods to the facts of the case.

Bibliography

Byrd JH, Norris P, Bradley-Siemens N. 2020. *Veterinary Forensic Medicine and Forensic Sciences*. Boca Raton, FL: Taylor & Francis.

Intarapanich NP, McCobb EC, Reisman RW, Rozanski EA, Intarapanich PP. Characterization and comparison of injuries caused by accidental and nonaccidental blunt force trauma in dogs and cats. *Journal of Forensic Sciences* 2016;61:993–999.

Merck M. 2012. *Veterinary Forensics*, 2nd Edition. Oxford: Wiley.

Tong LJ. Fracture characteristics to distinguish between accidental injury and nonaccidental injury in dogs. *The Veterinary Journal* 2014;199:392–398.

Touroo R, Baucom K, Kessler M, Smith-Blackmore M. Minimum standards and best practices for the clinical veterinary forensic examination of the suspected abused animal. *Forensic Science International: Reports* 2020;2:100150.

Postmortem Interval 18

MARTHA SMITH-BLACKMORE

Fundamentals of Postmortem Interval

The postmortem interval (PMI) is the time that has elapsed since an animal's death. When the time of death is not known, the interval may be estimated. Based on the estimated interval, an estimated time of death may be established. Unfortunately, as compared to human medicine, there are few validated or standard veterinary and scientific techniques supporting such estimations in animals.

Postmortem interval estimation can be an important factor in the investigation of animal cruelty incidents which cause death. An interval estimation may support the inclusion or rule out of certain suspects or to corroborate (or refute) witness accounts.

The variation in size and composition of animals (fur and skin thickness, subcutaneous and body cavity fat stores, muscle and bone composition, body mass:surface area ratio, gastrointestinal tract anatomy and contained matter) adds to the complexity of decomposition determination. This is in addition to already complex environmental influences such as temperature, sun exposure, wind velocity and humidity. Because of this, no single method can be reliably used to accurately estimate the PMI in animals.

Changes to the Body after Death

So long as an animal is alive, various cellular processes maintain homeostasis (a normal physiological state of being). Fluids are kept in their appropriate spaces (blood stays in the blood vessels for example). For the most part, bacterial and fungal growth are kept at bay, in warm-blooded animals the body thermoregulates (maintains their temperature within a narrow span) and the animal retains a supple, malleable condition. After death, the loss of normal function on an anatomic and cellular level allows a succession of changes.

DOI: 10.4324/9781003090762-18

Pallor Mortis

Pallor mortis is Latin for "the paleness of death". When the heart stops beating, and the blood vessels lose the normal tone that is maintained in life, a blanching of tissues becomes evident. In animals, since they may be heavily pigmented and/or furred or feathered, the place that is most convenient to note *pallor mortis* is the gums. In animals where the oral mucosa is heavily pigmented, the vaginal or penile mucosa may be another location to observe (Figures 18.1 and 18.2).

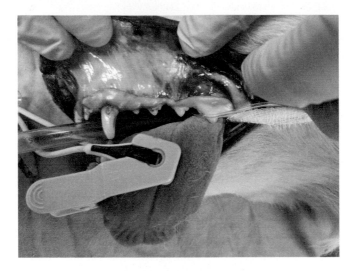

Figure 18.1 Normal healthy pink oral mucosa (gums).

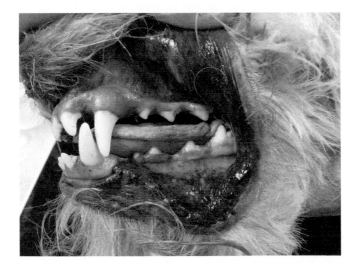

Figure 18.2 Normal postmortem mucosa. Note this tissue retains a pink color, somewhat more pale than the tissue shown in Figure 18.1.

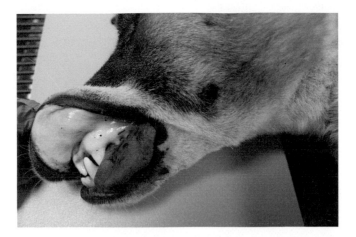

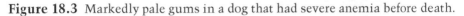

Figure 18.3 Markedly pale gums in a dog that had severe anemia before death.

An animal that was healthy prior to death, and that did not bleed to death, will ordinarily maintain some level of pink coloration. Animals that were anemic prior to death will be markedly more pale (Figure 18.3), animals that were jaundiced (also referred to as "icterus") will have a yellow coloration, animals that were hyperthermic may have brick red or a blue tinge, and other conditions may cause other color changes, such as "cherry red" color from cyanide poisoning (Figures 18.4 and 18.5). *Pallor mortis* is a somewhat subjective assessment and therefore is not very useful as a PMI assessment.

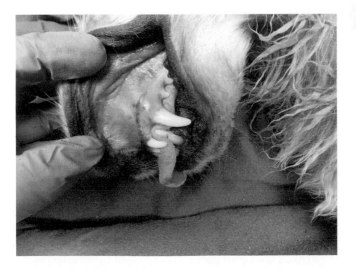

Figure 18.4 Yellow coloration to the gums may indicate liver disease, or diseases or toxins affecting the red blood cells.

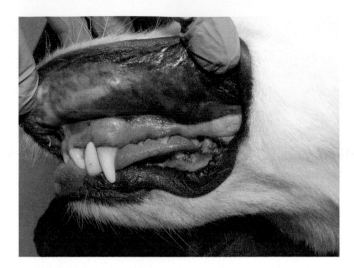

Figure 18.5 Blueish color may be seen in animals that have suffered hyperthermia, hypothermia or lack of oxygen.

Algor Mortis

Algor mortis is Latin for "the coldness of death". Upon cessation of normal life activity, the body loses the ability to maintain a normal temperature. For animals in environments that are cooler than the normal temperature of their body, the body will begin to cool. Studies looking at the average cooling time of humans after death vs that of animals demonstrate that the cooling rate for dogs is not the same as that for people.

One study in dogs demonstrated a steady, relatively constant decline in body temperature per hour. This study followed the cooling pattern in 16 dogs, so it is a small cohort and should be expanded in a larger study. The results may be considered a general guideline.

In the study, rectal, liver, brain and aural (ear) temperatures were recorded for approximately 32 hours, indoors in still air. The air temperature was approximately 70°F, and the ambient humidity was approximately 40%. The canine rectal temperature (with the thermometer inserted approximately 2 inches into the rectum) appeared to relay consistent results, with an average starting temperature of 100.4°F, 1 hour after death, and declining, on average 0.9°F/ hour. By way of contrast, people tend to cool at a rate of 1.5–2°F/ hour. The average healthy dog's resting temperature is 101°F–102.5°F, and this should be taken into account in any calculations. Note that obese or giant breed dogs are likely to cool slowly and very thin or toy breed animals will cool more quickly. This is due to the surface area-to-body mass ratio. In another study of *Algor mortis* in beagles, the rectal temperature of the dog was higher than the ambient room temperature for less than 1 day.

The early postmortem period can be divided into the early postmortem period and the late postmortem period based on body temperature. In the early postmortem period, the body temperature has not yet equilibrated with the temperature of the environment. In the late postmortem period, the body has the same temperature of the environment – ambient temperature is matched.

Rigor Mortis

Rigor mortis is Latin for "the stiffness of death". This temporary state of stiffness is due to chemical muscle activity. The stiffness will cause ongoing contraction of muscle until the molecular source of energy (adenosine triphosphate or ATP) is consumed. After this point, the muscles will remain contracted until the rigidity is disrupted by force, or early decomposition.

In people, rigor mortis sets in at approximately 2–6 hours after death and begins to relax after 36 hours. The timeline for Rigor mortis onset and relaxation is highly variable; however, depending on the ambient temperature, the animal's size, species and activity level, core body temperature and level of excitement before death. The stiffening is most evident in the small muscle groups of the body, then the jaw, the arms and then the legs (Figure 18.6). More muscular people and animals will display more prominent rigor, and young children, juvenile animals or the elderly may not express any observable rigor mortis. Birds enter a state of rigor mortis very quickly due to their relatively faster metabolic rate.

A study of rigor mortis in dogs reported the onset of rigor at less than 1 day, and persistence in the hind legs until 7 days after death. Again, this was a study in a small cohort of dogs, and in this study, the dogs were all beagles of similar size and body mass. For this reason, and for the other reasons mentioned above, rigor mortis can only be a general guideline, and further research is needed.

Livor Mortis

Livor mortis is Latin for "the wounds of death", referring to the deep purple-red or bruised appearance of blood pooling in gravity-dependent tissues (the underneath, or lowest positioned tissues of the animal's body in the position it was in after death). Lividity is not as pronounced in animals, and even after shaving fur it may be difficult to observe, depending on pigmentation.

In people, livor mortis sets in 1.5–2 hours after death, but timelines are not well established in animals. The earlier stages of livor mortis are due to pooling of blood within the gravity-dependent vessels. At this point, pressing

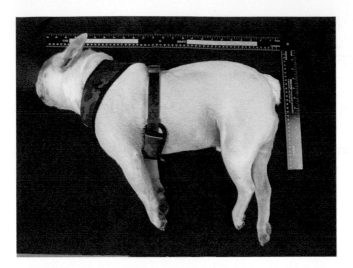

Figure 18.6 Dog exhibiting rigor mortis with evident stiffness and straightening of the forelimbs.

into a livor mortis discoloration will cause the blood to be pushed away, so the livor is said to be "nonfixed". Any objects the body was laying upon at the time of death, or wrinkling of skin may make a pattern of blanching that matches the surface or object the body was in contact with (Figure 18.7).

At about 8–12 hours postmortem in people, the breakdown of blood vessels and red blood cells causes the color to be throughout the tissue, not just held within vessels. At that time, pushing on the discolored tissue will not cause a blanching of the tissue and the livor mortis is said to be "fixed". Fixed livor mortis begins at about 8–72 hours postmortem.

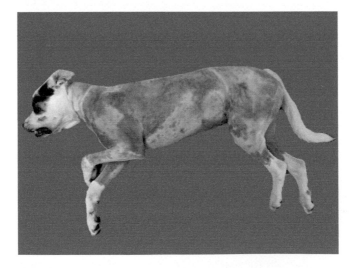

Figure 18.7 Animals with dense fur must be shaved to appreciate patterns of livor mortis.

One important aspect of lividity is that if it is seen on the top of the animal, or it is not consistent with the position the animal was in when discovered, it likely indicates that the body was moved some time after death. Internal organs may also demonstrate livor mortis and a necropsy may help to provide some additional insight on time since death, and body position after the time of death.

Decomposition

Decomposition is the reduction of soft tissue into simpler forms of matter, accompanied by a distinctive, strong and unpleasant odor. Decomposition is the result of autolysis or autodigestion (internal breakdown of cells and tissues of the body) and putrefaction (the overgrowth of bacteria, fungi and protozoa in the body). The bacterial overgrowth causes an accumulation of gases within the body, including the signature odor of cadaverine. The chemical processes of autolysis and putrefaction typically occur in a predictable order but within a variable timeframe, even within one individual.

There are a variety of published descriptions of the stages of decomposition that describe a number of stages (four-, five-, six- and even nine-stage decomposition schemes have been described). However, animal bodies will decompose at varying rates depending on numerous factors both intrinsic and extrinsic to the body, including body condition score (emaciated, thin, normal, overweight or obese), presence or absence of trauma, exposure to weather conditions (to include temperature degree days, humidity, sun exposure, rain), insect colonization and scavenging. All these factors influence the transitions through stages of decomposition. Bloating or a gray-green discoloration to the abdomen can be seen within 1 day of death. During this time, marbling may also be seen (Figure 18.8).

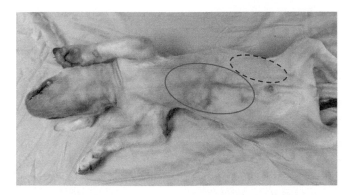

Figure 18.8 Green discoloration of this puppy's lower abdomen can be seen on the left side of the abdomen (dashed oval) and marbling of the veins can also be seen (solid line oval).

A SIX STAGE DECOMPOSITION DESCRIPTION SYSTEM	
Stage 1	**Fresh** Algor and rigor mortis. The skin is intact and hair is firmly attached.
Stage 2	**Primary bloat** Gas accumulates within the body, skin and hair loosen
Stage 3	**Secondary bloat** Limbs disarticulate, fluid purge, strong odor
Stage 4	**Active decay** Deflation, advanced disarticulation of limbs and head
Stage 5	**Advanced decay** Collapse of the abdomen, soft tissues liquified
Stage 6	**Skeletonization** Soft tissues and cartilage disappear

Figure 18.9 An example six-stage decomposition system.

Chemical processes during decomposition are complex and result in the breakdown of soft tissues, changes to constituent carbohydrates, proteins, and lipids resulting in transformations such as saponification (change of fat to a substance known as adipocere) or liquefaction (Figure 18.9). Additionally, an animal's body might be partially exposed to sun, and partly sheltered. In that case, it would not be unusual to have mummification at one end and bloat at another.

Desiccation or Mummification

When humidity is low in the environment, rather than a wet decomposition process, tissues may desiccate (dry out) in a mummification process. This is more likely to happen in the absence of insect activity and can happen in warm or cool temperatures. The mummified remains will have a brown or yellow appearance and leathery feel. Some remains can go through initial stages of decay, and after significant soft tissue is removed by scavenging or insect activity, the remaining skin, muscle and tendons may mummify leaving a hollow skeleton draped with hide and other dried out soft tissues (Figure 18.10). Mummification happens over a variable time-period depending on the presence or absence of air movement, ambient humidity and exposure to light. The PMI to the state of mummification of an animal is one that can be measured in weeks. A mummified animal cannot have a traditional necropsy as the leathery remains cannot be dissected; however, diagnostic imaging such as magnetic resonance imaging (MRI), computed tomography (CT) or radiographs (X-rays) can be helpful tools (Figure 18.11).

Insect Evidence

In addition to examining the body for pallor, algor, rigor, livor and signs of decomposition, the careful identification and collection of insect evidence may assist in establishing the PMI. An entomologist can determine the

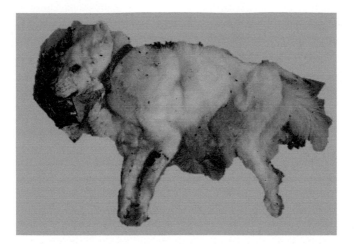

Figure 18.10 Mummified remains of a dog after insect activity has swept away all soft tissues under the skin.

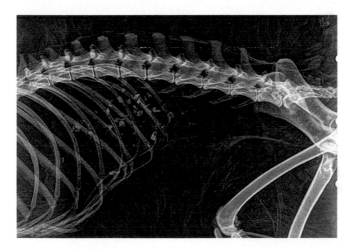

Figure 18.11 Radiograph of the same remains as in Figure 18.10. Even though the stomach is gone, radiographs demonstrate evidence of pica, foreign material left behind in the area where the stomach used to be. This is proof that the dog had an appetite and was able to chew and swallow at the time of death, refuting a defendant's claim the dog was deceased from terminal cancer when abandoned.

species collected through identifying the adults present and raising maggots. Knowledge of the represented species in combination with weather data can allow the entomologist to make an estimate of time since death. It is important to remember that insect colonization can happen before death in an untreated wound. This is more likely in a debilitated animal or an animal with heavy wool or a matted hair coat.

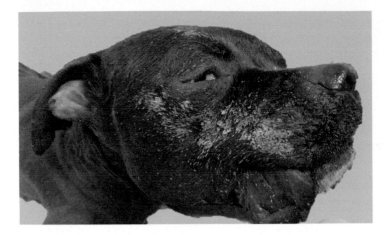

Figure 18.12 Fly eggs appear like fine off white specks, resembling sawdust.

Adult flying insects can be collected at the scene with an insect net and deposited into a vial of 70% ethanol (rubbing alcohol). Live maggots may be collected from the body, and a sample of living maggots can be preserved in a vial or jar with a layer of damp soil. A sample of the live maggots can also be preserved by first blanching them in very hot, but not boiling water, and then placing them in 70% ethanol. An investigator should aim to collect approximately 50 live and 50 preserved maggots if possible. A small amount of cat food or other meat can be placed on top of the soil to feed the maggots during transport to an entomologist. It is important to puncture the container of live samples with holes small enough to prevent escape but large enough to allow air circulation. Pupae or empty pupal cases, if present, should also be collected. They are generally brown to black elongated shell-like structures. They can go into a dry container; no ethanol or soil needed.

Insect eggs may be observed in clumps in the fur, resembling sawdust (Figure 18.12). These can be documented photographically if they cannot be collected at the scene. Containers of insect evidence should be labeled with the case and investigator information, time, date and location of collection. The entomologist will use the insect evidence and environmental data to report out the likely timeline (Figure 18.13).

Future Directions

Postmortem chemistry, such as sampling, the vitreous (eyeball fluid) for potassium levels and other biochemical markers is a future direction of research to help understand PMI. As postmortem time passes, the potassium

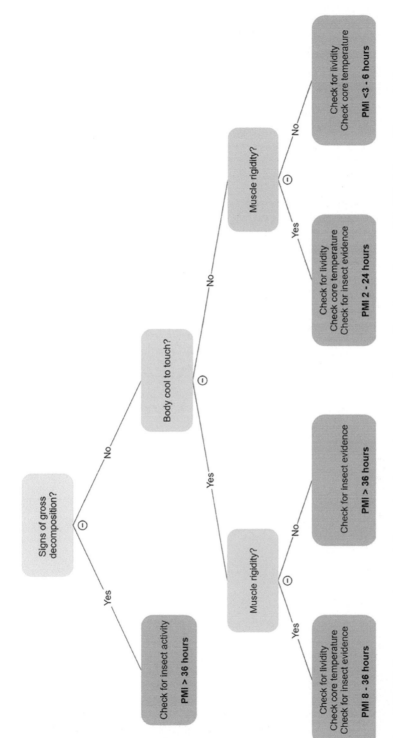

Figure 18.13 Postmortem interval determination and steps to take to refine the estimate. (Modified from Chapter 4 *Postmortem Changes and Estimating the Postmortem Interval in Veterinary Forensic Pathology*, Jason W. Brooks. Springer 2018.)

level in the vitreous increases. Studies have been done in people, but limited data exist in dogs and other animals.

Investigation into the degradation of DNA, RNA, microvesicles and exosomes also hold promise for forensic investigative techniques to determine PMI in animals. Investigators should bear in mind that the methods described here can only provide rough estimates, and caution should be taken in extrapolating from methods used to determine PMI in people.

Bibliography

Brooks JW. 2018. *Postmortem Changes and Estimating the Postmortem Interval in Veterinary Forensic Pathology*. Germany: Springer International Publishing.

Erlandsson M, Munro R. Estimation of the post-mortem interval in beagle dogs. *Science & Justice* 2007;47(4):150–154.

Janaway RC, Percival S, Wilson A. *Decomposition of Human Remains*. 2009. doi: 10.1007/978-1-59745-327-1_14.

Proctor KW, Kelch WJ, New JC. Estimating the time of death in domestic canines. *Journal of Forensic Sciences* 2009;54(6):1433–1437.

The Forensic Necropsy

19

MARTHA SMITH-BLACKMORE

The postmortem exam (also known as a "necropsy" in animals, or even "animal autopsy") is an important step for the documentation of suspected prior animal maltreatment in deceased animals. Postmortem exams may be performed by board-certified veterinary pathologist or general practitioner veterinarians. While veterinary pathologists have advanced training in the examination of deceased animals and tissues, they may not have training or familiarity with forensic practices. Some general practitioners have advanced veterinary forensic skills and will work in conjunction with veterinary pathologists when cases require microscopic examination of tissues. In most animal abuse cases, the gross necropsy will provide the necessary analysis to understand what happened to the animal. For this reason, forensic pathology is often referred to as a "naked-eye" discipline.

The purpose of a forensic necropsy is to detect and document nonaccidental injury, to provide estimates of how long a condition has been present, to determine or estimate postmortem interval and to investigate natural or disease conditions that may have contributed to the animal's condition. The forensic necropsy provides opportunity for a veterinarian to opine on degree and duration of suffering (from pain, hunger, air-hunger or other negative affective states.) Forensic necropsies may be performed at a university or other laboratory, veterinary clinic, animal shelter or in rare cases, in the field.

Before a necropsy is performed, the examiner should verify their legal authority to do so via consent, approved search warrant, or because the deceased animal has no known owner and was found on public property. The veterinarian performing the postmortem exam should review all available veterinary records, narrative reports, scene photos and diagrams before commencing the exam. There should be an understanding and agreement about what is going to happen with the remains at the conclusion of the exam, whether they are going to be maintained or disposed of, and who is responsible for the maintenance or disposal process.

Preparing the Body for Necropsy

After the animal has been documented at the scene, it should be packaged for a postmortem exam. The investigator should wear gloves whenever touching the

DOI: 10.4324/9781003090762-19

body. Ideally, the paws are bagged in paper bags, the body wrapped in a clean sheet and enclosed in a durable plastic bag, which is tightly sealed at the neck of the bag to prevent entry of insects or room air. It is important to evacuate as much air from the bag as possible as this will help slow decomposition. The bag should be labeled with a tag indicating the animal number, date, collection site and collector's agency and name of the person collecting the animal. The movement of the body should be accompanied by proper chain of custody processes.

Once the body is removed from the scene, the site where the animal was located should be inspected and photographed again to capture information that may be present under the animal's body. Opening the body bag should be avoided until the time of the forensic necropsy as re-introducing air into the bag can accelerate decomposition.

To Freeze or Not to Freeze?

Ideally, the body will move directly from the scene to the postmortem exam. Due to logistics, this is not typically possible. If the body cannot be examined immediately, but will be examined within 72 hours, it should be refrigerated as soon as possible and maintained in a refrigerated state until the postmortem exam. If it is not known when the exam will happen or if the exam will happen more than 72 hours after the body is collected, the remains should be frozen. While some microscopic detail will be lost due to freezing, that level of detail (and more) will also be lost due to decomposition, even in refrigerated conditions. Freezing a decomposing body helps to arrest the decomposition process and has the added benefits of reducing noxious odors after thawing and killing insects that may be present.

All remains of deceased animals suspected to be victims of maltreatment or found dead in questioned circumstances should undergo forensic necropsy. This is regardless of the level of decomposition or mummification. There is always the possibility of discovering some important information; if a necropsy is not performed, that important information will be missed.

Postmortem Examination

If the body has been frozen prior to exam, it can take up to several days to thaw, depending on the size of the animal. Thawing is slower in refrigeration than at room temperature. As a body is thawed, it should be turned every few hours to ensure even thawing. Turning should be done more frequently if the body is being thawed at room temperature, and once the body is malleable, it should be moved to refrigerated storage and necropsied as soon as possible. It is not necessary to open the bag to turn the body or feel it for malleability. Reopening a bag introduces oxygen and can contribute to the acceleration of decomposition.

Preliminary Steps

It is important to photograph the postmortem exam throughout the process for thorough documentation. This photography may be performed by the examining veterinarian, an assistant or a law enforcement officer. At the start of the postmortem examination, the unopened body bag should be photographed with a case card notating the date, start time, case number, agency the exam is being performed for, animal number, site of postmortem exam and initials of persons present. The identifying tag on the bag should be photographed, and the process of opening the bag and wrappings should be photographed at each step.

The examiner or an assistant should keep notes of the postmortem exam findings. The signalment of the animal should be recorded; this includes species, breed (or breed-type), markings, sex and neuter status, and age or estimated age. If the age is estimated, notes should be made regarding how the estimation was made (based on dentition, examination of the eyes, weight or other methods). The body should be weighed, and body condition scored, noting what body condition scoring system was used.

Anyone handling the body should be wearing gloves, and the gloves should be changed frequently, especially when they become soiled, or before collecting evidence that may contain DNA. Any material found on the animal such as harnesses, collars, ropes or ties should be photographed in place before removing. Any knotted cords should be cut at a point away from the knot and not untied. Duct tape or other adhesive tapes should be cut and placed sticky side down on a sheet of cellophane or plastic. All objects should be photographed, including both sides of tags, and packaged and preserved as evidence. The body should be scanned for a microchip, and if one is detected, the microchip number should be photographed on the screen of the scanner and noted on the record.

It is helpful to reference a checklist of steps taken in to ensure the necropsy is completed in detail. Body outline forms or sketches can assist in the notation of findings and measurements (See Appendix C for example forms).

External Examination

The condition of the body with regard to decomposition should be noted (e.g., fresh, early decomposition, advanced decomposition, skeletonized or mummified). Tissue changes related to decomposition such as marbling, color change, skin slippage, collapsed eye globes or bloating should be noted. Any odors noticed should be described. The presence of any insect evidence should be noted and samples collected.

The animal should be photographed on six sides ("like a dice" – overall views from the front, rear, each side, top and bottom/underside) as feasible. Any noted findings (e.g., injuries, trace evidence) should be photographed in

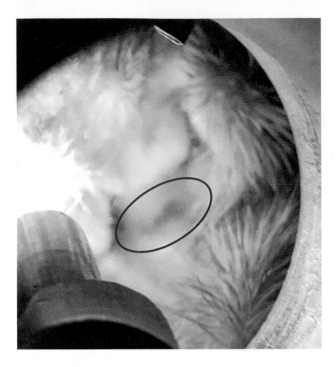

Figure 19.1 Otoscopic examination may reveal bruising in the ear canal that is indicative of head trauma.

context, from overall to mid-range to close up), with and without a scale present in the view before making any changes to the finding. The lesion or finding should be measured and located on the body with measurements taken from anatomical landmarks to help locate the position on the body. Any trace evidence should be collected and preserved as described in Chapter 6.

The body should be carefully examined externally, in the manner a clinical exam is performed on a living patient, to include oral, ophthalmoscopic and otoscopic exams to the extent possible (Figure 19.1). External palpation should include range of motion manipulation of all joints and palpation of the entire body, including long bones, skull, spine and ribs. The fur should be parted so that the skin can be examined for evidence of parasites or areas of interest.

Any lesions or wounds found should be photographed in the state they were found, before clipping fur or plucking feathers. This external exam will orient the veterinarian to the entire animal and reveal any areas requiring closer examination, specialized imaging or more extensive documentation.

Radiographs and Other Imaging

The entire animal should be radiographed (x-rayed) as there may be evidence of prior injury in areas of the body not suspected or previously known to be impacted. Additionally, radiographs can be useful illustrations to use in court when more graphic images may be disallowed by a judge. When head trauma is known or suspected to have occurred, computed tomography (CT scans) can provide better insight to the injuries over plain radiographs as the skull is a complex three-dimensional structure. Some CT systems can create three-dimensional reconstruction images and can be used as compelling illustrations in reports and testimony (Figures 19.2 and 19.3).

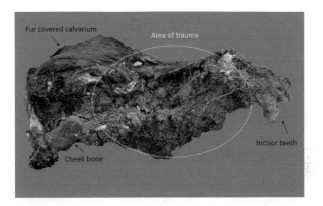

Figure 19.2 Exhumed dog skull of a dog reportedly killed by smoke inhalation in a house fire.

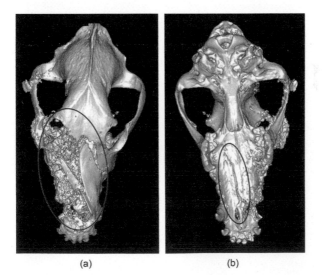

(a)   (b)

Figure 19.3 Three-dimensional reconstruction of a CT scan of the skull, revealing significant blunt trauma. The three dimensional CT reconstruction image can be rotated to observe trauma to the top of the skull (a) and the underside fo the skull (b). (CT image by The Ohio State University College of Veterinary Medicine.)

Dermal Inspection

Wounds should be photographed before changing their appearance, with and without a scale. After initial inspection and documentation, for suspected gunshot wounds, some fur samples should be gathered and preserved for analysis at a forensic laboratory for the presence of soot or gunshot residue. After initial documentation, wounds can be shaved to inspect the skin surface for associated marks such as gunpowder stippling or patterned injury (Figures 19.4–19.8).

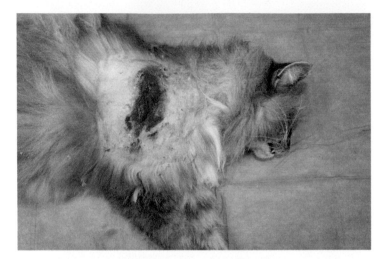

Figure 19.4 A wound should be documented on the animal in an overall view, far away enough to understand where it is located on an animal's body (midrange) and close up, before and after shaving, with and without a scale. This image demonstrates a wound on a cat's right shoulder. Prior photos were taken of the overall cat on all 6 sides, before shaving.

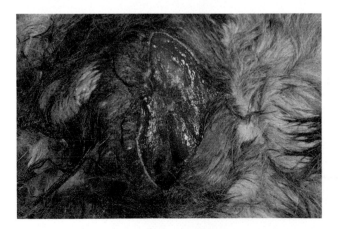

Figure 19.5 The wound, close up, before shaving.

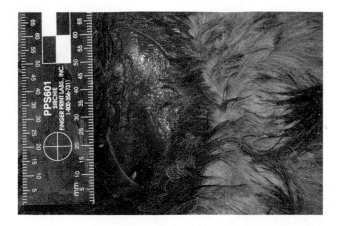

Figure 19.6 The wound, close up, prior to shaving, with a scale

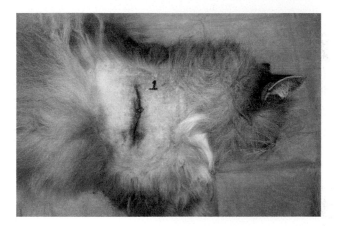

Figure 19.7 The wound, midrange, after shaving and numbering.

For animals with projectile wounds, the wound should be gently probed, and the direction of projectile travel (trajectory) determined. It is helpful to refer to radiographs at the same time as projectiles may leave a "comet tail" of metallic debris along their path. Entry wounds will often have barbered (cut) hairs at the margin of the wounds, and there may be a cuff abrasion to the circular wound. Exit wounds tend to be more irregular and larger than entry wounds, although close-range shots over bony regions may result in a stellate (star-shaped) entry wound. Projectiles that enter bone can cause shattering and fragments of bone may exit the skin creating shrapnel-type wounds that can be confused with entry and exit wounds. Documenting findings with photographs, drawings, diagrams, radiographs and CT exam provides ample visual support for a case, but certainly all modalities are not necessary to document a case. The investigator and veterinarian should work together to

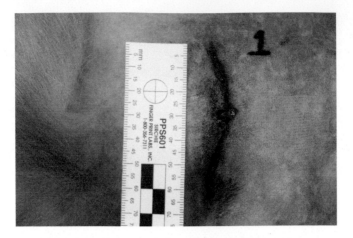

Figure 19.8 The wound close up, shaved, numbered and with a scale. There were three wounds on this cat, each treated similarly, an entry wound, a small nick wound made from the inside of the cat, and an exit wound. The wounds were determined to be made by a compound arrow passing through the cat from front to back.

determine which methods to use in a particular case, but photography and sketching with notes are expected minimum documentation. Original images must always be preserved, and if copies of images are used for illustration with annotations or contrast manipulation, that must be made clear when including images in reports or presenting them to the court (Figures 19.9–19.15).

For cases where practicality and the condition of the animal allows, the entire body should be shorn down to the skin with a #40 clipper blade. For animals with blood or fluid-soaked fur, heavy contamination with dirt or sand, or animals with skin slippage from decomposition changes, this may not be practical, or it may be reasonable to shave only specific regions depending on circumstances.

Shaving the animal allows for inspection of the skin for externally visible bruising and abrasions, and pattern injuries may be appreciated. For animals with multiple regions of marks, it is helpful to annotate directly on the animal's skin with a permanent marker. This helps to demonstrate the number of areas impacted and individuates one area of trauma from another in photography and notations (Figures 19.16–19.20).

After the external surface of the skin has been inspected, photographed (with and without scales, and in context with the overall anatomy), measured, and diagrammed in notes, the animal should be skinned so that the internal surface can be inspected. This process is also called "reflecting" the skin (Figures 19.21 and 19.22).

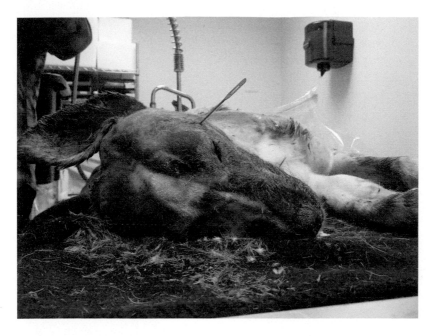

Figure 19.9 A dog was shot in the head by an individual claiming self-defense. The working photograph at necropsy may be too "gruesome" for the judge to allow as it may be considered "prejudicial" against a defendant.

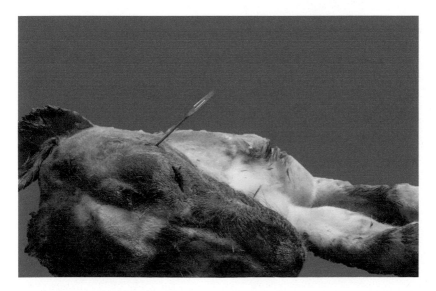

Figure 19.10 Dropping the background helps to clean up the image.

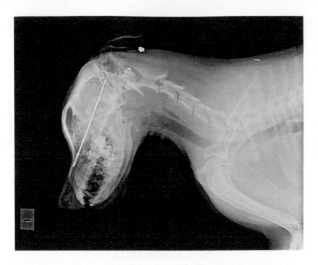

Figure 19.11 Radiographs with trajectory pin indicator help to demonstrate the direction or angle of the projectile without the judge or jury being subjected to a bloody image. A lateral view must be paired with a dorsoal ventral (or ventral dorsal view).

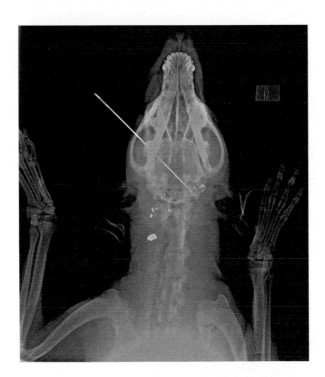

Figure 19.12 A dorsal ventral radiograph complements the lateral view in order to fully demonstrate the angle of the projectile trajectory.

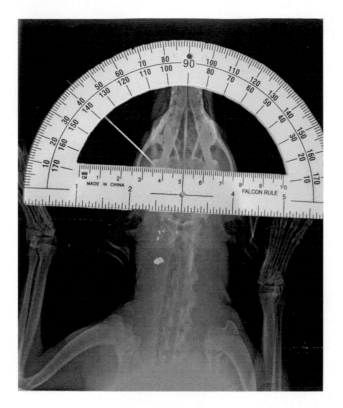
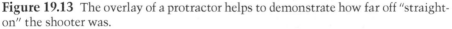

Figure 19.13 The overlay of a protractor helps to demonstrate how far off "straight-on" the shooter was.

Reflecting the skin helps to reveal deeper bruising. For many animals with thicker skin than people, a bruise may not be visible on the outer surface but can be quite remarkable on the interior surface of the skin. The inner surface of the removed hide (entirety of the hide, usually cut around distal limbs and tail so feet and tail skin are not included in the hide) should be photographed, and if injuries were noted on the external surface (e.g. A, B, C or 1, 2, 3), the corresponding inner surface of those wounds can be noted in photographs with small paper tags. The hide can be rolled up and placed in another bag within the body bag to keep it clean for future inspection by another expert.

Internal Exam

Most veterinarians perform necropsies on dogs, cats and other small animals in "lateral recumbency", meaning the animal is laid on its side. Some joints should be opened to inspect for signs of infection, bleeding or other

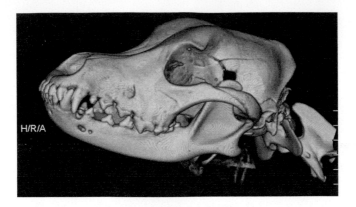

Figure 19.14 Three-dimensional CT images, if possible to obtain, give the best visual understanding of the path of the shot.

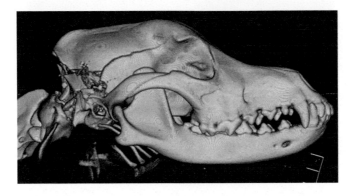

Figure 19.15 The three-dimensional CT image can be rotated in three axes, and still images captured that best illustrate the trauma, for use in reports or for exhibits in court.

abnormalities, and this helps to reflect the thoracic and pelvic limb to gain improved visualization within the body cavities.

The abdominal cavity can be opened for examination of the abdominal contents, and the diaphragm should be palpated to test for whether negative pressure is still present in the thorax. Conditions such as pneumothorax (collapsed lungs), hemo- or pyothorax (free blood or pus within the chest) will cause the diaphragm to be lax or have a "fluid wave".

Before disrupting the organs from their anatomical positions, open the thorax so that the open chest and abdomen can be appreciated and photographed overall. In animals that have been frozen and thawed, it is normal to have some watery red fluid present in both cavities, and within the pericardium. If there is frank blood, or blood clots present, these should be noted and measured. Postmortem blood clotting happens more slowly than in an acute bleed. For this reason, postmortem blood clots tend to have a "chicken fat", or

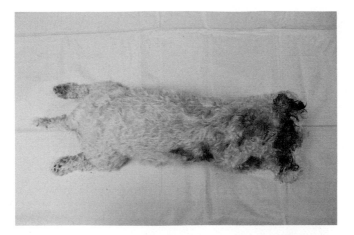

Figure 19.16 A dog was presented for necropsy with obvious head trauma.

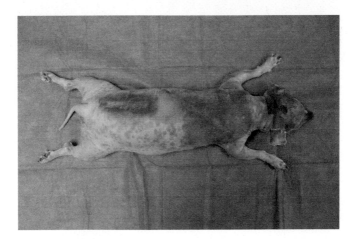

Figure 19.17 After shaving the body, tell-tale "train track" bruising consistent with blunt trauma from a long object was found. The defendant admitted to striking the dog three times with a baseball bat.

two-toned appearance with a dark red section and a yellow, more gelatinous section. Another important differentiator is that blood clots from a traumatic bleed will form outside of blood vessels (Figures 19.23 and 19.24).

The presence or absence of internal fat stores should be noted, as well as any unusual tissue coloration. Each solid abdominal organ should be removed, inspected, measured, and weighed, described, and photographed. Then they may be "bread-loafed" or cut into slices so that any interior abnormalities can be discovered. If an abnormality is questioned or likely to be related to the animal's condition, tissue samples may be taken and preserved in formalin for histopathology (inspection under a microscope by a pathologist). Each hollow organ should be opened so that the interior surface may be inspected and described. The ingesta (stomach contents) and digesta (intestinal contents) should be described, and the presence of lesions or parasites noted. In cases of suspected poisonings, samples should be taken and frozen. The stomach contents can be washed through a sieve to better understand what the animal's last meal may have been or what foreign objects they may have ingested (pica).

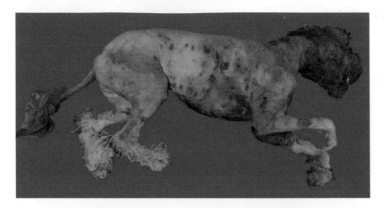

Figure 19.18 A dog was mauled by other dogs at a boarding facility, suffering hundreds of individual abrasions, contusions or puncture wounds from teeth and claw marks

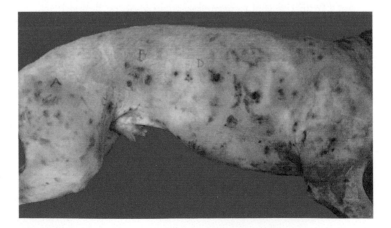

Figure 19.19 The dog was marked up into regions, each region was photographed, and the wounds within each region were annotated and counted.

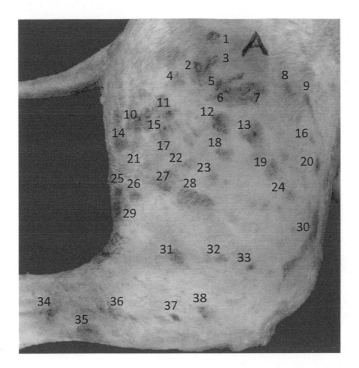

Figure 19.20 Photos of each region were entered into a spreadsheet, with the subtotals of noted lesions. The total number of lesions recorded was 473, and the report contained the statement "Dogs have 42 teeth, but not all teeth leave marks in a single bite. Bite marks are made by the teeth that make significant contact, enough to cause a bruise, abrasion, crush injury or puncture to the skin. Some bites will have four marks from the canine teeth only, while other bites will have marks from the incisors, premolars or molars, depending on the angle of the bite, the laxity of the flesh being bitten and the force exerted. As peppered as this dog's skin is with bite and claw marks, it is impossible to determine precisely how many bites were inflicted, or how many dogs were involved in inflicting the bites. The bites are estimated to number in the dozens".

The thoracic incision can be extended up to the mouth, and the entire "pluck" removed en bloc. This involves excising the tongue from the mandible, and removing the larynx, trachea, esophagus, heart and lungs all together (the stomach will already have been separated from the esophagus during the abdominal exploration). Then each organ can be inspected individually.

If death or injury by strangulation is suspected, careful dissection and inspection of the strap muscles of the neck, larynx, behind the angles of the mandibles ("corners" of the jaw) and under the skin of the occipital

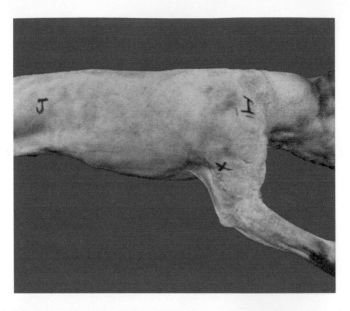

Figure 19.21 Sine external bruising is visible on the surface of the shaved dog.

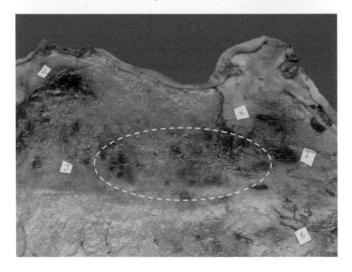

Figure 19.22 Note that on the inner surface, more extensive bruising is visible between the areas marked "I" and "J" on the outer surface.

protuberance (the point at the back of the skull) should be done, as these are the areas likely to be bruised or otherwise traumatized as the animal struggles against its own hanging weight.

The eyes and brain should be examined, and the spinal cord removed, if indicated. Other specific techniques to detect signs of particular types of trauma are outlined in veterinary forensic pathology literature and exceed the guidance provided here.

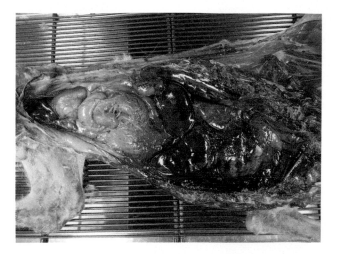

Figure 19.23 View of the open abdomen and thorax of an exmaciated German Shepherd dog. The owner claimed the dog died of "bloat" (gastric dilatation and volvulus, or "GDV") and buried the dog. The dog was later exhumed after a family member reported the defendant had starved the dog. Radiographs may have been "enough" to demonstrate a lack of GDV, but the anatomical photos more closely resemble the photograph of a case of GDV used for jury education.

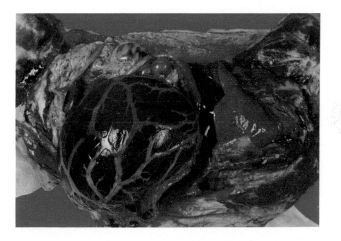

Figure 19.24 Similar view of a verified case of gastric dilatation and volvulus.

Final Thoughts

The bagged remains should be returned to storage (refrigerated, frozen or returned to the submitting agency. Photo logs should be created for all photos taken, noting findings highlighted as a memory aid. All materials should be reviewed, and a summary report written by the veterinarian with an opinion of the cause of death (natural, accidental, nonaccidental, euthanasia or undetermined) and estimates of the age of lesions, duration, nature and degree of suffering.

Bibliography

Brooks JW. 2018. *Veterinary Forensic Pathology*, Vols. 1 & 2. Germany: Springer.
Byrd JH, Norris P, Bradley-Siemens N. 2020. *Veterinary Forensic Medicine and Forensic Sciences*. Boca Raton, FL: CRC Press.
Veterinary Forensic Postmortem Examination Standards. https://www.ivfsa.org/wp-content/uploads/2020/12/IVFSA-Veterinary-Forensic-Postmortem-Exam-Standards_Approved-2020_with-authors.pdf.

Nonaccidental Injury 20

MARTHA SMITH-BLACKMORE

Fundamentals of Nonaccidental Injury (NAI)

Nonaccidental injury (NAI) is also known as "inflicted injury". These are harms to animals that occur when a deliberate action causes an injury to an animal. If an action is not deliberate, the injury is known as an accidental injury. NAI may also be referred to as "crimes of commission", or a crime when someone deliberately does something that harms an animal.

In some jurisdictions, this form of animal abuse may be considered a "specific intent statute", meaning that the person intended to inflict harm to the animal with the action. In other jurisdictions, it is interpreted as a "general intent statute"; in such cases, only the action that causes the harm is deliberate, and the harm caused to the animal does not have to be intended. In some jurisdictions, the intent of the offender may make the difference between a misdemeanor or felony charge. With a specific intent statute, there may be an obligation to prove the *mens rea*, or state of mind of the offender.

Some indications of a mindset to intentionally inflict harm on an animal could include restraining the animal to harm it, such as tying an animal to a fixed object in order to be able to strike the animal, striking the animal repeatedly or using a harmful instrument to strike an animal, such as a bat. In cases such as this, identifying signs of multiple blows, restraints or the implement used may be pivotal to the case. In other cases, the contents of the stomach may reveal that a bait was used to lure an animal to a place or position where it could be harmed (Figure 20.1).

Oftentimes, a person will claim an animal was the victim of a household accident ("fell down the stairs", "fell off the bed"), was accidentally hit by a motor vehicle or was a victim or a participant in an incidental dog fight. In those cases, an examination and opinion by a veterinarian may help to differentiate accidental from nonaccidental injury. The examination of the animal alone may not differentiate accidental from nonaccidental injury; the results of the examination must be considered in context with findings from the scene and witness accounts. For this reason, it is important to accurately capture the scene comprehensively through appropriate photographic and other documentation techniques. The veterinary expert is rarely at the scene at the time of initial scene examination and so the scene investigator has a responsibility to be able to convey the scene findings clearly, comprehensively and in context.

DOI: 10.4324/9781003090762-20

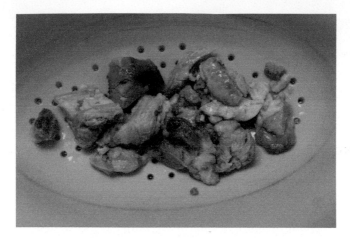

Figure 20.1 Washed stomach contents of a cat killed by a compound arrow were found to be consistent with chunks of rotisserie chicken. The perpetrator later admitted using this for bait.

Common Types of NAI

Common types of nonaccidental injury to animals include blunt and sharp trauma, burns (scalds, electrical, chemical and thermal), projectile injury (gunshot and arrows), drowning, strangulation or other nondrowning asphyxiation, staged animal fighting, animal sexual abuse (ASA) and poisoning. There may be cases where the circumstances are consistent with inflicted injury, but the postmortem exam cannot definitively pinpoint the cause of death. An example of this might be an animal bound with duct tape, submerged in a cage, weighed down by a cement block in a body of water. The postmortem exam may be "negative", meaning tissue damage from suffocation or drowning may not be visualized either grossly or under the microscope. However, these negative exams are important as they can refute a claim, rule out other causes of death and support other circumstantial information consistent with nonaccidental injury. A person might claim the animal died as the result of a hit by car accident, or disease, and this treatment of the body was intended as a "burial at sea"-type disposal. The absence of signs of hit by car trauma or natural disease will help refute those claims.

Funereal Abandonment

It is also important to bear in mind that a person may dispose of a deceased animal that died from natural or accidental causes in a public setting that is discovered later. The cause of the animal's death might not be a crime, and the intentions of the person abandoning the remains may even be to honor the animal. Cases like this can be referred to as "funereal abandonment". Often the body will be carefully wrapped or attended to, with objects of comfort such as blankets, beds or toys, and the bundle may be left in a public park, on the shore or at a human cemetery. Cases of funereal abandonment can be the last step of a criminally negligent decline, where the animal should have been provided veterinary care, a death after sudden illness or accidental death, or it may follow humane euthanasia in advance of an impending natural death (Figures 20.2–20.4).

Trauma to the Offender

Evidence of a violent interaction can help define nonaccidental injury. Marks of a struggle may be found on a perpetrator in the form of bites, scratches or bruises. As in any case of alleged violent interaction between people, the suspects' hands, arms, face, neck, abdomen, chest, back and legs should also be carefully examined as soon as possible for evidence of such injuries. In cases of bite or scratch wounds, DNA of the animal may be found in the wound if examined and swabbed while the wounds are still fresh. In delayed examination, bacteria found in older wounds may potentially be DNA typed and matched to the flora found in the mouth of the biting animal. Evidence of the inciting cause for the NAI may include a toileting accident, stolen food or an effort exerted by the abuser to demonstrate power and control.

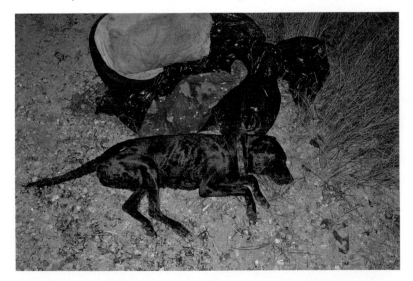

Figure 20.2 A dog was found in a bag on the shore with a dog bed and blanket, wearing a collar but with not tags, tattoo, microchip or other identifying information. A necrospy showed the dog had cancer and had been euthanized by a veterinarian. She was sick but not neglected, so the only crimes committed were related to illegal disposal. The keeping of items of comfort with the dog is consistent with funereal abandonment. (Courtesy of ACO Leslie Badger.)

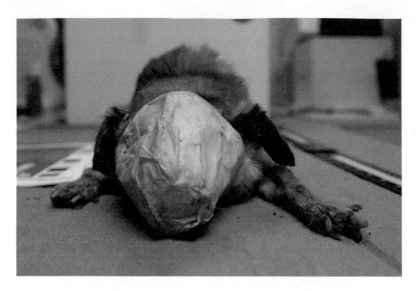

Figure 20.3 Another dog was found abandoned, wrapped in a bundle in a cemetery, with an elaborate masking tape mask over its face. Under the masking tape, a large erosive abscess was found, and coins had been inserted in the dog's eyes, under the eyelids after death, first noted on radiographs. This dog died of natural causes, but the abscess would have been painful, and the dog was emaciated, so it was consistent with neglect. The dogs in Figure 20.2 and 20.3 were unknown ("Dog Doe"s), and no suspects were found. The ritual with the dog at the cemetery is consistent with funereal abandonment.

Motive

The myriad reasons for harming an animal may be complex or indeterminable. The motive for harming an animal doesn't necessarily have to be known in order to prosecute animal cruelty, but it may help to build a theory of what happened. Likewise, a motive for harming an animal deliberately may or may not be exonerative, if self-defense can be articulated, and the measures taken are reasonable (Figures 20.5–20.7). In this chapter, we explore various types of NAI, leaving animal fighting, ASA and poisoning to separate chapters.

Blunt Trauma

Animal Evidence of BFT

The hallmarks of blunt trauma to animals can easily be remembered by the acronym CALF, which stands for Contusions, Abrasions, Lacerations and Fractures. Blunt trauma may be inflicted on an animal by an object striking the animal, either swung or thrown. Stomping and kicking injuries also inflict blunt trauma. If the animal is small enough and/or the perpetrator

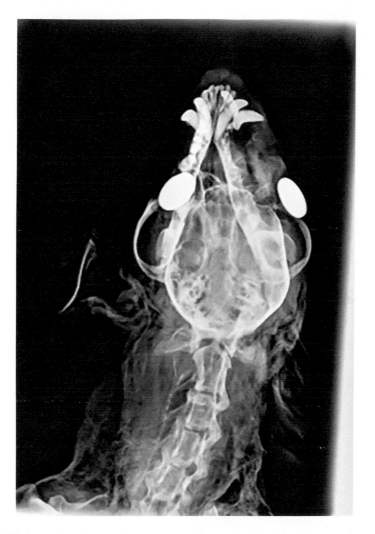

Figure 20.4 Under the masking tape, a large erosive abscess was found, and dimes had been inserted in the dog's eye sockets, under the eyelids after death, first noted on radiographs. This dog died of natural causes, but the abscess would have been painful, and the dog was emaciated, so it was consistent with neglect. In the cases illustrated in Figures 20.2–20.4, the dogs were unknown (considered to be examples of "Dog Doe"), and no suspect was found. The circumstances of keeping items of comfort with the dog on the shore and the ritual with the dog at the cemetery are consistent with funereal abandonment.

strong enough, the animal may be thrown or swung onto the floor, a wall or other fixed objects. Falls from a significant height ("high-rise syndrome") and being struck by a moving vehicle are examples of accidental blunt trauma (Figures 20.8 and 20.9).

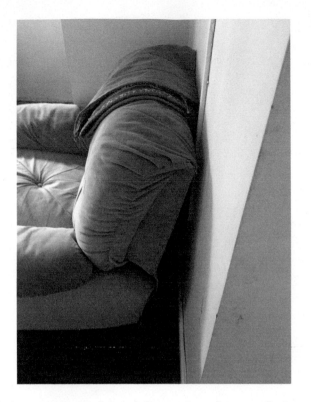

Figure 20.5 A perpetrator claimed frustration after a toileting accident and claimed to kick a recliner that accidentally crushed the puppy against the wall. The recliner cannot make contact with the wall at the close-to-floor level of a chihuahua puppy. There were significant blood stains in the middle of the room with no blood trail from the area of the chair. (Courtesy of ACO Jason Costa.)

In general, contusions are not easily visualized on animals as they may be obscured by fur and pigmentation. In many species, the skin is thicker than that of people, and so a contusion may only be visualized on the reflected (peeled back) inner surface of the skin in the deceased patient.

When blunt trauma is suspected, the patient should be photographed before and after shaving (Figures 20.10 and 20.11). A veterinarian's exam should include whole-body radiographs and palpation of the head and body for symmetry. Soft tissue swellings may be present that are consistent with bruising; these may not photograph well but can sometimes be documented in radiographs. Sometimes, the outline of an object used to strike an animal may be visible. This type of injury is referred to as a patterned injury. Patterned injuries may be abrasions, welts or contusions in the shape or contours of the surface of the object that impacted the animal.

A linear object used to strike an animal, such as a bat or stick, may leave a pattern injury described as "train tracks". These parallel lines represent

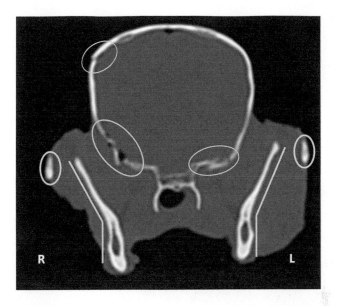

Figure 20.6 A "slice" view of a CT scan. The blue circles demonstrate the intact cheek bones, the green lines parallel the intact jaw bones and the yellow ovals circle skull fractures. Had the puppy's head been crushed between two hard surfaces, the outermost bones of the head, the cheekbones, would have been crushed.

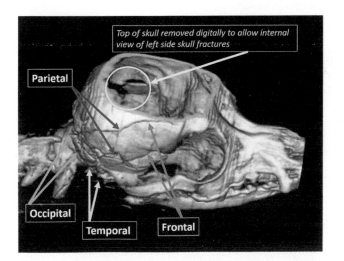

Figure 20.7 The 3D image of the skull further illustrates the skull fractures which are consistent with manual crushing. Manual crushing is squeezing the puppy's head with a hand; this form of nonaccidental trauma left the cheekbones still intact. Lower fractures on the skull are consistent with indenting from fingertips, and there is shattering of the back of the skull where it meets the cervical vertebrae. This death may have been the result of a failed attempted neck wringing.

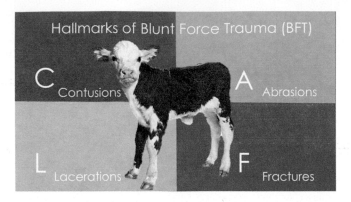

Figure 20.8 Hallmarks of blunt force trauma are contusions, abrasions, lacerations and fractures, CALF.

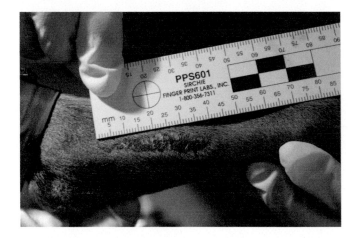

Figure 20.9 An abrasion is a partial thickness rubbing or wearing away of the skin.

broken blood vessels, and the blanched middle between the parallel lines represents where the object struck the animal. The action of impacting the animal with a linear object forces the blood out of the area of greatest impact to the skin to either side. The sudden increase in volume of blood to the capillary beds results in the parallel linear bruises (see Figure 19.17).

The force from an object striking an animal may travel through soft tissues, causing solid organs (such as the liver) to fracture, resulting in internal abdominal bleeding (Figure 20.12). When an animal is struck over a bony surface, the force does not dissipate as easily, and the skin splits or tears over the hard surface. This tearing type of skin defect is referred to as a laceration (Figure 20.13).

At times, lacerations can be difficult to differentiate from sharp force, or incised wounds (cuts). One hallmark of a laceration is a "tissue bridge", a tiny strand or strands of tissue which traverse the skin defect. This occurs when the

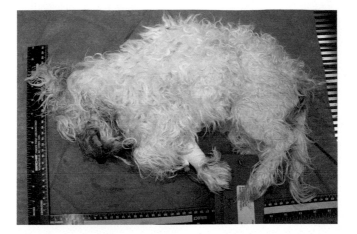

Figure 20.10 The body of a dog that suffered multiple blunt force trauma, before shaving.

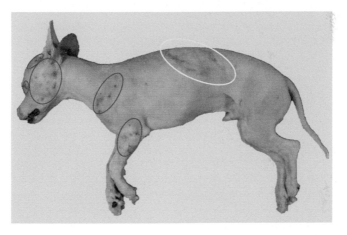

Figure 20.11 The same dog, after shaving. A patterned injury can be seen over the dog's back where he had been whipped by a looped extension cord.

skin tears, but the force is not strong enough to also tear nerves, blood vessels or strands of muscle tissue. Tissue bridges may also persist across crush injuries, such as across a bite wound that at first inspection appears to be a true puncture.

When an animal is kicked hard in the chest, the ribs may break. This breakage is generally at the middle of the rib and only affects one or two ribs (Figure 20.14). When animals suffer broken ribs because they are hit by a car, the rib fractures tend to be high on the rib, near where they attach to the spine (at the "insertion"). This is because the broad and sudden lateral force abruptly pushes one side of the ribcage in, and the forces snap the ribs where the resistance is greatest. Additionally, when animals suffer broken ribs from an accident, the fractures are generally only on one side of the chest. Animals that have been battered (repeatedly struck) may have broken ribs on both sides of the chest (Figure 20.15).

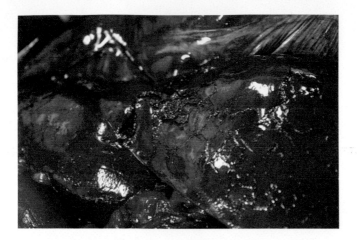

Figure 20.12 Multiple blunt trauma to the abdomen caused liver fractures and internal bleeding.

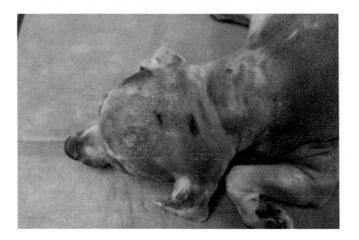

Figure 20.13 Multiple blunt trauma to the head caused skull fractures and lacerations.

Blows to the chest can also cause collapsed lungs, bruising to the lungs, torn blood vessels within the chest or tears to the muscles between the ribs (the "intercostal" muscles). These injuries can cause difficulty breathing, which is a struggling sensation. Cats (and less commonly dogs) will sometimes develop subcutaneous emphysema, or air trapped under the skin, due to blunt trauma to the chest that causes tears in the trachea (windpipe) or the bronchi. Animals with this condition may feel like crisped rice cereal when touched ("crepitus") (Figure 20.16).

Different forces to the bone will result in different types of bone fractures. A twisting force (sometimes seen in swinging injuries) will cause a long spiral fracture. Compression injuries will cause crush fractures. Pulling injuries can cause avulsions. It is appropriate for an investigator to inquire of

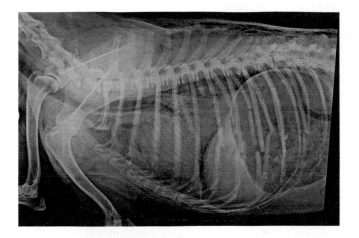

Figure 20.14 Multiple rib fractures.

the veterinarian or radiologist about what type of forces could be responsible for a particular fracture type. This type of inquiry may help to orient the veterinarian to the investigation in a thoughtful way.

Animal Experience of BFT

Blunt trauma causes pain. Blunt trauma that causes fractures or deep contusions causes severe and lasting pain. Intensity of pain felt is correlated with the intensity of force applied. Repeated blunt trauma causes pain and anxiety related to the anticipation of further blows. An animal that is restrained so that blows may be inflicted also experience frustration over the inability to escape the violence. Blunt trauma that causes significant internal bleeding may cause a sensation of weakness, and blunt trauma that causes the lungs to collapse causes the additional suffering of dyspnea (a sensation of "breathlessness" or "air hunger" with difficulty breathing).

Potential Scene Evidence of BFT

Blunt force trauma may be inflicted with an instrument such as a baseball bat or golf club. Items such as this may bear DNA of the victim at the end that impacted the animal, and of the perpetrator at the grip end. Blunt force trauma may cause cast blood or saliva spatter. Animals thrown against the wall may leave adhered strands of fur, footprints or imprints of the portion of their body that strikes the surface. Animals thrown into other objects (such as a window) may break the object and leave blood evidence with the broken items. If these items are too large to collect, they may be swabbed for species detection and individual profile generation. Some scenes of BFT may be in disarray due to the melee that preceded or was part of the violence. There may be tracking of kitty litter, feces, urine, saliva or blood droplets, or other evidence of a track or trail of activity.

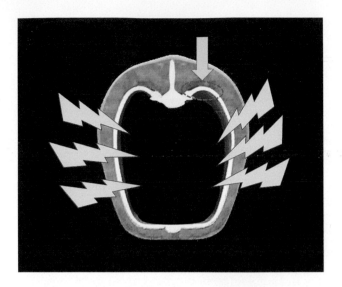

Figure 20.15 This is a "bread loaf slice" or "transverse" view of a dog's chest. Broken ribs from a hit by car accident tend to be up high and one-sided, in the area of the green arrow and oval. Nonaccidental rib fractures tend to be along the length of the ribs, on the side of the chest. If multiple fractures, they are likely to be at different levels and may be on both sides of the animal, as indicated by the "lightning bolt" shapes.

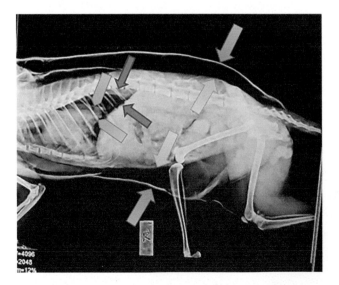

Figure 20.16 Radiograph of a cat shows significant amounts of air trapped under the skin (orange arrows show the skin of the cat; the black area under the skin is trapped air) and collapsed lungs. The dark blue arrows indicate where the lung tissue should expand to, in normal circumstances. The light blue arrows indicate the visible borders of the collapsed lung tissue.

Sharp Trauma

Animal Evidence of SFT

Nonaccidental sharp trauma includes incised wounds caused by edged instruments resulting in stab wounds, incised wounds or chop wounds. Stab wounds are deeper than they are long. Incised wounds (cuts) are longer than they are deep. Chop wounds are the result of a combination of blunt and sharp force. Edged instruments include knives, razors, scissors, machetes and crossbow arrowheads.

Accidental or natural causes of sharp injury include animal interactions or predation resulting in bite wounds, scratches or goring injuries. Animals may accidentally impact broken boards or wires in their environments that cause injuries that mimic stab, incised or chop injuries. Discerning whether an injury is accidental or nonaccidental requires consideration of the placement of the wound, the nature of the wound and correlation with a reported history and other circumstantial information. Animals becoming injured in dangerously cluttered environments may fall outside the reasonable definition of "accident" because the injury was predictable and preventable.

Nonaccidental sharp trauma to an awake animal is painful and may result in complex shaped wounds due to the coursing of the instrument and movements of the animal. The size and shape of the instrument and the thickness and elasticity of the skin also influence the resulting shape and size of injury. Simple wounds are linear or crescent-shaped, affecting the skin and superficial soft tissues. Complex wounds result from dynamic interaction. They are generally deeper, may impact internal organs or bones, and may have an "M", "X", "Y" or "L" shape, reflecting movement of either the instrument, the animal or both. In accidental circumstances, animals may create a complex wound struggling against a fixed object or with other animals (Figures 20.17 and 20.18).

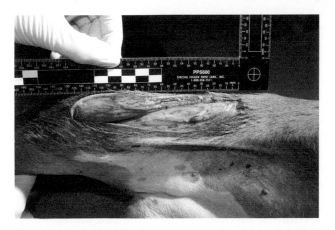

Figure 20.17 Long incised wound.

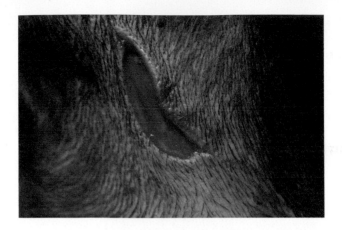

Figure 20.18 "Three-corner" wounds may be made by the blade moving, the animal moving or both.

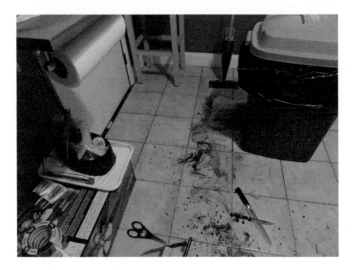

Figure 20.19 A scene of a violent killing of a dog by multiple sharp trauma featuring scattered sharp instruments, blood spatter, cast and swipe marks.

At the scene of a sharp force injury, there may be obvious or occult blood evidence, as well as evidence of a struggle, with swipe marks in the blood from the animal's body, paws or tail. There may be obvious or hidden edged instruments that may bear the DNA of the injured animal and possibly the perpetrator too (Figure 20.19).

The injured animal is also evidence, and the wounds should be carefully measured, described and documented. The sides of the wounds are known as "margins", and the ends of the wounds are "angles". If the animal is deceased, a forensic necropsy can describe the depth of the wounds, the wound tract and impacted organs.

In the live sedated or anesthetized animal, a wound exploration by the veterinarian should be documented in the medical record, and if possible photographed before and after shaving. The wounds should be measured and documented using anatomical reference points and sketched on an appropriate body diagram (See Appendix C for example forms). Due to the elasticity of the skin, the measurements of a wound may not correlate perfectly to a particular instrument.

When there are multiple wounds to a single animal, it is helpful to designate each wound with a letter or number, and the reference number may be written directly on the shaved animal with a permanent marker for demonstration purposes in the photographs (Figures 20.19–20.21).

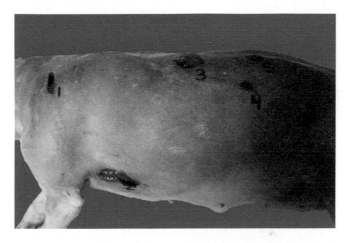

Figure 20.20 Annotated stab wounds on the from the scene in Figure 20.19. Wound #2 has herniated lung tissue.

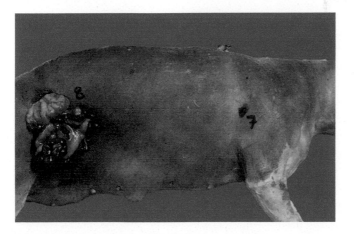

Figure 20.21 Wound #8 has herniated intestines. The presence of stab wounds on three sides of the animal and bruising consistent with grab marks are a testament to the intentionality, intensity and duration of the attack.

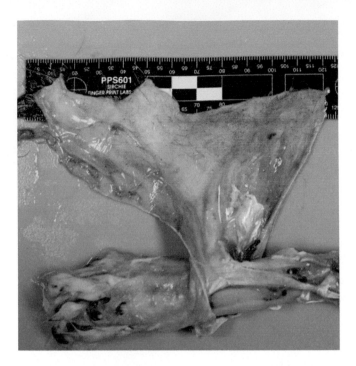

Figure 20.22 Scalloped skin edges of a cat limb left behind after coyote predation.

It is important to know that predators (e.g., birds of prey, foxes, coyotes) inflict injuries that can very closely mimic nonaccidental sharp force trauma. Predators may leave body parts behind with sharply demarcated, often "scalloped" skin edges. The fur or skin of such body parts can be carefully examined for dried saliva marks and DNA evidence (Figure 20.22).

Burns

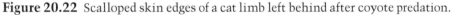

A burn is an injury resulting from exposure to heat, caustic chemicals, electricity or some forms of radiation. The degree of injury is dependent upon factors such as intensity of the injury process, distance from the heat source and duration of exposure or contact. There may be varying degrees of fur, feather and skin destruction. A heat source involving flames is said to be "incendiary".

Heat can transfer from a source to another object or a victim by convection, conduction or radiation. Convection is heat transfer between a surface and adjacent gas (including air) or fluid. Conduction is the direct flow of heat through a material resulting from physical contact. Radiation requires no transfer medium; it is the transfer of thermal energy through space by electromagnetic waves.

Burns can be accidental, such as a puppy chewing on an electrical cord, spilled hot drinks or accidentally spraying an animal from a hose that has been lying in the hot sun. Nonaccidental burn injuries may be inflicted while an animal is restrained, and negligent injury such as solar burns may occur when animals are not provided adequate shelter.

Animal Evidence of Burns

When a deceased animal is discovered with evidence of burn injury, it is vital to establish if the animal was dead or alive at the time of burning. This may be accomplished with a full postmortem exam. Animals that are fully charred externally may be relatively unscathed internally, and a cause of death may be established based on gross and microscopic analysis of the internal organs. The examination of a burn margin under the microscope (histology) may also elucidate vital (during life) versus postmortem changes.

Animals alive in a fire scene will inhale smoke, and particulate matter (soot) may be found in the airways or the stomach at postmortem exam. Superheated gases may also cause burns to the respiratory tissues. Animals that were deceased before the fire activity may have preserved undamaged tissues in the axillae (armpits), under the neck or at other skin folds (Figure 20.23).

Scalds are burns caused by hot liquid exposure. Akin to intentional scalding of children, animals may be held in hot water ("dunked"). These injuries will be uniform and well demarcated between injured and noninjured tissues. Accidental scalds will have irregular margins due to the movement of the animal and the splashing fluid.

Small animals may be burned in conventional or microwave ovens. Animals burned in conventional ovens may have burns to foot pads and broken nails from struggling to escape and heat injury to airways. Microwave ovens cause burning to tissues at different layered levels, with some tissues burned internally with spared tissue externally.

Electrocution injuries involve contact with a source of electricity such as exposed wires, tasers, jumper cables, lightening or stray voltage (electricity traveling from an electrical source through damp ground or equipment). Accidental electrocution from chewing on an electrical cord may cause burns at the back corners of the mouth (the "commissures"), the roof of the mouth or the tongue. There may be other points of trauma where the electrical current exits the body (Figure 20.24).

In cases of burns, animals should be photographed before and after shaving, and for surviving animals, monitored during the recovery process as the tissue trauma may become more evident with the passage of time, before

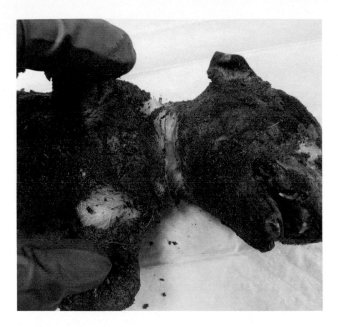

Figure 20.23 A puppy found in a fire pit at a beach. Internal exam was consistent with natural disease. External exam shows unburned fur in the neck fold and axillae (armpits) – areas that would have been exposed to combustion if the puppy was awake and moving.

healing. Injuries should also be measured, described in shape and relation to anatomical landmarks and sketched on body diagrams.

Adverse reactions to vaccines or medications, snake or insect bites and some disease processes may trigger dermal reactions that closely mimic the appearance of burns. In such cases, biopsy samples will assist in the differentiation between natural disease and burns. Biopsies should be taken from healthy tissue, at the margin of the defect and from within the defect (Figure 20.25).

Potential Scene Evidence of Nonaccidental Burn Injuries

Many state agencies and fire departments have designated and specially trained arson investigators. It may be appropriate to consult with them before examining a scene where an animal or animals have been subject to incendiary trauma, or other types of burn injury.

Devices to ignite a fire, such as matches, or lighters may be present. If accelerant dowsing is suspected, samples of fur near the burned area should be plucked and preserved in a new, airtight container such as an unused, unlined paint can, which can be purchased from a hardware store. Avoid the use of shaving or cutting instruments that have been lubricated with

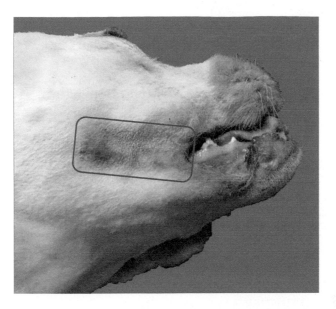

Figure 20.24 Burns at the corners of the mouth of a puppy, caused by the puppy chewing on a live extension cord.

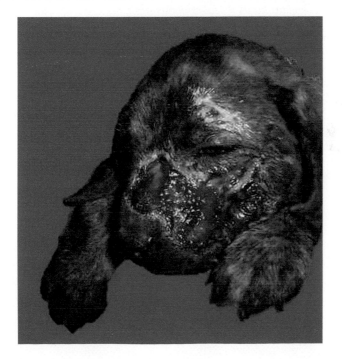

Figure 20.25 A large ulcerative erosive lesion developed on this puppy's face, secondary to a severe case of juvenile cellulitis ("puppy strangles"), a naturally occurring disease condition not to be confused with nonaccidental trauma. (Photo courtesy of Mark Vespucci.)

petroleum-based products or other chemicals as these may alter the evidence. Comparison samples of fur should also be submitted from an unaffected area.

When accelerants or caustic chemicals are used, original or secondary containers may be found at the scene, as well as liquid residue. Accelerants may not be completely consumed by fire, as it is the volatile gas that burns, not the liquid itself. If there is sufficient liquid present, this may be absorbed with a sterile cotton ball or gauze pad and sealed in a can to be analyzed at the forensic laboratory.

Bodies are not easily destroyed by fire, even those of small animals. In order to reduce a human body to ash, it must be burned at 1800–2000°F for several hours. Even then, bone fragments and teeth will be left behind. Smaller animals will be consumed faster, but often, significant physical evidence will remain at a fire scene, even when directly doused with accelerant.

In nonaccidental electrocution cases, there may be extension cords altered with bare wires or clips attached, car batteries or other modified apparatus to allow the application of electricity directly to an animal, to a pool of water or to a metal conduction surface.

Metallic items, heated and applied to animals in branding injuries may retain tissue fragments or fur on the injuring end, and the DNA of the perpetrator on the handled end. Metallic deposits may be seen on the surface of both thermal contact burn and electrocution lesions, termed "thermal metallization". Healed skin may have scar formation or white hairs in the shape of the burn.

Projectile Injury

Animal Evidence of Projectile Injury

Projectile injuries may be caused by firearms (explosive or gas powered), arrows (fixed and compound), darts or less commonly by a machinery accident (e.g., a lawn mower throwing debris). Firearms may inflict injury with metallic projectiles (bullets, pellets, shot) or "nonlethal" projectiles (paintballs, gel pellets, bean bags) that cause serious injury or death to animals.

A projectile injury may be penetrating or perforating. Penetrating injuries enter the animal, the projectile creates an entry wound and is retained in the body; perforating injuries are through-and-through, with both an entry and an exit wound. Animals may have multiple projectile injuries with a combination of penetrating and perforating injuries.

An odd number of wounds is suggestive of one or more penetrating injuries with a retained projectile. Full body radiographs can help discern wound tracts and projectiles. Even in perforating injuries, there may be a "comet tail" pattern of metallic dust from bullet fragments seen in radiographs (Figures 20.26 and 20.27).

Projectile injuries may be difficult to locate, particularly if there is a lack of external bleeding. The best approach in evaluating an animal with suspected projectile injury is to first perform full body radiographs to highlight the projectile (if present) and wound tract, followed by close inspection for wounds with the information from the radiographs for orientation.

All wounds should be photographed, measured and documented using anatomical reference points and sketched on an appropriate body diagram. It can be difficult to differentiate entry wounds from exit wounds, but in general, the entry wound is smaller than the exit wound. The entry wound is usually sharply marginated and may have a burned or abraded margin of skin (collar). When asymmetrical, the collar helps to indicate the direction of the projectile's approach. A single projectile may cause both perforating and penetrating injuries if it first passes through a body part and then re-enters the animal. In such cases, the second entry wound may lack some of the distinct collaring and hot gas-related trauma seen in the initial entry wound (Figure 20.28).

Contact wounds, or close wounds, may have singed fur or soot in the fur, or they may leave a muzzle imprint. Fur should be collected and preserved from the wound margin before shaving the wound. This fur may be examined at the laboratory for the presence of gunpowder which may be typed and matched to a source. Fur may be carried into the wound upon entry, and hairs may be cut by the projectile at the exit wound. The exit wound tends to be more irregular in shape, may be stellate (star shaped) and may have eversion (turning out) of tissue; however, it is important to note that some contact shots over bony surfaces can cause stellate entry wounds.

Firearm projectiles cause trauma along the wound tract from the projectile itself, from the heated gases and shock waves that travel with the bullet that create a temporary cavity (the bullet itself causes a permanent cavity by destroying tissues in its path). Both the bullet and cavitation can cause significant organ trauma. A veterinarian can carefully probe projectile tracts to help determine trajectory, and trajectory rods or pins may be used to better illustrate the projectile pathway in photographs and radiographs. Trajectory determinations are especially important in claims of self- defense and use of force investigations. The scatter or spread of shotgun pellets may refute or support a claim of a certain distance when the weapon was fired (Figures 20.29 and 20.30).

Postmortem or surgical projectile recovery should be performed with gloved fingers or plastic instruments in order to avoid marring any identifying marks that may be present on the projectile.

Once collected, projectile fragments collected from an animal may be rinsed under running water without scrubbing. Different protocols exist as to whether the bullet should be rinsed (but never scrubbed) or submitted "as is", without rinsing. The investigator should determine a protocol based on

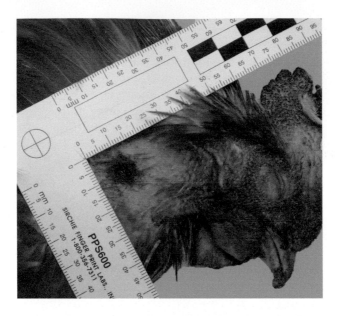

Figure 20.26 An air pellet was shot through a rooster's neck, leaving entry and exit wounds.

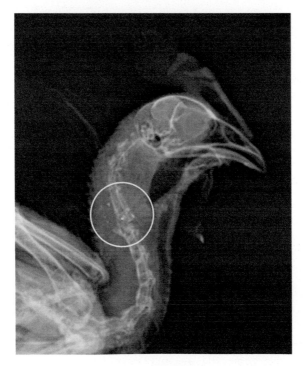

Figure 20.27 Metallic debris and a broken 5th cervical vertebra can be seen on the radiograph. This injury caused a slow death (as compared to a high cervical dislocation) because the injury was not high enough on the cervical spinal cord to cause immediate loss of consciousness.

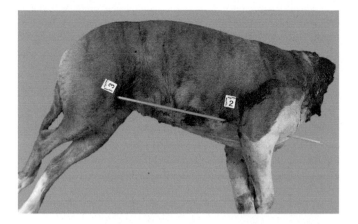

Figure 20.28 A dog was killed by a gunshot wound by a police officer, claimed to be in self-defense. The head was removed prior to necropsy for a "head test", to determine if the dog was rabid. The necropsy revealed two entry wounds and one exit wound, with a projectile retained in the body. The positions of the wounds were consistent with the officer's report that the dog was facing and may have been moving toward the officer when he shot. The report for this case contained the following statement: "Nothing in the exam is inconsistent with the officer's description of events. The actions of the shooting officer were ostensibly, in the moment they were taken, an application of force by an officer who apparently had a fear of an imminent threat of serious bodily harm or threat to his life. Whether this fear was reasonable is not within our purview to determine. However, since 1936, no officer has been killed in the line of duty by a canine attack. The documented canine-related death of an officer in 1936 and four other dog-related deaths prior to the 1936 attack were caused by rabies infection, not mauling injuries. The totality of circumstances in this case suggests that the city should invest in appropriate training of animal control officers and police officers with regard to enforcement of negligent dog owner behaviors, response to reports of loose dogs and the practice of field euthanasia by gunshot".

the priorities of the local police and firearms examiner and convey this to the examining veterinarian. If rinsed, metallic fragments should be dry prior to packaging to reduce the risk of corrosion or rusting, as advised by the ballistics examiner. Air dry the bullets or blot them with a soft dry facial or toilet tissue. Once dry, the fragments should be wrapped in soft tissue paper and sealed in a labeled paper envelope or cardboard box. Sealing a damp bullet in an airtight package can cause corrosion of identifiable detail.

Potential Scene Evidence with Projectile Injuries

The location and condition of firearms and related evidence at a crime scene should be diagrammed and photographed before recovering and securing them. In some circumstances, it may be possible to determine the position of a shooter by the location of ejected cartridge casings. Scene sketching

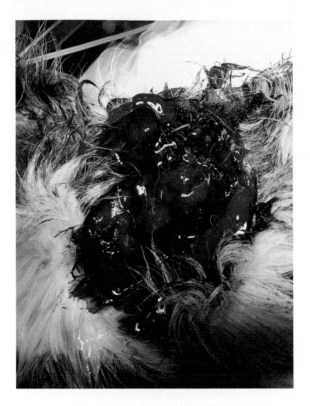

Figure 20.29 A photograph of a shotgun wound to the neck of a stray hunting breed dog, found near a hunting reserve. (Photograph courtesy of Dr. Elizabeth Rozanski, DVM, DACVIM, DACVECC.)

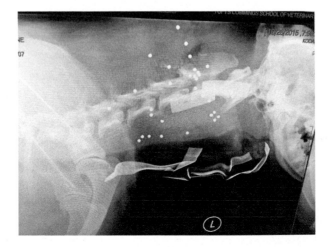

Figure 20.30 A radiograph of the same wound. Shotgun pellets and radio-opaque wound dressing strips can be seen. While the wound may have been accidental, the discharge of the firearm was not reported, and no one claimed the dog. The dog survived and was adopted. (Radiograph courtesy of Dr. Elizabeth Rozanski, DVM, DACVIM, DACVECC.)

should be performed with measurements of the location of fired cartridge cases. When a shotgun is fired, the wads travel along with, or behind, the shot charge for a short distance. In cases involving close shots, wadding may be found in the fur or wound of the animal. Package each item separately and mark the packages with the pertinent information.

Animals that are illegally hunted (poached) may be found discarded in the woods or on other public lands with trophy body parts removed such as head (for antlers) or pelt. Poached coyotes may be found with no head or pelt, and the finding party may report that they have found a skinned dog. While the remains are canid, foot pad arrangement, and if present, skull shape differences can help determine coyote vs. domestic dog. Stomach contents of a coyote will likely contain fur or bones from rabbits or other small prey. Genetic analysis may also be performed to confirm species identification (Figure 20.31). Poaching is generally an illegal activity, and there may be charges related to leaving a carcass behind.

Asphyxia

Asphyxia is the deprivation of oxygen. This may result in brain injury or death. Additionally, strangulating forms of asphyxia may also cause broken blood vessels in the eyes or other mucous membranes due to increased blood pressure to the head. There are both accidental and nonaccidental causes of

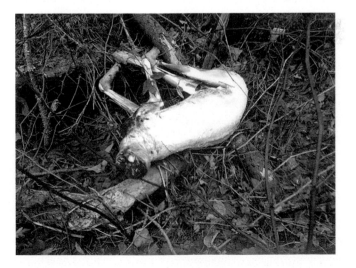

Figure 20.31 A typical poaching carcass found discarded in the woods. (Photo courtesy of Massachusetts Department of Conservation & Recreation Lt. M. O'Bannon.)

asphyxia. Asphyxia may be caused by drowning, strangulation, positional restriction, inert gas inhalation or smothering.

Drowning

Drowning is the process of experiencing respiratory impairment from submersion (the body is completely under water) or immersion (the body is partially covered by water, and the airway is affected) in water or another liquid. Drowning may result in death, or injury. In some cases, animals may experience the trauma of attempted, or "near drowning" that causes significant suffering during the event, with or without long-term harm depending on the duration of hypoxia and possible tissue damage.

Animal Evidence of Drowning

When a body is found submerged or immersed, the big question to answer is whether the animal was alive when they entered the water. Animals found dead in water may have drowned accidentally, deliberately or they may have been disposed of in a body of water after death. Scavengers and postmortem changes due to immersion can cloud the picture. As in people, the diagnosis of drowning in animals is usually one of exclusion, made after considering all scene findings, witness accounts and an examination of the body to rule out other causes of death.

Accidental causes of drowning may include epilepsy, ataxia (stumbling or staggering due to a medical condition), accidental electrocution or other trauma causing an animal to fall into the water, entrapment or entanglement. Some species of animals, such as opossums, cannot swim. Animals may fall through thin ice. Drowning may follow exhaustion or hypothermia as the animal fails in a prolonged attempt to stay afloat.

Since many animals are small enough to be easily moved after death, some bodies found at dry locations may be victims of drowning. A wet body enclosed within a secured plastic bag must raise the index of suspicion for drowning. A body disposed of in the open air may be dry on the upper surface and wet on the dependent (down) side. The fur may dry in clumps, or points, consistent with having been wet without the animal shaking or grooming out the fur (Figures 20.32 and 20.33).

Animals that have been forcibly held under water, particularly in a domestic setting (sink, toilet, tub), may have bruising found under the skin, over the bony prominences such as the tops of the spine bones, the scapular spine and the shoulders. There may be oval-shaped fingertip bruises. Animals that have been drowned within a cage may have injuries to the lips, teeth, paws or claws from struggling against the enclosure.

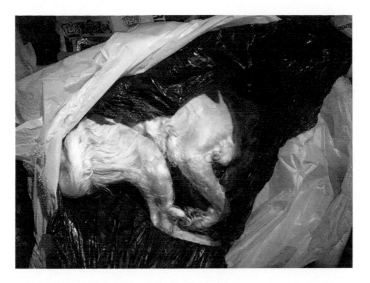

Figure 20.32 A wet dog found in a dumpster in a sealed plastic bag. The dog also had bruises over bony prominences, consistent with being forcibly struck or pinned against a hard surface. A bathroom in the residence where the dog had lived was described as being in disarray with water all over the floor. (Photo courtesy of ACO Darleen Wood)

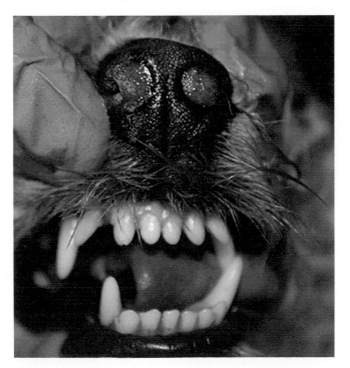

Figure 20.33 The dog also had red-tinged foam in her airway, a finding consisten with asphyxia.

Wildlife may be drowned in traps because they are perceived to be "nuisance animals" and unwanted puppies or kittens may be drowned as a method of disposal, often enclosed in a cloth sack or pillowcase tied shut and containing rocks, bricks or other heavy object used to weigh the bag down. While some people believe drowning to be free from suffering, this is not true. According to the American Veterinary Medical Association, drowning is not an acceptable means of euthanasia and is inhumane.

Drowning dogs struggle violently for the first minute and a half of drowning, and deep inspiratory gasping can last for more than 3 minutes in a conscious animal. Water may enter the lungs, or it may be prevented from entering the lungs due to spasms of the larynx; this may be referred to as "dry drowning". Water may be swallowed during the drowning event, followed by violent vomiting. Death generally occurs within 5 to 10 minutes of submersion or immersion drowning.

Potential Scene Evidence of Drowning

Scene findings of deliberate drowning events may include a vessel large enough to be filled with water and submerse an animal in a cage. There may be signs of a struggle, with water spilled in an area or injuries to the person causing the drowning event. There may be animal hairs or tissue inside of a trap or bag that can be matched to an individual using DNA techniques. The fur of an animal drowned in a body of water and moved to another scene may have sand or other trace evidence associated with the drowning event in their fur.

Strangulation and Wringing Injury

Manual strangulation ("throttling") is asphyxia using hands on the neck, and ligature strangulation is asphyxia using a rope, wire or cord. Strangulation causes decreased oxygen delivery to the brain by compression of cervical blood vessels or tracheal occlusion. The term "choking" is used colloquially to describe manual strangulation, but this is inaccurate – choking is internal obstruction of the airway, usually by a foreign object.

With strangulation, there may be broken blood vessels in the whites of the eyes, the pink tissues of the eyes or mouth, or there may be no external evidence of strangulation. Animals that are hanged and removed from the hanging position shortly after death may have no external signs of hanging. Animals that hang for a period of time after death may have congestion (increased presence of blood in the blood vessels) in the caudal half of the body, or the lower half when in a hanging position. This may be marked by increased redness seen in the caudal (lower) abdomen. The animal may have a deep groove around the high neck, under the jaw and behind the ears. Because of the strong nuchal ligament (the ligament from the back of the head to the spine) in quadrupeds, death by hanging is more difficult to accomplish in animals than it is in people. When hanged, dogs struggle against the hanging; they may cause abrasions to the occipital protuberance (bump on the back of the head) as they struggle against the taut rope. During hanging strangulation, animals may be able to protect their airway by arching their neck until they are exhausted. Dogs and cats also have abundant collateral circulation to the brain. For these reasons, loss of consciousness in animal hangings may take 15 minutes or more.

At necropsy, a careful dissection of the strap muscles of the neck and the back of the neck is important to detect signs of ligature strangulation. Bruising may be evident in the underside of the skin and the muscles underlying the ligature. Knots may be "signatures", unique to the person who tied them, so ligatures should be removed by cutting at a point away from knots, preserving the knots for further analysis. Ropes may retain the DNA of the perpetrator or embedded hairs from the victim animal.

Accidental strangulation hangings may happen when a dog is on a tether long enough to allow them to jump a fence or other barrier but not long enough to allow the dog to bear weight on the ground. Dogs improperly restrained and inadequately supervised at a grooming facility may die of strangulation hanging by jumping or falling off the grooming table. In those cases, the animal may have the forward noose around their neck but not the secondary restraint around the waist.

Wringing is the breaking of the neck by grasping the head in one hand and the body in another and twisting. Wringing is a method of poultry slaughter that is used on small farms, and done expertly, it can avoid suffering. Unfortunately, there is usually a learning curve for this method, and the initial birds killed this way may suffer terribly. Some perpetrators of animal cruelty will inappropriately attempt wringing other species such as small dogs, puppies, cats, kittens or rabbits. These events can cause pain and suffering as death is generally not achieved swiftly. In order to be effective, the wringing injury must be high on the cervical spine and rapid.

Smothering, Gagging, Inert Gas, and Positional Asphyxia

Smothering is blocking the external upper airway (nose and mouth) to prevent adequate air exchange; this may be achieved manually or by using objects such as a pillow. Gagging is asphyxia caused by covering the face or placing of a foreign object in the mouth and restricting the muzzle from opening. Inert gas smothering occurs in oxygen-deprived environments where oxygen is replaced by other gases (e.g., methane, carbon dioxide, neon, nitrogen and helium). Toxic gas smothering is complicated by harmful gases in addition to lack of oxygen (e.g., carbon monoxide and hydrogen sulfide).

Animals confined in airtight spaces will exhaust the available oxygen and eventually smother, and this may also be exacerbated by increasing environmental temperatures and humidity. Positional asphyxia happens when an animal can't get enough air to breathe due to the positioning of their body. This happens most often when their chest may be unable to fully expand, from entrapment in a too-small space (Figure 20.34).

Animal Experience of Asphyxia

During asphyxiation, an animal will develop a sensation of a strong urge to breathe or a feeling of severe breathlessness. This sensation is also known as "air hunger", a primal phenomenon accompanied by anxiety, frustration, fear and panic. People who have survived asphyxia events report a painful burning sensation in the chest.

Dryer Injury

Animals can be hurt or killed accidentally or nonaccidentally in washing machines and dryers. In the case of both machines, tumbling may cause multiple blunt trauma especially in empty machines. Cats may crawl into a

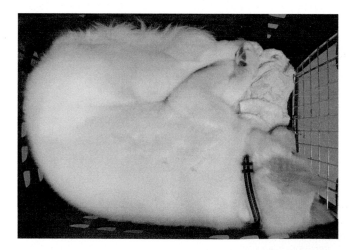

Figure 20.34 This dog became hypoxic and hyperthermic after struggling to sit in a hunched position overnight and was found in her too-small crate at a boarding facility by employees in the morning. It was claimed the dog simply "died in her sleep", but the necropsy revealed signs consistent with hypoxia and hyperthermia that entailed significant suffering. This is a view of the dog from the top of the crate with the crate top removed. Her body is simultaneously in firm contact with all four sides. The legs are in an unnatural position and the curve to her lower back is exaggerated.

dryer when the door has been left open, particularly when there is warm, dry laundry to nest in. Determining whether a laundry machine injury is accidental or nonaccidental depends on careful interviewing and understanding of circumstantial evidence.

Animals may have broken teeth, facial trauma and crush injuries to the dorsal spinous processes (the bones that can be felt on the midline on the top of the animal), whip injuries to the tip of the tail and nail or foot pad trauma. Cloth material, if present, may cause smothering. Washing machines may cause drowning, and dryers can cause asphyxiation and airway burns due to dry heat or steam injury.

Potential Scene Evidence of Washer or Dryer Injury

The lint filters may have excessive fur in the trap. There may be blood, urine or feces within the barrel of the machine.

Bibliography

Wohlsein P, Peters M, Schulze C, Baumgärtner W. Thermal injuries in veterinary forensic pathology. *Veterinary Pathology*. 2016;53(5):1001–1017.

Neglect and Hoarding 21

MARTHA SMITH-BLACKMORE

Fundamentals of Neglect

Animal neglect is the failure to provide adequate food, water or shelter from the weather (e.g., excessively hot or cold temperatures, precipitation and solar radiation), grooming and veterinary care to the extent that a reasonable and prudent animal caretaker should have known the animal needed. Typically, these cases involve passive maltreatment, meaning that it is a failure to act, rather an action that harms the animal.

Animal neglect, while having distinct legal definitions in different jurisdictions, can be thought of in general as any failure to provide an animal with appropriate sustenance for comfort and for life. These types of crimes are sometimes referred to as "crimes of omission". The animal cruelty laws of all states have provisions stipulating minimal care standards (e.g., food, shelter, veterinary care and sanitary conditions) for animals.

While neglect is a passive form of animal abuse, it must be acknowledged that the harms and trauma from neglect can be as painful and cause as much or more suffering compared to some forms of nonaccidental injury. Neglected animals may suffer from a variety of painful or suffering conditions due to starvation, morbid obesity, parasitism, dehydration, skin infections or wounds, ear and eye conditions, embedded collars or nails, overgrown hooves, severe dental disease, hypo- or hyperthermia, untreated injuries or infections, very large tumors or other painful or debilitating medical conditions.

Additionally, neglect may happen in the presence of adequate food, water and shelter. For instance, if the animals are crowded enough to be fighting with one another, if they are deprived of light 24 hours a day, or if they are kept in an environment where a lack of enrichment or interaction with other animals causes mental anguish, these may be criminal offenses. While a challenge to prove or prosecute, there are instances when it is appropriate to bring charges for neglect not related to food, water, shelter, veterinary or grooming care. It is helpful to such cases to have a veterinarian, or another suitable expert describe the suffering endured by the animals because of a failure to provide specific aspects of care. With regard to mental anguish, veterinarians often make behavioral diagnosis and prescribe psychoactive medications to

DOI: 10.4324/9781003090762-21

treat mental illnesses. Therefore, it is not a stretch to acknowledge mental suffering in animals as a condition that can be treated and alleviated. A failure to treat or alleviate a suffering emotional or mental condition can also be viewed as criminal neglect.

Compound conditions increase the misery of suffering. An animal that is cold, dehydrated, starving **and** in pain suffers considerably more than one that is cold, starving, dehydrated **or** in pain. When conditions are compounded, each aspect may be more debilitating and miserable than if it was endured singly (Figure 21.1).

Contributing causes or cited reasons for neglect by a responsible individual may include a lack of caring, ignorance, economic hardship, lack of awareness of available resources, mental illness or cognitive decline, cultural beliefs or practices, or greed. In cases of animal hoarding or greed-driven breeding, the numbers of animals (and potential squalor) on scene can be overwhelming. A lack of recognition of the neglect by the perpetrator is not exculpatory and intervening in a case of animal neglect may be the only effective pathway to stop or correct the animal maltreatment. A criminal process does not necessarily result in a criminal outcome. With the criminal process, a defendant may not necessarily be convicted of a crime, and yet there can be relief provided for the animals and potentially interventions provided for the humans in need as well.

A failure to prosecute based on an investigator's perception of the perpetrator's circumstances can contribute to future claims of *selective prosecution* on the part of defendants who are charged with similar crimes. In a claim

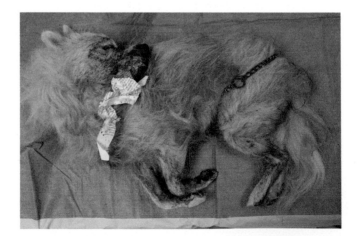

Figure 21.1 A deceased, emaciated dog was found entrapped in a closet of an object hoarding house. The dog had been heavily infested with fleas and was anemic. This anemia may have contributed to weakness and the inability of the dog to escape from the closet after stacks of debris tipped over and trapped the dog. The collar of the dog slipped to the level of the hips, reflecting the duration of weight loss and struggle.

of selective prosecution, a defendant argues that they should not be held criminally responsible for breaking the law, as the criminal justice system discriminated against them by choosing to prosecute, when they have failed to prosecute similar cases because of bias.

A Failure to Provide Care as Intentional Abuse

When "neglect" requires intentional action to perpetrate, it may indeed be legally defined as abuse rather than carelessness or negligence. This distinction may require an understanding and proof of the offender's *mens rea* (state of mind, or intent), and in some jurisdictions, the difference may be the dividing line between misdemeanor and felony. For example, a person who gathers animals and deliberately cages them without providing adequate food, water, sanitation and mental stimulation may in fact be committing a deliberate action to harm animals. In rare cases, some animals at a particular scene will be provided adequate care while others are denied basic needs. When animals are singled out and deliberately denied access to food and water, the act may be termed "starvation abuse" as opposed to neglect. A case of "neglect" on face value may also have elements that qualify for evaluation as torture (Figures 21.2 and 21.3).

Borderline Care

Investigators or veterinarians might encounter "borderline care" of animals. In these instances, it is appropriate to exercise the due diligence of educating the animal's caregiver as to standards of adequate care and allow them an opportunity to improve the animal's condition. Reasonable deadlines for improvement should be set, and expectations should be documented. If the caregiver then fails to show up for a recheck appointment, or if the animal is no better off at recheck, a criminal investigation may ensue. Once a perpetrator has been informed of appropriate care, ignorance cannot be used as a defense. That said, ignorance is not necessarily a legal defense in the first place.

Failure to Provide Adequate Food or Water

Animal Evidence of Starvation and Dehydration

Animals are deemed "starved" when they are in an emaciated poor body condition due to a prolonged negative energy balance. This may be due to a lack of accessible, nutritious or species-appropriate food. Animals may be starved in the presence of food, if the available food is spoiled, still sealed in packaging, in a feeder, trough or bowl the animal cannot reach, if the food is of no nutritional value to a particular species, or if there is insufficient feeding opportunity for less dominant animals (Figures 21.4–21.7).

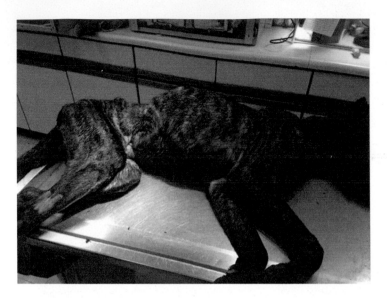

Figure 21.2 An emaciated dog was brought in near-death condition to a veterinarian's office where he latere died. A subsequent investigation found two other dogs in good condition in the home.

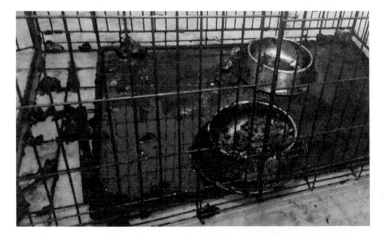

Figure 21.3 The filthy crate where the emaciated dog was kept. The fact that the other dogs were regularly brought to the veterinarian for routine preventive care, and care for illnesses supported the theory that this dog was deliberately neglected. This form of animal maltreatment may be referred to as "starvation abuse", a deliberate choice to abuse an animal through the withholding of nutrition.

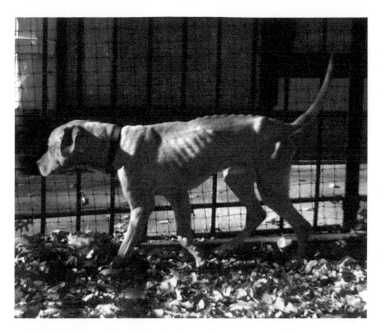

Figure 21.4 A young dog was starved in the presence of food because his companion Cocker Spaniel dog would attack him if he tried to eat any of the food that was provided to them. This dog was too thin, and the spaniel was obese.

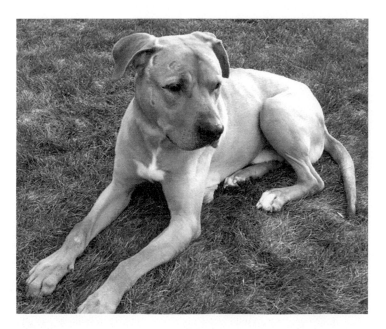

Figure 21.5 The young dog regained good body condition after being removed from that situation. He continued to bear scars fro the prior attacks by the food aggressive Cocker Spaniel. (Photo courtesy of Lauren Youngquist)

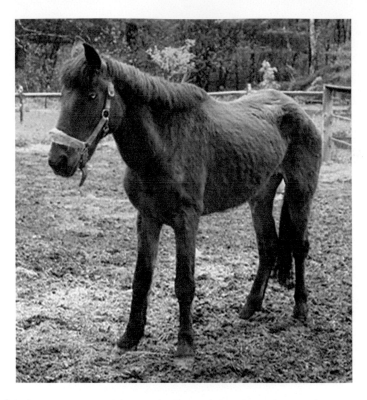

Figure 21.6 An emaciated horse that was fed only stale bread, iceberg lettuce and Oreo cookies, an insufficient diet for horses. (Figure 21.6 courtesy of ACO Hilary Cohen.)

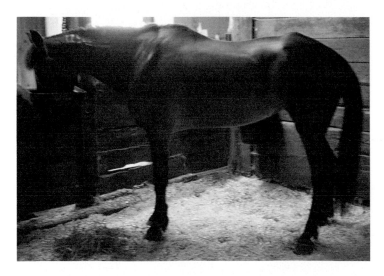

Figure 21.7 The horse showing an approved appearance a few months into feeding an appropriate diet. (Figure 21.7 courtesy of ACO Hilary Cohen.)

Starvation is a diagnosis of exclusion, meaning that there is no evidence of any other medical reason for the emaciation. A live animal can be deemed to have been starved if they subsequently respond to feeding an appropriate type and amount of food and regain a normal body condition without any other medical intervention. It is important to maintain records and photographs of the animals as they regain condition over time. This record can help to refute claims that an animal was in poor condition because it refused to eat or because it had cancer.

Starvation causes gastric pangs, which are painful. When starvation is of a longer duration, the abdomen itself starts to have painful contractions which occur with greater frequency and intensity over time. One way to help alleviate this pain is to put something – anything – into the stomach. Animals who are starving will ingest nonnutritive substances (non-food items) to achieve this goal. This activity is called pica. Pica is evidence that an animal had the desire to eat, and the ability to chew and swallow. If foreign matter is detected within the gastrointestinal tract or feces, that is evidence that the GI tract had normal motility, the ability to move ingested matter along the pathway of digestion. If the animal has demonstrated pica, the veterinarian should note this in the report because it indicates that the animal had an interest in eating, thus reducing the likelihood that inappetence from disease led to emaciation. Feces found on scene with large amounts of foreign material in them are evidence of pica from starvation (Figures 21.8 and 21.9).

For animals previously kept as pets, it must be acknowledged that there is emotional suffering related to the isolation of abandonment. Animals

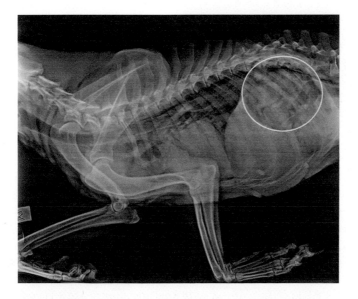

Figure 21.8 A radiograph of an emaciated dog shows a collection of foreign material in the stomach.

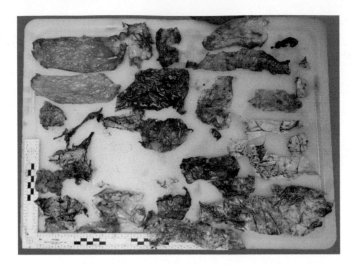

Figure 21.9 At necropsy, the matter seen in the stomach in the radiograph in Figure 21.8 was found to be paper and plastic.

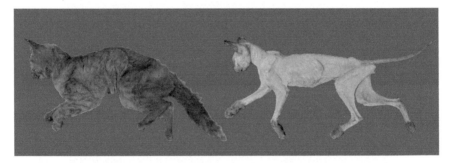

Figure 21.10 A starved cat before and after shaving. The contours of the emaciation are more obvious in the shaved animal. Photographs of the shaved starved animal often better document the condition for future testimony in court, where the "finders of fact" (judge or jury) will not have opportunity to touch the animal.

enclosed in spaces without access to food may pace or dig or chew at corners, walls, window frames or doorways out of frustration, hunger or in an attempt to escape, leaving claw or chew marks from their efforts. Animals in late-stage starvation will be too weak to stand or reposition themselves, and the skin may be more vulnerable to trauma. These animals may suffer from pressure sores over bony prominences, urine scald or flystrike with maggot activity (Figures 21.10–21.12).

For animals that were once in a normal body condition and are starved *absolutely* (meaning no food is available whatsoever) but who have water available, it takes weeks to succumb to starvation, generally 3 to 5 weeks. If no water is available, the animal will more likely die of dehydration within days, before it can starve to death and before the body shows significant signs

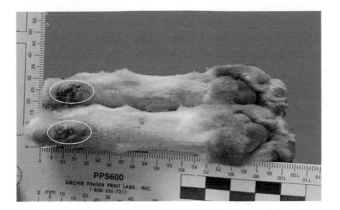

Figure 21.11 This cat had pressure sores on her hocks (heels), which is a common finding in the starved cat, indicating long periods of time spent in a hunched position. The lack of protein in the starved animal weakens tissues and the immune system, making them more vulnerable to tissue breakdown, infections and other complications. A starved animal may have ulcerations (similar to "bed sores") over bony prominences on one side of the body, suggesting that they were too weak or debilitated to stand up or change positions.

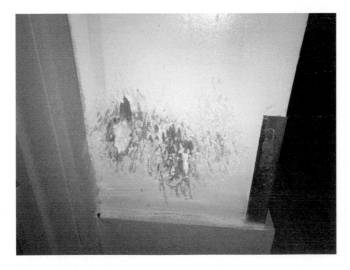

Figure 21.12 The plaster walls in an apartment where a dog had been abandoned without food bear marks of the dog's desperate actions. (Photo courtesy of T. J. O'Connor Animal Control Officer Tracy Rondinello.)

of starvation. Obese cats that are suddenly denied access to food may develop hepatic lipidosis, an acute condition of liver failure. Cats with advanced hepatic lipidosis will have a distinct yellow tinge to the sclera (the whites of the eyes) and mucous membranes (gums and other ordinarily pink tissues). These are common findings in animals left behind, enclosed in a house or apartment after an eviction, foreclosure or abandonment.

Animals that have access to intermittent food, inappropriate or poor-quality food, may maintain an emaciated body condition for a protracted period of months or even years. This level of poor or insufficient nutrition may lead to an eventual death from starvation or may weaken the animal to the point that they die from parasitism or an infection that they might have otherwise been able to withstand.

It is important to note and record at such scenes whether there is any available water, including in the toilet bowl. Note if the toilet lid is up or down, whether water is present in the bowl and whether an animal would have access to that water. A short dog may not be able to reach toilet water, but a cat could presumably jump up to the rim or seat to drink out of the bowl. We know from the human condition that dehydration causes headaches and muscle cramps, and additionally, dehydrated animals are more susceptible to hyperthermia.

Animals discovered at scenes without access to clean water should be videotaped when water is offered for the first time. A prolonged drinking of water recorded visually can be very impactful in court.

Caution should be taken when offering food, however. Some species of animals are vulnerable to "refeeding syndrome", a life-threatening condition that occurs when a starved animal is offered food that is excessive or too rich for them initially, due to damage to the intestines during starvation. Emaciated animals, especially ones known to have been starved absolutely should be re-fed carefully under the direction of a veterinarian. Starved animals that have had intermittent access to food, or access to poor-quality nutrition, are less vulnerable to refeeding syndrome.

A veterinarian can also perform clinical laboratory tests to help determine if an animal is suffering from a disease condition or starvation. Low blood albumin ("hypoalbuminemia") is a common finding in animals that have suffered starvation. Other common findings include an elevated blood urea nitrogen (BUN) level, because of protein catabolism (breaking muscle tissue down for energy, which is an abnormal finding seen in starvation). Additionally, a complete blood count (CBC) may reveal findings such as anemia and low white blood cell count. These laboratory results are not specific for starvation, but they support that diagnosis in the absence of any other disease. If an animal was ill from malnutrition, the laboratory values can be repeated in a few weeks' time after instituting a healthy diet, and the findings should be improved.

Animals suspected of being denied adequate nutrition should be body condition scored by a veterinarian or another individual appropriately trained in body condition scoring for the species involved. Most body condition scoring systems are on a scale of 1 to 5, where a 1 is the thinnest condition possible and a 5 is the most obese an animal can be. Purina has a body condition scoring system for dogs and another for cats that runs from 1 to 9, where 1 is the thinnest condition possible and 9 is the most obese an animal can be. The body condition should be reassessed regularly, along with weights as the animal regains a good body condition. It is important to note what body condition scoring system was used. If fur obscures the body condition of the animal, shaving the body helps to illustrate advanced emaciation.

In cases of emaciated deceased animals, a postmortem examination by a veterinarian will help to diagnose any disease conditions that could account for the animal's emaciated condition. Many medical conditions can cause emaciation; it is important to recognize that an emaciated animal isn't necessarily a starved animal. The failure to recognize and seek veterinary treatment for an emaciated animal may be neglect. Generally, the bar for neglect is a condition that any reasonable and prudent animal owner should have recognized and corrected.

At a scene of an enclosed abandonment, note and record the presence or absence of food and water, and their quality. Note the condition of these and the presence of any empty food or water containers. Note the presence of feces, and whether they have foreign matter contained within them. Try to count or approximate the number of bowel movements in the environment as this helps to address the chronicity of abandonment. Overall photographs of the scene will support the estimate, and other marks of distress created by the frustrated animal. A sampling of "fresh" feces (still moist) can be collected for analysis for the presence of parasite eggs. A "fecal egg count" should be requested from the laboratory if parasite eggs are detected, in order to quantify the burden parasites present.

At the opposite end of the spectrum, obesity can be a suffering condition that may require or benefit from an investigation and documentation. Similarly, the responsible parties can be counseled on the need for the animal to lose weight and should be directed to a veterinarian for assistance in developing a weight loss program, as well as to ensure that a medical condition such as hypothyroidism is not playing a role (Figure 21.13).

Failure to Provide Adequate Sanitation

It is important to record subjective observations such as describing the smell at a scene, or the odor of an animal. The feel of the texture of the haircoat, and the color of fur that would ordinarily be white should be noted. If there is an accumulation of feces on the premises, the depth should be noted, and photographs should be taken of the overall scene depicting the feces and body fluids in place, as well as some closer photography. The character of any accumulated squalor can be described as either wet or dry squalor. Some social workers will describe squalor in degrees of squalor (Figure 21.14).

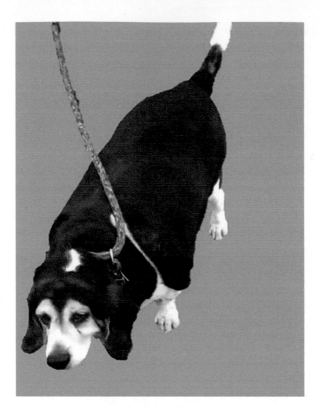

Figure 21.13 An obese Bassett Hound was monitored by animal control after his owner was warned that the obesity was causing immobility and suffering. While not visible in this view, the dog's abdomen (belly) made contact with the ground when he was standing. The dog was eventually surrendered to animal control by the owner because of a failure to help him lose weight. The dog was placed in an adoptive home where he successfully lost weight and regained mobility. (Photo courtesy of the City of Boston.)

Degree of squalor	Description
1st degree (dry)	Piles of clutter accumulating, out of the way of traffic. Normal use of rooms and facilities is not impeded.
2nd degree (dry)	Household areas are not useable due to accumulation of clutter (eg bed, desk, dining table, counters). Normal movement through the residence or use of facilities is impeded.
3rd degree (wet)	Features of above, plus the presence of rotting food and animal feces or urine in the house. Lapsed household repairs.
4th degree (wet)	Features of above, plus the presence of human feces and/or urine that is not in the toilet.

Figure 21.14 Degrees of squalor.

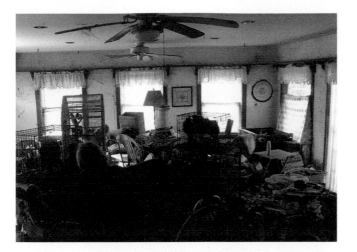

Figure 21.15 A typical hoarding scene with both caged and free roaming animals.

Dry squalor exists without the presence of decay and is characterized by the uncleanliness and poor maintenance of the residence. Dry squalor is often characterized by accumulation of papers, empty food containers and other debris. Wet squalor is characterized by decay and foul odors from the stockpiling of household garbage, rotting foodstuffs, infestation of vermin and pests, animal waste, and makeshift arrangements for human waste disposal. Dry squalor can become wet squalor when a building structure is allowed to decay sufficiently to allow entrance of water (Figure 21.15).

Failure to Provide Veterinary Care

Animals may have injuries, conditions or illnesses that are long standing that should have been treated. An animal owner might claim that the injury "just happened". A veterinarian can refute that claim by examining the wound or wounds and describing the presence of infection or tissues that indicate a time period of healing, such as "granulation tissue" and "re-epithelialization". Biopsies and measurements of wounds can help provide a timeline.

A "granulation bed" is the first healing tissue to cover a wound; it is bright pink and has an orange peel-type texture. Biopsies can be performed on wounds that have granulation tissue and the granulation tissue measured to estimate the time since injury. In general, a granulation bed forms within 5 days after injury. It begins at the edges of the wound and creeps across the wound at a rate of 0.5 to 1 mm/ per day. The next phase of healing is re-epithelialization, and this is characterized by a light-colored rim of new skin tissue at the border of the wound. Re-epithelialization eventually

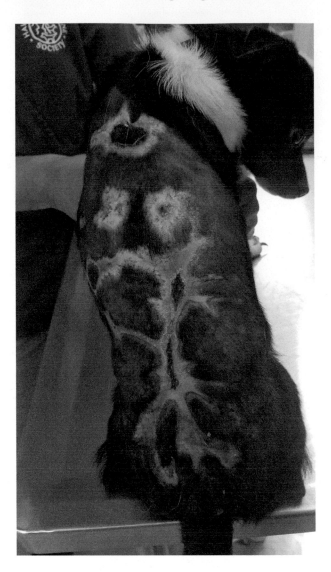

Figure 21.16 A healing burn wound on the back of a dog shows progress in healing with re-epithelialization (pale scar tissue type skin) and contracture. The central red scabbed areas are mature granulation tissue. This wound is nearly healed, likely several weeks into the healing process. (Figure 21.16 courtesy of the Hawaiian Humane Society.)

closes a wound by "creeping" across the granulation bed, and this process happens at a fairly predictable rate. After re-epithelialization, the wound will undergo contracture, which will cause wrinkling of the wound. Biopsies of healing tissue can help to establish the age of a wound, but even taking serial pictures of a healing wound with a ruler in the picture can help a veterinarian estimate how long the wound has been present, at a minimum (Figures 21.16–21.18). Malnutrition can prolong healing.

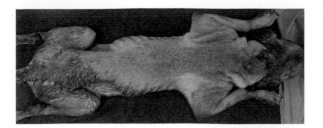

Figure 21.17 A mastiff type tody was brought to an animal shelter in a near-death condition, thin, pale, dehydrated and exuding a puss-like fluid from her vulva. A witness reported that the dog had been "on and off sick" for a few months after giving birth to a litter of puppies, and they had urged the owner to seek veterinary care.

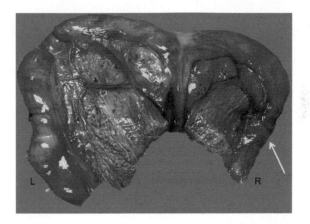

Figure 21.18 The dog was euthanized due to her poor prognosis. On postmortem exam she was found to have a long-standing uterine infection, with scarring that was consistent with a prior uterine rupture. This finding was consistent with the report that the dog had been sick, recovered somewhat and subsequently became morbidly ill.

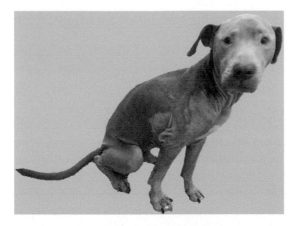

Figure 21.19 A typical ventral distribution (affecting the underside) of dermatitis from overkenneling, with prolonged direct exposure to filth.

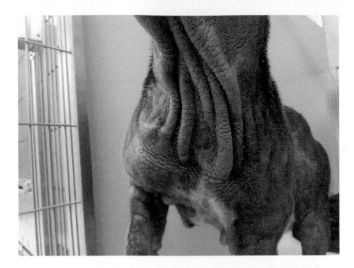

Figure 21.20 The lichenified skin of a dog with a long standing, untreated skin infection. This thick, bumpy appearance is often referred to as "pachydermatitis" or "elephant skin".

Skin conditions are very common in neglected animals, especially animals that are neglected in filth. The skin conditions may or may not entail external parasites such as fleas, ticks or mites. Animals that are "overkenneled" ("overcrated") and forced to sit in their own excrement will often have a "tide line" of yellow or yellow-brown staining of the fur, or a dermatitis affecting the skin most consistently in contact with the excrement (Figure 21.19). Animals that have been overcrated may have weak, flat feet that splay out like starfish. These should be photographed and monitored as the animals (and their feet) return to physical fitness.

Chronic (long-standing) skin infections can cause thickening of the skin, and a rough, pebbled appearance referred to as "lichenification". This is also sometimes referred to as pachydermatitis, or "elephant skin". Skin infections are painful (Figure 21.20).

Untreated cancers can cause large and painful tumor masses. Bone cancer is particularly painful, and bones affected by bone cancer are vulnerable to "pathological fractures", basically the diseased bone breaking under the normal weight and activities of the animal. Painful oral conditions, including severe dental disease and cancers, may prevent an animal from eating and will contribute to an emaciated state. Additionally, cancer is very metabolically active, burning more calories than healthy tissue, causing animals to become cachexic ("wasting"). Other illnesses of the liver, intestines or kidneys can cause increased losses of protein, leading to thin conditions. An overly thin animal can be suffering from a multitude of conditions and requires a veterinary exam with laboratory analysis of the blood and urine, and often radiographs (X-rays) to determine the cause or causes of the animal's condition (Figure 21.21).

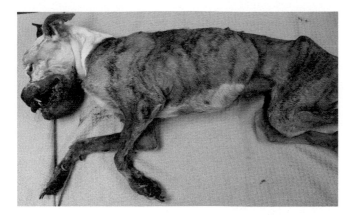

Figure 21.21 This deceased dog was found in the woods, enclosed in a laundry bag, in a shopping cart. The body was emaciated, and a large tumor affected the jaw. Decomposition precluded a determination of the exact cause of death, but it was clear the dog had not been provided adequate care. The identity of this Dog Doe was not determined.

Failure to Provide Adequate Grooming Care

Animals may suffer from a lack of adequate grooming care, such as over-grown hooves, overgrown teeth or beaks, embedded nails or heavily matted hair coats. Matted hair coats can be severe enough to prevent the normal range of motion of limbs or cover the anus preventing normal defecation causing a "fecal dam". There may be painful moist dermatitis under mats, and even maggots ("myiasis").

Severe cases of matting can strangulate a limb, cut into the skin and other soft tissues, and even cause traumatic amputation. Animals may have very serious corneal ulceration secondary to neglect, even as severe as rup-tured globes (eyeballs), that are caused and obscured by facial hair mats. Overgrown toenails can circle back to embed in the paw pads, making walk-ing painful and difficult. Overgrown hooves can cause severe lameness, pain and even an inability to move to access food and water, leading to starvation in the presence of food.

Enclosed and Open Air Thermal Stress

Animals may suffer from hypo- or hyperthermia if left exposed to cold or hot conditions. Obese and flat-faced ("brachycephalic") animals are more vul-nerable to hyperthermia, as are older dogs suffering from conditions such as laryngeal paralysis or tracheal collapse. A lack of available drinking water also intensifies the effects of hyperthermia, and so scenes where animals

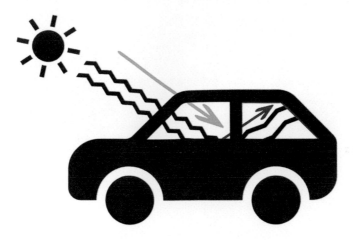

Figure 21.22 Short-wave energy enters the vehicle through the glass and is converted to long-wave energy released by the heated interior of the vehicle. The long-wave energy cannot escape.

are found dead from suspected hyperthermia, an effort should be made to document water sources. Hyperthermia is exacerbated by humid air, and any respiratory condition will also make hyperthermia worse. Animals can become hyperthermic on days that are not especially hot particularly when enclosed or in direct sun with no ability to escape it.

Dog in Hot Car

The hyperthermia that occurs in a vehicle can happen very quickly. The vehicle's interior is heated by the short-wave solar rays that enter the vehicle through the glass. The heated interior releases long-wave energy that cannot pass back out through the glass or escape the vehicle, so the vehicle is a heat trap (Figure 21.22). Vehicles can absorb solar energy on even overcast days. The exact rate at which a vehicle gains heat is variable, based on many factors such as the color of the vehicle, the ratio of the volume of the vehicle interior to glass surface area and angle of the sun relative to the glass.

If a window has been left open a "crack", a laser thermometer can be used to measure the temperature of various surfaces of the interior, and measurements should be recorded on various surfaces, in the sun and in the shade of the interior of the vehicle. A laser thermometer used on a closed window will only return the surface temperature of the glass. Additionally, an animal breathing in a vehicle will increase the humidity of the air, causing it to worsen the hyperthermia.

Open Air Hyperthermia

Dogs that are penned or tied out without shade are vulnerable to hyperthermia. It is important to note that sun exposure will change with the position of the sun, and the scene should be documented at various times of day (Figures 21.23 and 21.24).

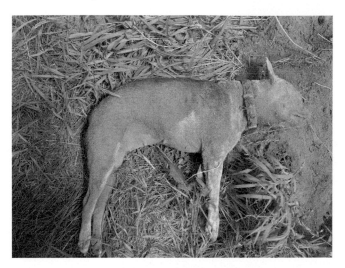

Figure 21.23 A Boston Terrier died from hyperthermia ("heat stroke") because it was tethered to a railing by asphalt driveway, with no shade. The owner buried the dog, and it was later exhumed on a search warrant. Rigor mortis (stiffness of death) sets in relatively more quickly in cases of hyperthermia. (Figure 21.23 courtesy of ACO Emanuel Maciel.)

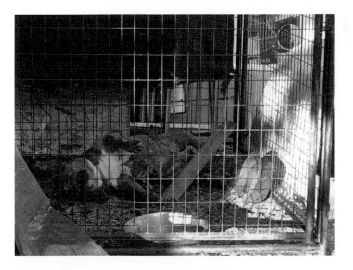

Figure 21.24 While this deceased dog was in shade in the late afternoon when the scene was documented, earlier in the day, he was in the full sun with no shade. (Figure 20.24 courtesy of ACO Christopher Husgen.)

Hypothermia

Thin, neonatal and elderly animals are more susceptible to hypothermia than other animals. Small animals have an increased surface area-to-body mass ratio, and so they become cold more quickly. Animals that have matted hair coats cannot insulate against the cold as well, and wind contributes to cooling. Adequate shelter from the cold must be insulated, elevated off the ground, of a proper size related to the animal, with minimal exposure to air movement, and contain dry bedding.

Animal Hoarding

The *Diagnostic and Statistical Manual of Mental Disorders* describes animal hoarding as a condition associated with hoarding disorder and defined by "the accumulation of a large number of animals and a failure to provide minimal standards of nutrition, sanitation, and veterinary care and to act on the deteriorating condition of the animals (e.g., disease, starvation, death) and the environment (e.g., severe overcrowding, extremely unsanitary conditions)". The consequences of animal hoarding include starvation, illness, and death of animals, neglect of self and others, and household destruction.

The destructive nature of animal hoarding in a home environment is dramatic, featuring large numbers of sick, dying or dead animals, crammed into the hoarder's property. These animals may be in individual cages, or they may freely roam the house or grounds. Often urine and feces cover and saturate floors, counters, furniture, walls and other surfaces, creating high concentrations of ammonia and aerosolized organic contaminants that pose serious health risks to occupants.

The home and other structures may be hazardous for other reasons, such as the risk of rotted floorboards breaking underfoot, toppling of stacks of debris, decaying or damaged electrical wiring, blocked exits and insect or rodent infestation. It is not uncommon for the animal hoarder's property to lack running water or electricity due to a failure to pay bills or repair broken items. Human toileting may occur in locations other than the toilet. Some animal hoarders suffer from paranoid delusions and may have unsecured weapons, trip wires or other "booby traps" on their property or within buildings. All searches must be conducted with these risks in mind. Preparing for a search and seizure of hoarded animals must include careful advance planning as detailed in Chapter 8. The scene documentation of animal hoarding will benefit from a coordinated Incident Command System approach.

Animals of any species may be hoarded. It is advisable to have a species specialist (e.g., a veterinarian, reputable farmer or breeder familiar with the type of animal) on scene during the search. This will help with triage of animals in need of urgent care, and with the identification of salient evidence that might otherwise be overlooked.

Understanding the Behavior of Typical Animal Hoarders

Animal hoarding can be viewed as a mental disorder, and people who hoard animals may be referred to more accurately as people with animal hoarding disorder. Regardless of any psychiatric diagnosis, the negligent suffering created by people with animal hoarding disorder is generally considered a criminal activity. For ease of discussion, we use the term "animal hoarder" as shorthand for people with animal hoarding disorder.

It is helpful to understand the animal hoarder in context of their motivations – they break down into three general types: the Overwhelmed Caregiver, the Rescue Hoarder and the Exploiter Hoarder. These personality types are not intended as diagnoses, but a guide to help responders understand the animal hoarder's motivation and sometimes bizarre behavior. A general rule of thumb when planning a seizure of hoarded animals is that there is likely to be triple or quadruple the number of animals present that a hoarder claims or admits.

The Overwhelmed Caregiver

The "Overwhelmed Caregiver" may have started as a hobby pet breeder or engaged in another activity where they initially provided adequate care to a number of animals. In most cases, the Overwhelmed Caregiver suffers a life change, perhaps due to cognitive decline, the loss of a job or a spouse. At some point, the needs of the animals outstrip the Overwhelmed Caregiver's ability to provide adequate care and the animals slip into suffering conditions. The Overwhelmed Caregiver likely has a passive attitude, and they may present as helpless. In general, the Overwhelmed Caregiver is receptive to intervention or assistance and is more willing to part with animals to improve the quality of life for all involved. In interviews with Overwhelmed Caregiver animal hoarders, they may point to individual animals and assign names and relationships to other animals in the setting. If pressed however, this "knowledge" of the population often breaks down, and they will offer different stories if presented with the same animal several different times.

The Rescue Hoarder

The "Rescue Hoarder" is more difficult to work with as compared to the Overwhelmed Caregiver. They may consider themselves valiant mission-driven lifesavers. The Rescue Hoarder's acquisition of animals is more active, they will seek to collect animals from "free to a good home" advertisements and other avenues, far beyond their own capacity to provide humane care to the collection. The primary challenge with the "Rescue Hoarder" is that they are reluctant to part with the animals they have accumulated, believing that no one will care for their animals better than they can. They will often have impossible to pass screening tests for prospective adopters (e.g., requiring a 6-foot fence in the backyard, requiring an adult be at home with the animal 24 hours a day or requiring 6 months of volunteer work before being eligible to adopt). Rescue Hoarders may have an extensive network of enablers who also believe the heroic Rescue Hoarder is doing incredibly good work, while failing to see the suffering of animals who live endlessly caged lives. These well-intentioned supporters can enable the ongoing "shelter hoarder", and they may engage in subterfuge, hiding animals or otherwise assisting the Rescue Hoarder achieve their mission.

Legitimate shelters, rescue groups or sanctuaries put the needs of the animals first, recognizing when capacity to provide care could be exceeded, and will take the required steps (either stopping intake, increasing adoption, increasing staff or resources) in order to provide proper care. Rescue Hoarders do not sufficiently enact such responses; the needs of the animal are secondary to the need of the Rescue Hoarder to be in control. When dealing with a Rescue Hoarder, you are likely dealing with someone who believes they know best, and any external involvement is an insult.

The Exploiter Hoarder

The "Exploiter Hoarder" is the most difficult personality. This type of animal hoarder tends to use animals for personal gain, whether financial or otherwise. They tend to have characteristics of antisocial personality disorder. They tend to view animals and other people as tools to be used to advance their own cause or satisfy their own needs. This type of animal hoarder can choose to be charming and convincing, or they can be extraordinarily confrontational and vexatious. It is common for the Exploiter Hoarder to engage in legal abuse, frequently and repeatedly filing unwarranted or improper lawsuits with malicious intentions. This is a tactic that can keep landlords, town officials and others on the defensive and at bay, so the Exploiter Hoarder can continue their criminal conduct uninterrupted.

The Hoarded Animal

From the perspective of the animal, it does not matter what behavior the hoarder exhibits, and animal hoarders may exhibit characteristics of more than one classification. Animal hoarding causes suffering, and intervention should be focused on documenting evidence, and rescuing the animals. Once a collection of hoarded animals has been seized, they remain evidence and property of the owner. They must remain in the care and custody of the seizing authority until released by a legal process. "Custody" indicates that the seizing authority can present the animals if required by the court; it does not preclude the seizing authority from placing the animals in foster homes. Once the animals start to receive adequate care, their status of evidence has changed. For this reason, prompt detailed documentation of each individual animal is essential at the outset of the seizure. Planning for search warrant affidavits in animal hoarding scenes is detailed in Chapter 8.

Documenting the Scene and Evidence

The squalid and chaotic living conditions of animal hoarders complicate investigations. Filth and debris are compounded by potentially unbreathable air and potentially by the actions and vocalizations of dozens (or more animals). Investigators must be prepared to wear appropriate personal protective equipment, and entry should be conducted in consultation with the Department of Public Health and the Fire Department. There may be very high levels of ammonia gas, aerosolized biohazards (*E. coli* cell wall "dust" from dried fecal matter that can cause flu-like symptoms if inhaled), mold and other fungi, and high levels of bacteria present.

Documenting the Environment

Environmental ammonia levels should be measured with an ammonia meter before the building is ventilated. Ventilation of the building must be undertaken with care, recognizing that some animals may escape. Ammonia readings should be taken at or near floor levels as this is where the relatively heavy ammonia gas settles, and it is where the animals are breathing. The same holds true for taking environmental temperature readings – the readings should be taken in the animal's primary enclosure, as the temperature of the entire room can be very different than that within a cage or crate.

Once the scene has been made safe or measures have been taken to protect people entering the scene, teams may process the scene and animals. The scene should be diagrammed and photographed as described in Chapters 5 and 8. In certain cases, it may be prudent to leave food and water, in humane traps, and revisit the property for several days to ensure all animals have been captured and removed.

It is important to note the condition of the interior of the animal's enclosure, food bowls and water receptacles, and whether the food is edible, and the water fit to drink. While it may not be practical to seize every cage, it is recommended to take samples of crates, furniture cushions and rugs as exemplar evidence that preserves the odor and squalor.

Documenting the Animals

After the preliminary scene and animal documentation, comprehensive over-all photographs should be taken of each animal, capturing multiple views: from the top, each side, front and back and, if possible, the underside. This is often done at the same time as the veterinary evaluation which is described in Chapter 17.

It is important that each animal has an individual exam and record list-ing the various conditions affecting the animal. Once the population has been described in individual exams and photographs, it is helpful to create a spread-sheet that identifies each condition so that aggregate numbers can be gathered (i.e., how many animals have dermatitis, dental disease, embedded nails and so forth). Spreadsheets are also helpful to track animals' recovery and restora-tion of good health by recording weights and body conditions over time.

Documentation

In animal hoarding cases, it is important to create order out of chaos and to follow all ordinary crime scene documentation practices. Additionally, tracking ongoing care delivered to the animals will provide a record of what was done. These documents can be used to put a dollar value on the care given to the animals during their rehabilitation for civil redress or for bond and forfeiture procedures.

Helpful forms include memoranda of understanding between a lead agency and assisting agencies detailing who is responsible for what parts of the response, an animal inventory form to record all living and deceased animal removed, chain of custody for multiple animal forms, exam forms, transport logs, evidence cage cards and a service tracking sheet for purposes of restitution.

Final Thoughts

Neglected animals can endure a variety of forms of suffering. Animal hoard-ing scenes can be thought of as neglect on a large scale. When an animal neglect scene is examined, it is important to note the totality of squalor and general conditions, while also documenting each individual animal, live or deceased. Even an animal in a state of advanced decomposition may have evi-dentiary value and should be documented and recovered for possible exami-nation by a veterinarian. If a long bone (femur or humerus, the upper bones of the legs) is still moist, it can be submitted to a laboratory for bone marrow fat analysis. This test can help to support a diagnosis of a death by starvation. Bones may have signs of traumatic injury or chronic infections. Neglect can cause tremendous, long-standing suffering, and the appropriately detailed investigation of these cases can help relieve severe animal suffering. It is possible that some people will be helped by the intervention as well, including the responsible party or parties.

Bibliography

Banerjee S, Halliday G, Snowdon J. 2012. *Severe Domestic Squalor*. Cambridge: Cambridge University Press.

FEMA. NIMS implementation and training. https://www.fema.gov/emergency-managers/nims/implementation-training.

Gregory NG. *Physiology and Behaviour of Animal Suffering* [VitalSource Bookshelf version]. 2008. Blackwell: Oxford.

Ian Freckelton SC. Severe domestic squalor by John Snowdon, Graeme Halliday, and Sube Banerjee. *Psychiatry, Psychology and Law.* 2013;20(1):152–155, doi: 10.1080/13218719.2013.761743.

Patronek GJ, Loar L, Nathanson JN, eds. *Animal Hoarding: Structuring Interdisciplinary Responses to Help People, Animals, and Communities at Risk.* Hoarding of Animals Research Consortium. 2006. https://vet.tufts.edu/wp-content/uploads/AngellReport.pdf. Accessed July 8, 2021.

Animal Sexual Abuse 22

MARTHA SMITH-BLACKMORE

Fundamentals of Animal Sexual Abuse

Defined simply, animal sexual abuse (ASA) is the intentional sexual contact between a person and an animal. The legal definition differs by jurisdiction. Typical statutory language for sexual contact is "(a) any act between a person and an animal that involves contact between the sex organs or anus of one and the mouth, anus or sex organs of the other; (b) touching or fondling by a person of the sex organs or anus of an animal, either directly or through clothing, without a bona fide veterinary or animal husbandry purpose; (c) any transfer or transmission of semen by the person upon any part of the animal; or (d) the insertion, however slight, of any part of a person's body or any object into the vaginal or anal opening of an animal or the insertion of any part of the animal's body into the vaginal or anal opening of the person".

The distribution or possession of ASA-involved pornography is often illegal as well. ASA in the presence of minors and coercion of a minor or mentally disabled individual to engage in sex acts with animals are usually distinct criminal acts. In the few jurisdictions where ASA is not specifically illegal, any physical harm inflicted on an animal during an ASA act still falls under animal cruelty statutes. In these jurisdictions, acts performed in the presence of children or coercing children to engage sexually with animals will be covered under other sexual offenses.

Forceful acts of ASA may be performed with physical restraints such as rope, duct tape or straps, with blows to the head to stun the animal or with the use of psychoactive agents (drugs or sedatives) to disorient the animal. Alternatively, ASA may be achieved through conditioning (training for desired compliance or behaviors using positive reinforcement).

Types of Evidence

At the scene where ASA is alleged to have occurred, there may be corroborating evidence such as materials with DNA evidence, video or photographic evidence, restraints or drugs. Additionally, there may be evidence at the scene such as scratches on the floor or broken objects, resulting from animal's

DOI: 10.4324/9781003090762-22

struggles. There may be large amounts of lubricant and cloth used for cleanup may contain DNA evidence from the perpetrator and the victim animal. Animal hair may be embedded in ropes used to restrain animals. Condoms, if present, should be collected. Used condoms may contain the DNA of the perpetrator and the animal victim. Unused condoms may be used for reference to lubricant found on swabs taken from the assaulted animal.

When potential DNA samples are located on smaller items such as clothing or weapons, the entire object should be placed in a paper envelope or bag and transported or shipped to a laboratory at room temperature. Blood frozen in snow and ice should be collected into a tightly sealed tube and, if possible, kept frozen. Bloodstains on items that cannot be shipped can be collected using a clean lightly moistened cotton swab. Allow the swab to air-dry and then seal it in a paper envelope and ship at room temperature.

Because animals may bite or scratch while resisting attempted ASA, suspects should be examined for evidence of bites or scratches, and the claws of the victim animal can be swabbed for the presence of human DNA.

Evaluation of the Victims

The type and degree of physical injury inflicted on an animal victim depend upon the methods of control and restraint employed, the force used and anatomic size differentials. In addition to head trauma and trauma from physical restraints, there may be fissures (or tears) to the anus or vaginal opening (Figures 22.1 and 22.2). There may be bruising to the perineum (the area around the anus and vulva or scrotum, or around the tail base, and the tail may be traumatically luxated (dislocated)). There may be fingertip bruises on the inside of the rear legs.

Animals that are too small to be physically penetrated may have the perineal skin invaginated (pushed in) through the pelvis without entry into the vagina or anus. Friction to the invaginated tissues may create a "target sign" on the animal with a large circular area of wet fur or abraded (rubbed off) fur or feathers centered on the attempted point of entry. Internally, there may be tears to the rectum, colon or vaginal wall. Foreign objects used to penetrate an animal may be retained in the animal, within the gastrointestinal or reproductive tract, or the foreign objects may be forced through the organs and deposited within the abdomen.

During a physical exam, it is important to have a veterinarian consider what other types of activity might cause conditions or trauma that mimic ASA. Impacted anal glands or parasitic worms can cause animals to scoot or rub their hind end, causing abrasions. Normal and abnormal hormone-driven changes can cause prominent appearance to the anus or vulva that may mimic trauma from ASA, or there may be ulcerative diseases of the anus (Figures 22.3 and 22.4).

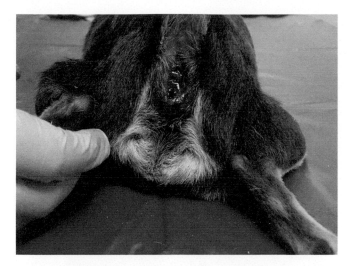

Figure 22.1 Dilated anus with radial tears.

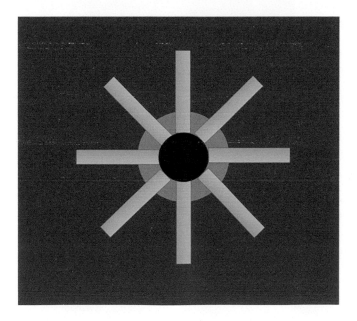

Figure 22.2 Diagram demonstrating potential positions of radial tears.

The animal's temperature should not be taken with a rectal thermometer until after the forensic examination is completed, and no lubricant should be used on equipment until after swabs are taken. Slow and gentle insertion of equipment should be performed for the animal's comfort and to avoid iatrogenic injury (injury caused by a medical process).

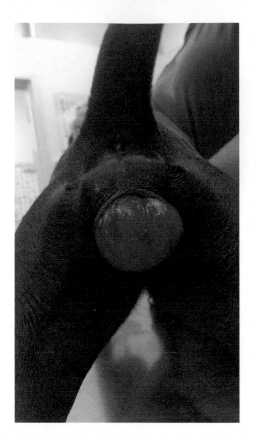

Figure 22.3 Vaginal hypertrophy with prolapse is a naturally occurring condition in an intact female dog that can erroneously be identified as evidence of sexual abuse.

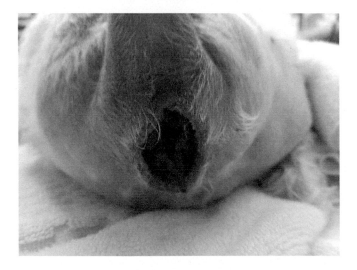

Figure 22.4 A rim of inflamed tissue around the anus after a fecal dam is removed and can mimic ASA trauma.

If possible, animals should have an Elizabethan collar (lampshade style cone) placed prior to transport to minimize the amount of grooming they do on themselves. This may help preserve important evidence. Also, if small enough, animals should be placed in a clean transport carrier for transportation to the site where the physical exam and sexual assault exam are to take place. This reduces the risk of introducing contamination or confounding materials on the animal. Animals should not be offered food or water until the forensic examination, if reasonable to do so.

Animals should have a fecal floatation analysis for the detection (or ruling out) of parasitic worms. The presence of a natural or disease condition does not exclude ASA as a possibility, but this should cause the veterinarian to consider why or why not the condition may be a contributing reason for the appearance of the animal. For a veterinarian, ASA should be a differential diagnosis in any case of genital or anorectal injury or trauma.

A commercial human sexual assault victim evidence collection kit, obtained from a forensic supply warehouse, may be used for the examination of the animal victim. If this kit is not immediately available, one may be obtained from the sexual assault nurse examiner at a local hospital emergency room, or one may be assembled from available materials, employing the same principles for examination, detection and collection of evidence.

The animal should be examined over a double set of clean sheets. The upper sheet collects material that may fall from them during the examination and the bottom sheet prevents contaminants from the floor inadvertently being collected onto the top sheet. A regular nose-to-tail exam should triage any necessary medical response for pain or injuries before proceeding with evidence collection and documentation.

Animals who have been conditioned to perform sexually may exhibit sexualized behaviors during the examination, such as assuming the position of lordosis (lowering the front of the body and raising the hind end) or pelvic thrusting. These behaviors should be described in notes and captured on videotape if possible.

All injuries should be documented; measure and describe injuries indicating the location of the injuries. Use a species-appropriate body diagram and photographically document the injuries as well. If a species-appropriate body diagram is not available, the position of the injury in relationship to an orifice can be described in clock-face fashion, such as "an abrasion was noted at the 8 o'clock position on the anus". Exemplar forms are offered in Appendix C.

Examination and Sample Collection

Ideally, the animal is examined, and evidence collected as soon as possible after the alleged assault. Personal protection equipment should be employed while collecting evidence to protect the collector from exposure to human body fluids and to prevent the contamination of collected materials.

Equipment and supplies should be prepared in advance to facilitate uninterrupted examination. Supplies include speculum (an otoscopic cone may be employed if a veterinarian does not have a vaginal speculum), swabs, envelopes, swab boxes, sterile water, extra sets of powder-free gloves, blood drawing supplies, supplies to assess vital signs (at least a stethoscope), a ruler or calipers, a permanent marker, a stable stand for holding and drying swabs, paper envelopes and bags for evidence packaging.

Equipment specific for a sexual assault exam would include a colposcope, toluidine blue dye, an alternate light source and a camera for photography. The preferred alternate source wavelength to detect human semen is 420–450 nm, viewed through orange lenses. The Bluemaxx BM500 (Sirchie; Medford, NJ) is recommended as a more specific light source to detect human semen than a Woods Lamp which emits a light with a wavelength of 300–400 nm. However, most veterinary clinics do have a Woods Lamp; this ultraviolet light source can aid in the detection of foreign materials, especially when enhanced with orange lenses (Figures 22.5 and 22.6).

Swabs and swab boxes or envelopes may be used for DNA evidence collection. Envelopes or boxes should be labeled before placing evidence inside. This minimizes the destruction of evidence and prevents the mix-up of evidence samples. If a dry area is to be swabbed, the cotton tip swab should first be moistened with sterile water. Use one or two swabs per hand depending on the amount of visible debris. Place these swabs in a stable stand and let air-dry. Once dried, place swabs in a prelabeled envelope. If swabs are collected

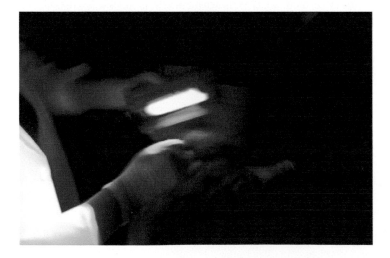

Figure 22.5 Woods lamp can be used to examine an animal for seminal fluid. Fluorescence (glowing) is suggestive of proteinaceous material, and samples should be collected for further analysis.

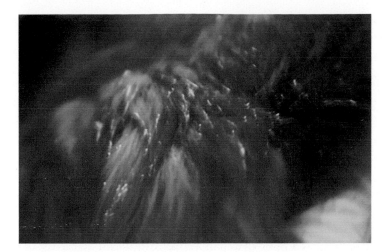

Figure 22.6 Fluorescent matter was collected from the fur on this dog and was later proven to be semen.

from claws on both front feet, package swabs from the left and right paws separately, with clear indication of where the sample was collected.

Once an exam is started, the examiner is responsible for "Chain of Custody", and the integrity of the collected evidence. The examiner must stay with the evidence collected during the exam until all evidence has been properly sealed and secured.

If a drug facilitated assault is suspected, the urine should be collected and preserved. Urine may be collected up to 94 hours post assault. Urine may be collected by free catch or cystocentesis. Catheterization should be avoided until after complete internal examination is performed. The urine specimen container or cup should be labeled with patient information and securely sealed.

A fresh sample of blood should be collected into an anticoagulant tube and refrigerated for reference DNA profiling. If the patient is deceased, a small sample of muscle tissue can be collected and frozen for the reference DNA. Frozen samples must be delivered by overnight courier.

Species each have their own specific primers for DNA testing. Samples to be tested for animal DNA must go to a veterinary genetics laboratory, and samples to be tested for human DNA must be submitted to the crime lab or other certified forensic laboratory.

Oral Exam

Inspect the oral cavity, documenting any injuries and photograph noted injuries. If oral penetration is reported or suspected, swab the gumline, the margin between the gums and cheek, crevices between teeth, and under the tongue with cotton swabs, dry and place in the "Oral Swab" labeled envelope or swab box.

Genital Exam

Place the patient in the appropriate position to optimally allow the vaginal/ penile/rectal exam. Inspect the external genitalia and rectal area for visual signs of trauma. If an animal has been chronically or repeatedly abused, broken hairs, abrasions, or callusing may be present.

Observed injuries should be indicated on a body diagram and injuries photographed before obtaining any swab collection. After inspection and sample collection, the tissues may be painted with Toludine blue dye to potentially enhance lacerations that may not have been detected.

Toluidine blue is a basic dye with a high affinity for acidic tissue components. The epithelium does not have nucleated cells and prevents uptake of stain by nuclei. Where the epithelium is damaged, the underlying nucleated cells are exposed, and the nuclei will stain blue. Application of toluidine blue dye (1%) and its subsequent removal with a destaining reagent, such as diluted acetic acid or a lubricant, will increase the detection rate of lacerations. This process does not interfere with the detection of DNA. If lacerations are detected in an area that was not yet swabbed, the newly detected laceration areas should also be swabbed (Figure 22.7).

Hair Combing

The perineal fur, or fur where an animal is manually restrained, may contain dried secretions from drainage or ejaculation. Be sure to inspect the fur on the

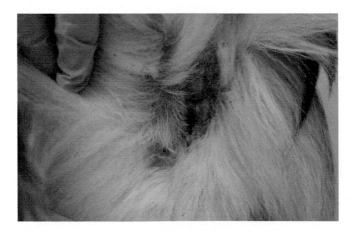

Figure 22.7 Broken hairs, the abrasion and calluses found around this dog's anus were consistent with alleged chronic ASA.

entire animal but especially around the anus and perineum, on the underside of the tail where it contacts the perineum, and the fur of the scruff of the neck. If hair is matted, representative samples should be cut and packaged in a prelabeled envelope. Clearly mark on the envelope what was collected and from where.

Anal Swabs

If rectal penetration is reported or suspected, inspect the anal area first. Examination and evidence collection of the anal area is performed prior to the genital area because this area can be contaminated when inspecting and collecting vaginal specimens.

Inspect the rectal area for injury and document any noted injuries prior to obtaining swabs. Remove any foreign bodies and let air dry before placing it in an envelope. Clearly document on the envelope where the evidence was obtained from. Two separate swabs may be taken from the exterior anal surface and then two from within the orifice. Perform swabbing on swab at a time and use the entire surface of each cotton-tip swab to maximize the amount of sample collected. If particulate matter/fibers are on the swab, do not remove it or them from the swab.

Mark the first swab obtained with a permanent marker on the distal wooden portion of the swab stick. Place the swabs in a stable stand and let the swabs air dry. Once dried, place all swabs into an envelope or swab box labeled "Anal Swabs".

Vaginal and Cervical Swabs

If vaginal penetration is reported or suspected, examine the vaginal area for injury. Document injuries on a body diagram prior to inserting the speculum. Insert the speculum and inspect for injury or foreign bodies. Document any injury within the vaginal canal. Documentation by colposcopy (if available) should be done before obtaining any swabs.

Remove any foreign bodies and let air-dry before placing in a marked envelope. Clearly document on the envelope where the evidence was obtained from. Obtain swabs of the vaginal area. Indicate on the envelope whether the swabs are collected from the external genitalia or from within the orifice. If swabs are obtained from both areas, package in separate envelopes or swab boxes and clearly mark where the evidence was collected.

Do one swab at a time; use the entire surface of the cotton tip swab to collect the maximum available sample. Mark the first swab obtained. If possible, examine the area of the cervix for injury. Colposcopy documentation should be done prior to obtaining any swabs. Obtain swabs of the cervical os with cotton swabs, one swab at a time until four swabs have been collected. Again, mark the first swab obtained, allow to air-dry and, once dried, place into an envelope or box marked "Cervical Swabs".

Male Genitalia Swabs

Collect penile, scrotum and urethral opening swabs. Using four swabs, one at a time, swab the primary sources of potential foreign DNA. This may include the penile shaft, the pocket of the prepuce, the scrotum or urethral opening. Allow swabs to air dry. Once dried, place all -swabs into an envelope or swab box labeled "Male Genitalia".

Miscellaneous Evidence

If there is any other evidence such as blood, dried secretions, human hairs, material fibers, environmental debris (vegetation, dirt, gravel and glass), collect, dry and place in an evidence fold and place in an envelope labeled "Miscellaneous".

If it is reported that the animal was licked or bitten, use swabs moistened with sterile water to collect samples from the patient's body where contact was reported. Alternate light source or Woods Lamp ultraviolet lighting may help visualize body fluid.

Sample Packaging

Plastic bags should never be used for packaging evidence. Plastic retains moisture which causes degradation of biological fluids; use paper packaging only. The top floor sheet should be folded inward into small squares to contain debris or loose evidence and placed in a paper bag labeled "Floor Sheet". Fold the top of the bag over twice and staple across the final fold. Place this secured bag in a larger brown bag that will ultimately contain all of the collected evidence.

All swabs must be air-dried prior to packaging. Do not use heat to dry. Any envelopes to be sealed by moisture should be sealed using a damp paper towel or water-moistened gloved finger; never lick evidence envelopes! Tape across the sealed flap of the envelope. The examiner must initial and date across the tape so that the writing overlaps from the tape onto the envelopes. Place all swab boxes or envelopes in one larger paper envelope or bag. Clearly indicate on the outside larger bag the contents as separate items on the item list. Seal as above.

Urine and blood samples must be submitted separately. If the urine is to be tested for toxicology and also submitted for DNA analysis, the sample must be divided, appropriately labeled and submitted to the proper labs (veterinary toxicology and human forensic/crime lab).

Final Thoughts

Animal victims of ASA may show physical or behavioral signs of the abuse, and they may have been manipulated with drugs or other intoxicants. A thorough exam is vital, and natural causes of unusual appearing tissues must be considered. While it might be tempting for the veterinarian to analyze collected evidence in the clinic laboratory, this should not be done. The veterinary practice is not a certified crime laboratory, and this could invalidate the evidence.

Bibliography

Bradley N, Rasile K. Addressing animal sexual abuse. Clinician's Brief, April 2014, p. 77 https://files.brief.vet/migration/article/18041/addressing-animal-sexual-abuse-18041-article.pdf.

New Mexico SAEK Instructions. 2005. http://www.ncdsv.org/images/SexAssault EvidenceKitInstructions.pdf.

Stern AW, Smith-Blackmore M. Veterinary forensic pathology of animal sexual abuse. *Veterinary Pathology*. 2016;53(5):1057–1066. doi: 10.1177/0300985816643574.

Animal Fighting

23

MARTHA SMITH-BLACKMORE

Fundamentals of Animal Fighting and Other "Blood Sports"

Organized animal fighting is an exhibition of antagonistic engagement between animals. The typical and most frequent types of animal fighting are dog-fighting and chicken-fighting (aka cock-fighting). The fighting of these animals is done for a variety of reasons to include wagering, greed, reinforcing gang affiliation with clandestine activities and for the self-aggrandizement for the owner of the "winning" animal. Conversely, the owner of the losing animal may take it as a personal affront, and they may cruelly kill the animal in a demonstration of force and to "save face". The financial benefits to the "winning" dog owner include prize money and the increased value of the offspring from champions.

There are federal prohibitions against animal fighting. Under the Animal Welfare Act, Title 7, Chapter 54, Section 2156 of the United States Code, animal fighting ventures that involve interstate or foreign commerce are prohibited. There is also a ban against attending fighting events and an additional penalty for bringing minors to fighting events. The "interstate or foreign commerce" constraint gives the federal court jurisdiction over an activity that would otherwise be regulated by a state, such as the transportation of animals across state lines for the purpose of fighting. It is a violation of federal law to use the U.S. postal service to mail implements used for animal fighting, such as gaffs (a sharp hooked blade that is fastened to a rooster's leg to make the sparring more lethal).

State prohibitions may be specifically against stipulated types of engagement, such as dog-fighting and hog-dog-fighting, or they may ban staged animal fights in general without articulating the species of animals involved. Other forms of the so-called blood sports include bull baiting, and horse, fish and finch fighting. Even where specific forms of animal fighting are not prohibited, the failure to provide an animal adequate veterinary care after being injured in a fight could constitute animal abuse.

Animal fighting is often a gang activity and associated with other crimes such as illegal weapons possession, drug dealing, racketeering, human trafficking and financial crimes. Federal law defines the term "gang" as "an

DOI: 10.4324/9781003090762-23

ongoing group, club, organization or association of five or more persons: that has as one of its primary purposes the commission of one or more…criminal offenses….; the members of which engage, or have engaged within the past five years, in a continuing series of offenses…which affect interstate or foreign commerce" (US Code Title 18, Chapter 26, Section 521a).

Depending on the elements of state law, the animal fighters may have to be witnessed engaging in the act of animal fighting in order to be prosecuted. In these jurisdictions, the infiltration of a gang by undercover agents may be the only avenue to interrupting these cruel events. These can be very dangerous efforts, requiring information gathered from confidential informants and careful surveillance. In other states, it may be illegal to possess paraphernalia associated with animal fighting, such as training equipment (treadmills, spring poles and jennys), break sticks (used to separate fighting dogs in training bouts) and forced breeding stands (also known as "rape stands", used to breed female fighting dogs while preventing her from attacking the male dog). It would not be illegal to own any one item of these types, so the association with animal fighting would have to be proven based on the totality of the information generated by the investigation and circumstances discovered.

Indications

The finding of discarded dead animals may be the first sign that animal fighting is happening in a given community. For this reason, it is beneficial to have dead dogs found on the side of the road, floating in a body of water or discarded on public lands examined by a veterinarian for determination of the cause of death. Other small animals may be used for "bait", to increase aggression in the dogs, without the risk that the victim animal will cause harm to the fighting dog.

Deceased dogs discarded with puncture wounds from bite marks may be erroneously interpreted as having been shot. Dogs may be fought to death, or they may die hours or days after a fight from shock, kidney failure (from muscle damage) or sepsis (systemic infection). After losing a fight, dogs may be executed by gunshot, electrocution, drowning, hanging, "slamming" against the ground or by other brutal methods (Figures 23.1–23.4).

In an urban setting, dog fighting generally occurs in basements, and the sounds of dog fighting may be muffled or disguised by very loud music with a driving beat. In suburban or rural settings, dog fights may be staged in plywood lined "pits" with carpeted or dirt floors in a backyard, in an outbuilding or in the woods. Animal fights may be highly organized and professionally run, or they may be informal gatherings of a few individuals.

Dog "yards" are outdoor spaces where dogs are kept, restrained on tethers within close proximity to other dogs. This spacing helps to increase dog aggression and frustration. Each dog may have an individual shelter such as a

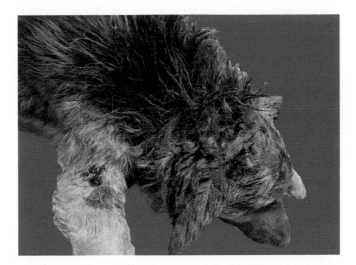

Figure 23.1 A dog was believed to have been shot to death in his backyard from the nearby wooded land, and police combed the area for projectiles.

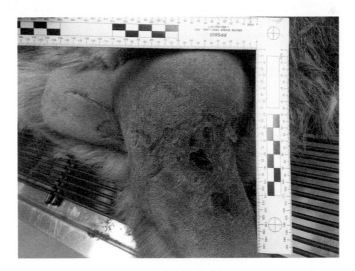

Figure 23.2 The same dog, after shaving. Wounds are not perforating (through and through injuries), and there are no retained projectiles. The fur around the neck was wet and clumped consistent with saliva deposition. It was determined that the dog was killed by other dogs kept in the same yard.

plywood doghouse or 50-gallon barrel with an opening cut into the side. Dog yards are generally established under the canopy of trees so that they cannot easily be observed from unmanned aircraft systems (drones) or other aerial surveillance.

Similarly, cock-fighting may be highly organized or an informal local event. Fighting bird yards also feature closely spaced shelters, usually small

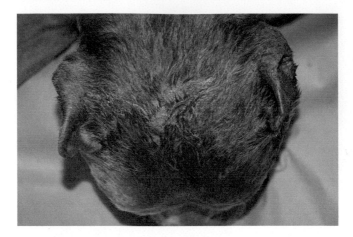

Figure 23.3 In another case, law enforcement issued a call for information leading to the arrest of anyone having shot dogs found dead in the woods. It was thought the wound on this dog's head was a gunshot graze wound, but this was a laceration inflicted by a tooth. This dog was peppered with other puncture wounds and abrasions in a distribution consistent with organized dog fighting.

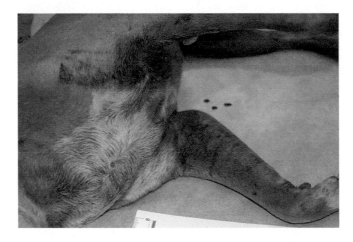

Figure 23.4 Typical organized dog-fighting wounds are typically clustered on the front and underside of the dog. Linear wounds encircling the limbs are consistent with the bitten dog pulling their leg out of the mouth of the biting dog. Dogs that have been trained to fight will bite, hold on and tear, causing significantly more trauma than can initially be seen from the exterior of the dog.

plywood A-frames to which the roosters are tethered. In dog fighting, both female and male dogs are subjected to fights; in cock, finch, betta fish and horse fighting, only males will engage in the agonistic behaviors, and for some species, only in the presence of a female of the species. Some small bird fighting cages are specifically designed with an attached chamber for a female bird to be contained in, to incentivize the male fighting birds.

Scene Documentation and Evidence Collection

Items that can be found at a dog fighting scene include the "pit," generally constructed of plywood walls and a carpet floor. The walls and floor of the pit may be heavily contaminated with blood and saliva evidence. The distribution of blood evidence may include spatter from tail whips and ear shakes, transfer from body rubs, arterial spurting or expectorated (coughed) blood. There may be paw prints or nose prints in blood on the pit walls, as well as claw marks. The carpet may be heavily saturated with blood. Dogs may salivate heavily while being restrained before the fight, and there may be drool marks on dividers or walls. Samples from discrete blood droplets may be taken for DNA to match with seized victim dogs, which can be cheek-swabbed.

These samples must go to a veterinary genetics laboratory for analysis as human crime labs lack the appropriate primers. It is advisable to use an International Standards Organization and International Electrotechnical Commission (ISO/IEC) accredited laboratory; this accreditation is issued by the American National Standards Institute's (ANSI) National Accreditation Board (ANAB). Accreditation assures that the laboratory is committed to a rigorous quality program that promotes acceptance of test results in legal proceedings.

At a fighting scene, there may also be wash tubs and sponges for washing the dogs prior to a match. Depending on the prevailing rules, trainers may swap dogs to wash any possible caustic materials off the opponent before beginning the fight. There may be breeding records or fight records with championship histories, scales to weigh the dogs, wound treatments and surgical equipment, medications, vitamins and performance-enhancing drugs.

Chickens are also fought in pits, and there will be gaffs (blades that are affixed to the roosters' legs with leather, twine, or other strap or cord materials), scales and carriers for transporting the birds. In cockfights, it is more frequent that the birds fight to the death, and there may be a large pile of discarded birds or significant amounts of bones from carcasses.

At training sites, there may be slat or carpet mills (homemade treadmills), jennys (devices used to space dogs and keep them running in circles), weights for strength training (usually hung around the neck on chains), spring poles (a "tug of war" device that the dog will jump off the ground to grasp and hold on to a cloth or toy to strengthen jaw muscles and encourage "bite, hold and tear" behaviors) and kennels. Fighting birds are trained with boxing glove-type implements instead of blades so that they will survive training bouts.

Clinical and Postmortem Exam Findings

Typical injuries to staged dog fighting victims include a pattern of abrasions, puncture wounds and scars on the front legs, chest, neck and face. Wounds may be anywhere on the body, but they tend to be more prominent at the front of the dog. Some lacerations may be present on the front legs from a dog twisting their leg out of the bite of another dog. These wounds may be so deep as to scar the bones. Dogs may be missing chunks of facial tissue. There can be significant tissue under the skin from crush injuries, and the bite wounds may be significantly worse than they appear on the surface.

Bite wounds are crush injuries that include punctures from individual teeth. Circular lesions may mimic gunshot or pellet wounds, but on closer inspection, tissue bridges may be appreciated. Tissue bridges are strands of nerves or blood vessels that transverse the wounds. These tissue bridges do not appear as a feature of projectile wounds. Gastric contents may include ingested tissue from other dogs, including furred skin, fur, ears or lips.

If dogs have survived a fight, but sustained substantial injuries, they may have significant blood loss or infection that can become life-threatening if untreated. The crushed muscle tissue releases myoglobin, a protein that can clog the kidneys and cause acute kidney failure. Dogs may also succumb to shock hours after a fight.

Fighting birds may have wounds or scars to the chest, wings, neck and face, particularly around the eyes. There may be linear marks on bones from the gaff injuries. Birds may have bands on their legs with a numbering system that correlates to records.

Various tissues and body fluids can be collected from the living or deceased animal by a veterinarian for analysis by a toxicology laboratory for performance-enhancing substances such as anabolic steroids, methamphetamines, cocaine and epinephrine.

Canine "CODIS"

The University of California Davis Veterinary Genetics Diagnostic Laboratory maintains a Combined DNA Index System ("Canine CODIS") database with individual DNA profiles from dogs that have been seized during dog fighting investigations as well as profiles from unknown samples collected at suspected dog fighting venues. The DNA reference materials are used to identify relationships between dogs and thereby allow investigators to expand their investigations to those who breed and train dogs for fighting, sometimes across state lines.

Final Thoughts

Animal fighting is a brutal crime that inflicts painful injuries to animals. The offense is often accompanied by other violent criminal activities. Animal fighting desensitizes children and adults in attendance to violence and causes social harm.

Animal fighting ventures are often complex, clandestine and difficult to penetrate. Investigators must plan for safety and the extraction of large numbers of animals. While fighting animals are usually trained to be aggressive to other animals and gentle with people, this isn't always the case and due caution must be exercised at all times.

Bibliography

Intarapanich NP, Touroo RM, Rozanski EA, Reisman RW, Intarapanich PP, McCobb EC. Characterization and comparison of injuries caused by spontaneous versus organized dogfighting. *Journal of the American Veterinary Medical Association.* 2016;251, doi: 10.2460/javma.251.12.1424.

Lockwood R. 2011. *Dogfighting Tool Kit for Law Enforcement: Addressing Dogfighting in Your Community.* Washington, DC: Community Oriented Policing Services, U.S. Department of Justice, pp. 8–20.

Merck M. 2013. Animal fighting. In *Veterinary Forensics: Animal Cruelty Investigations,* 2nd Edition. Merck M (Ed.). Ames, IA: Wiley-Blackwell, pp. 243–254.

UC Davis. Using a CODIS (Combined DNA Index System) to fight dog fighting. Veterinary Genetics Laboratory. https://vgl.ucdavis.edu/forensics/canine-codis.

Forensic Toxicology 24

MARTHA SMITH-BLACKMORE

Fundamentals of Toxicology and Poisoning

Poison is a substance that can cause death or illness in living organisms by chemical action. Malicious poisoning of animals is a deliberate act, most commonly done by delivering a toxic substance in a bait (in tempting food, for example). Accidental poisonings are much more common than deliberate poisonings, as animals will often ingest whatever they might be able to access, or they may become contaminated with toxins they encounter in the environment. Environmental contamination with a toxin may be a criminal or civil matter, depending on the circumstances and prevailing laws. Poisonings may be a regulatory issue if the food supply has been contaminated, or a civil matter for insurance litigation.

Toxicology is the study of the adverse effects of substances on biological systems. When poisoning of animals is suspected, forensic toxicologists may perform tests to document the presence of toxins or poisons in trace or minute amounts. These traces may be detected in collected tissues, body fluids or from environments where poisoning is suspected.

Poisonings may be accomplished by a single overwhelming dose that causes immediate death, or from repeated small doses that accumulate over time. As a criminal matter, poisoning is not specifically mentioned in many state animal cruelty laws; however, it is covered by broad language of "injury" or "harm". When developing the crime scene search strategy, some information regarding the case will be known, but regardless, the search must be conducted with an open mind to all possible evidence; when using the information, it is critical to ensure it is as accurate and objective as possible. Searching with preconceived notions about the evidence that will be of use introduces bias to the search and could ultimately hinder the success of the investigation.

Malicious poisonings have been estimated to account for less than 0.5% of all potential cases of animal poisoning reported to animal poison control centers. Common accidental exposures are to prescription drugs, over-the-counter medications, substances of abuse, xylitol (a sweetener found in some sugar-free gum and lower calorie foods), mushrooms and ethylene glycol (antifreeze, as an accidental spill). Some outbreaks of viral disease, especially in an unvaccinated population, can cause a die-off that is first misinterpreted as a poisoning event.

DOI: 10.4324/9781003090762-24

Dogs and chickens used for organized animal fighting may be subject to the use of substances that the animal fighter believes will have performance-enhancing qualities, such as cocaine, methamphetamine, testosterone and other substances. Racing commissions will routinely test racing horses and racing dogs for performance-enhancing drugs. Animal sexual abusers may manipulate their victims with drugs or other substances to facilitate compliance with activities. The use of substances in these cases may have an unintended but still illegal toxic outcome for the animal.

In malicious poisonings, the toxin used varies on what is available or accessible to the poisoner. The most common poisons used deliberately on animals are ethylene glycol, insecticides and rodenticides (anticoagulant and strychnine), while herbicides, heavy metals, household products and pharmaceutical substances have also been used. Dogs are most commonly the target of deliberate poisonings, followed by cats, horses, livestock, exotic animals and wildlife. The oral route is most common, but toxic substances can be inhaled, injected or absorbed across the skin. The poisoners may act in a targeted fashion, with the intent to harm specific animals, or they may maliciously scatter tainted bait in a public setting, with the intent to harm a population of animals.

Indications

The finding of multiple animals suddenly dead, especially animals of a variety of species, around a common food or water source should raise the index of suspicion of an intoxicant, either accidental or deliberate. In enclosed spaces, the investigator must be wary of hazardous accumulations of gasses, such as carbon monoxide, which is odorless and colorless. Additionally, occurrences such as die offs from algal blooms or botulism in stagnant water may cause sudden, unexpected or multiple deaths.

A poison causes negative effects on the body by damaging normal chemical reactions. If a poisoning has occurred, it is possible that the source of the poison or traces of the poison will be found at the scene. Additionally, traces of the poison may be detected in fluid or tissues of the affected animal(s). Body fluids commonly collected at necropsy for analysis include urine, blood, stomach contents, vitreous humor and bile. Tissues to be collected include liver, kidney, lung, brain and adipose tissue (fat).

In cases of deliberate poisoning, there may be multiple scenes, such as where the victim was found, where the poison was procured, prepared, administered and where residual matter may have been disposed of. Motivations for poisoning may be diverse and obscure. Poisoners may not like the animal or species, they may be annoyed by barking or other animal behaviors they consider to be a nuisance, they may have a vendetta with the animal's owner or they may act out of pure sadism. Some cases have been identified as akin to Munchausen's by proxy, where an owner is deliberately poisoning their own animal for attention or for some other perverse motivation. A suicidal owner may seek to kill their own pets in advance of a planned suicide. An owner may commit "iatrogenic intoxication" by using human medication on an animal, not knowing of the toxic effects.

Interviews and Scene Documentation

The behavior of the poisoned animal will vary, depending on the substance used. It is important to interview the owner or caretaker about their feeding practices, where the food is kept, how it is fed, etc. The owner or caretaker should be asked about previous veterinary care, vaccinations and episodes of illness and where the animal has access or has been walked. Any witnesses to the animal's onset and progress of illness should be interviewed for a time-line and observed behaviors of the affected animal(s). Common symptoms of some types of poisoning include "SLUDGE" signs: salivation (drooling), lacrimation (tearing/watery eyes), urination, defecation, gastrointestinal disturbances and excitement. Other significant signs include nervousness, anxiety, hyperactivity, dilated pupils, hypothermia (low body temperature), hyperthermia (high body temperature, perhaps marked by excessive pant-ing), difficulty breathing, tremors, twitches and seizures.

Traces of toxin may be found in bait such as hot dog segments, or scat-tered birdseed. As in any suspected crime scene, the environment and spe-cific findings should be documented through photography (overall to close) before collecting evidence.

Sample Collection

Possible containers, food bowls and wrappers should be collected from the environment. Bear in mind that a wrapper may have fingerprint evidence or DNA evidence linking to a suspect, as well as trace amounts of poisons. Food and water samples, vomit, feces and urine may be collected if left on a surface that allows collection. Rodenticides may be in a treated substrate, looking like brightly colored (usually blue or green) bird seed or pellets. Any fine matter should be carefully collected into a pharmaceutical fold following standard collection techniques.

Various tissues and body fluids can be collected from the living or deceased animal by a veterinarian for analysis by a toxicology laboratory. Other indicators of poisoning a veterinarian might note include irritated tis-sues (nasal planum, foot pads, oral cavity, esophagus or stomach tissues) or other characteristic findings (e.g., cyanide gives off an almond-like odor and

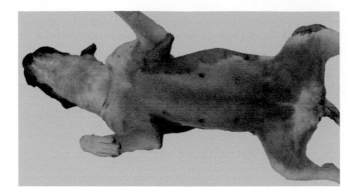

Figure 24.1 Cherry red tissue color changes in a dog suspected to be killed by cyanide poisoning.

causes a "cherry red" tissue color change (Figure 24.1); acetaminophen causes a brick red to blue change of color to the mucous membranes) .

Additionally, gastric contents may include wrappers, visible bits of toxic materials or other evidence that can provide linkage to a suspect, scene or material used. The veterinarian should confer with the forensic toxicologist, if possible, on amounts of tissues to collect, how to preserve and ship. In all cases, chain of custody documentation should be generated to move with the samples and document points of transfer until ultimate analysis (Figure 24.2).

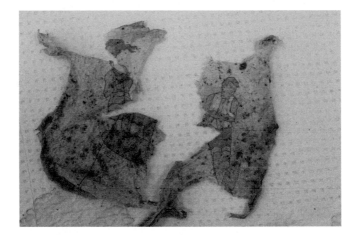

Figure 24.2 Paper towel with a distinctive pattern was found in the stomach of the dog. The owner did not have this type of paper towel, and another person had threatened to kill the dog with cyanide. No cyanide was detected in tissue and stomach content sampling;. This is not unusual for cyanide as it "off gasses", and it may not be detectable after a period of time. This patient had been frozen and thawed prior to necropsy, and the necropsy was delayed by several days.

Sample Analysis

The careful examination of scenes and collection of evidence will deliver samples to be analyzed by a forensic toxicologist. There is no single test to detect all poisons, and thousands of compounds may be used as a poison. There may be a limited amount of material available for testing, or limited financial resources to pay for testing. Information gathered from the scene investigation and findings related to the animals will help to narrow the list of tests to request.

The forensic toxicologist may be able to detect and document a substance or substances present, they may be able to opine on the volume ingested and they can detail the effects of the toxins on various biochemical processes. The veterinarian will be able to opine on pain and suffering endured by the animal based on viewing any available footage, reviewing witness statements of animal behavior before death and due to the findings on postmortem exam.

Final Thoughts

Depending on the resources of the investigating agency and the particulars of the case, samples collected may be submitted to the city or state crime lab, the FBI lab or a private forensic toxicology laboratory. In cases where animals have been harmed, it is appropriate to involve a veterinarian to document the signs the animals exhibit and to assist in sample collection.

Bibliography

ASPCA. Poison control top 10 toxins of 2019. https://www.aspca.org/news/announcing-top-10-pet-toxins.

Dinovo EC, Cravey RH. Forensic toxicology in death investigation. https://www.ojp.gov/pdffiles1/Digitization/44096NCJRS.pdf.

Gwaltney-Brant SM. Veterinary forensic toxicology. *Veterinary Pathology*. 2016;53(5):1067–1077. doi: 10.1177/0300985816641994. https://journals.sagepub.com/doi/full/10.1177/0300985816641994

Trestrail JH. 2007. *Criminal Positioning: Investigational Guide for Law Enforcement, Toxicologists, Forensic Scientists, and Attorneys. Criminal Positioning.* Springer. https://www.springer.com/gp/book/9781588298218.

Report Writing and Court Testimony

25

VIRGINIA M. MAXWELL AND
MARTHA SMITH-BLACKMORE

Introduction

The diligent work of the crime scene investigators and veterinarians is ultimately reduced into a written report. This report is retained in case files and distributed to the relevant parties involved in a case, such as attorneys and lead investigators or unit heads. Though it will be seen that a lot of information contained in a report duplicates other forms of documentation such as scene photographs and videos, all forms of documentation are necessary and complement each other. A report should not simply refer the reader to a photograph to understand the size of contents of a room, but it should also describe it and mention the major objects contained in it, especially those where evidence was located. This report will form the basis of courtroom testimony by the submitting investigator, examiner or veterinarian.

Many agencies will have a specified report format that must be followed, while others may offer a less formulaic approach, though all will ultimately provide the same information. Veterinary medical records and necropsy reports may also vary in their format depending on veterinarian preference, training and experience. Summary reports, written in simple lay terms, are helpful to convey the totality of animal suffering to the court. Some forensic veterinarians chose to illustrate these reports with selected annotated photographs that are representative of the conditions that affected the animals. All notes, reports, diagrams, sketches, photographs, interviews and other materials considered while composing the summary report must be listed and made available for examination. This chapter discusses the general approach to writing a comprehensive report from both the crime scene and veterinary viewpoint.

Crime Scene Reports

Regardless of whether a specified format for the crime scene report is required by an agency, all crime scene reports must present similar information and are best broken down into different sections for clarity.

DOI: 10.4324/9781003090762-25

1. Section 1: General case information

   The information that should be at the start of a report includes the case number, lead investigator, scene location, incident type, victim information, suspect information, date/time of initial incident report, date/time of scene processing (both start and completion) and date of report writing. This section can also include additional general information such as weather conditions or further important information about the scene.

2. Section 2: Body of report

   After providing the important identifying information about the case and crime scene, this section is a narrative that describes the initial actions and provides a detailed description of the scene but stops short of the specific evidence and actions in regard to that. The early part of this section will cover the initial report of an incident, the information received and initial scene briefings. It then addresses issues related to the search warrant and any justification for why a warrantless search was appropriate. Beyond the search legality, consent for the removal of any live animals should be included along with the determination of legal ownership that allowed consent to be obtained from a specific person. Any plan developed for removal, veterinary care and housing of seized animals can be included.

   Once these topics have been covered, the scene itself is described in detail, including any measurements and room dimensions. While the evidence itself is not covered in this section, any item where evidence was located, such as a dog crate, should be included along with relevant measurements and placement in a location. In animal cruelty cases, excuses are often made as to how animals received injuries, for example, blunt force trauma may be attributed to a fall down some stairs rather than a blow from a weapon. With this in mind, the measurements, heights and location of relevant objects should be included.

   Having described the scene in detail, the report must now address all the evidence located and the actions that were taken regarding each piece of evidence. This will include any interaction with ALS, any screening tests, with results, how the evidence was collected and packaged, and its disposition at the scene. Any measurements that relate to the items of evidence or its location should be included. If circumstances require that any actions vary from typical scene procedures, for example, if the weather forces an outdoor scene to progress in a different order, then this should be addressed with the reason for the deviation from standard procedure clearly articulated.

   If any findings at the scene lead to a new scene, this must be explained in the report though a separate report must be generated for the next scene.

3. Section 3: Evidence collected

Once the narrative sections of the report are complete, providing a complete listing of the evidence collected is a useful reference section over and above the discussion of each item of evidence in the report body. The inventory of evidence in the report includes the assigned number, description of the evidence (including any measurements if they were not in the report body), location, packaging and the disposition, for example, "evidence room" or "submitted to laboratory".

4. Section 4: Latent print evidence

Some investigators include a separate section in their report that lists the evidence that was processed for latent prints. This is also a useful reference section that complements the report body which will also include these items along with all other observations and evidence. If included, this section would provide the evidence number, description, latent print processing method and whether identifiable prints were developed.

When multiple scenes exist in the same case, each scene should have a separate report. In these cases, investigators must ensure that evidence numbers are not inadvertently duplicated in different scenes. Reports are usually written by the lead investigator, or a designee with firsthand knowledge of the scene; thus, if a secondary scene is developed and processed contiguously, responsibility for that scene report must be assigned to one of the investigators at that scene.

Veterinary Reports

The report written by the veterinarian is for the purposes of helping the criminal justice system understand what the veterinarian knows or believes to be likely, based on their professional opinion. The report is more than the veterinary medical record or notes; it should be written in a clear lay language so that it can be understood by other investigators, attorneys, judges and others involved in the judicial process who may lack knowledge of medical and veterinary terminology.

The report should include the veterinarian's name, the name of the practice or facility where they work, and a brief synopsis of how they became involved in the case. Similar to the investigator's report, the veterinarian's report should include the basic information related to the case as listed in Section 1.

The veterinary report serves to convey an understanding of what the veterinarian did (e.g., physical exam or necropsy, laboratory and imaging tests), what diagnoses were made and what conclusions were drawn, based on this information. The veterinarian should list all materials reviewed in advance of producing the report such as scene photos, narrative reports and witness accounts.

The report should conclude with the veterinarian's professional opinion as to whether the animal's condition is consistent with natural disease, accidental injury or nonaccidental injury and why.

Trial Testimony

In the absence of a plea or any other pretrial disposition of a case, the final stage is a trial. During a trial, both the prosecution and defense present a variety of witnesses to provide testimony regarding the incident in question, including investigators and veterinarians. The specific roles of investigators and veterinarians in court proceedings may vary as veterinarians may not always have been present at the crime scene nor had the opportunity to examine the animal victim, living or dead. If the veterinarian did perform an exam, they may serve as both fact and expert witnesses.

A veterinarian who did not perform an exam on an animal, but rather reviewed documents and work done by other professionals and veterinarians, serves as an expert witness only and if the judge admits the witness as an expert. Rules of evidence allow expert witnesses to testify in the form of an opinion, provided their opinion is based on scientific, technical or other specialized knowledge that will help the trier of the fact to understand the evidence or to determine a fact in issue. The testimony must be based on sufficient facts or data.

If providing testimony for the prosecution, a veterinarian should submit their resume or CV and prepare for trial in a meeting with the prosecutor. Pretrial meetings serve to review findings and opinion and determine what questions will be asked, in what order.

Veterinarians can help attorneys develop predicate questions. These questions help lay the foundation for the veterinarian to be admitted as an expert witness. Typical questions include: What is your occupation/profession and educational background? What degrees, certificates or licenses do you have? Have you attended or conducted continuing education seminars, conferences and related training? Are you a member in any professional organizations/societies? Have you received any awards or other professional recognition? Have you published articles in your field? How many cases involving [animals of this species] have you examined? How many years have you worked in this field? Once a judge makes the determination that a veterinarian may serve as an expert witness, testimony via direct examination and cross-examination may begin.

Direct and Cross-Examination

During a trial, the prosecutor will ask witnesses' questions about what they saw, did or know about a case, and when the witness is an expert witness, they will also ask questions about their opinion and how it was formed. This is called direct examination. In direct examination, attorneys are generally not allowed to ask leading questions.

Following direct examination, the defense attorney has the opportunity to ask questions of the witness to test or challenge the credibility of what was said or the opinions that have been formed and expressed. If acting as a witness for the defense, the prosecutor will cross-examine the witness. Whichever attorney has called the witness will be the direct examiner, to be followed by a cross from the opposing side. The cross-examining attorney is permitted to ask leading questions.

Credibility is the most important aspect for the witness. Answers should be concise and address the content of the question. Be sure to listen to the entire question. It is appropriate to pause before answering, think about the question and answer. During this pause, an attorney may object to a question, and the judge may agree, in which case the answer to the question is moot. If the question is multipart, or confusing, you may ask for the question to be rephrased. The witness does not argue a case; that is the attorney's job.

Think before you answer; if you do not recall, say so. If counsel asks a question you do not understand, or asks a question with multiple parts, ask them to repeat the question one part at a time, or to reword the question. Do not answer unless you are absolutely sure what the question is. Don't accept facts stated by opposing counsel if you do not know the fact to be true. Don't try to figure out why a particular question is being asked. Sometimes, questions are asked just to stall for time while the attorney is thinking about what their next question might be. It goes without saying that you should always tell the truth. You may ask the judge for permission to reference your notes before answering. Don't allow yourself to be drawn into an argument, and know that if the attorney is becoming emotional or aggressive, it is because you are doing a good job and your testimony is frustrating to them. Beware the very friendly cross-examination – they may be trying to lure you down a head-nodding path of agreeing with them. Pay attention, be cooperative and take your time. Know that the judge or jury want to hear what you have to say because they want to understand the veterinarian's perspective.

If you misspeak, correct your inaccuracy. If you are asked why you didn't do a particular test, a useful response (if correct) is "because I didn't think it was necessary". If you are being pushed to answer a question with a "yes" or "no" only, and you can't, respond that you can only answer the question with an explanation. If the interrogator interrupts your answer, it may be because they do not want your answer to be entered into the record – ask the judge for permission to finish your answer. Look at the person who is asking you the question while they are asking it, and then turn to address the judge or the jury with your answer as they are the ones who need to hear and understand your answer. After cross-examination, the initial attorney has an opportunity to re-direct or ask some clarifying or follow-up questions.

If you are thirsty, you can ask for water. If you are tired or unwell, you can ask for a recess. At all times, be truthful, polite and cooperative. The role of the witness is to illuminate the truth; the goal of a trial is to find the truth, not to achieve a conviction. If there is a guilty finding, the sentencing may occur at the trial or in a separate proceeding.

Final Thoughts

Whether in a crime scene report or a veterinary report, it is important to avoid the use of either subjective or ambiguous terms. In the same vein, testimony should be accurate and unbiased; it is not the role of the expert witness to determine the guilt or innocence of a defendant no matter how heinous the case is. The role of the investigator or veterinarian is to provide the facts, or related opinion, from which the judge or jury will make their decision. This appropriately fulfills the roles of criminal investigator and forensic veterinarian in providing evidence in cases of animal maltreatment.

Appendix A
Evidence Collection and Packaging Summary

Evidence Type	Collection	Packaging	Labeling Notes	Miscellaneous
Chemical Evidence				
Accelerants	Debris should be placed into container until no more than half full. Liquid samples should be decanted or pipetted into glass jars.	Clean unused, metal paint cans or glass jars with metal lids.	Ensure location of sample is stated on label.	Do not use plastic to package evidence, including plastic bags or containers and lids with plastic coatings. Ensure lids of glass jars are not coated.
Acids	Decant from larger container. Sample pooled liquid with plastic pipette.	Glass bottle and plastic cap. Cushion bottle with packing material. Hydrofluoric acid must be in a plastic bottle.	Label as "ACIDS, GLASS, CORROSIVE" in addition to normal labels.	A sample approximately 1 mL in volume is sufficient for analysis. Safety glasses are highly recommended.
Alkali/bases	Decant from larger container. Sample pooled liquid with plastic pipette. Use clean wood or plastic spatula to obtain solid samples.	Glass bottle and plastic cap for liquid samples, glass or plastic vial with plastic top for solid samples.	Label as "ALKALI, GLASS, CORROSIVE" in addition to normal labels.	Includes bleach, ammonia and caustic soda. Safety glasses are highly recommended.

(Continued)

Evidence Type	Collection	Packaging	Labeling Notes	Miscellaneous
Explosives/ firecrackers	Live explosives – call for assistance. Debris – collect as much as possible.	Debris should be packaged in glass container with no plastic liner.	Clearly label as explosive material.	
Lubricants	Obtain sample using clean gauze or swab.	Clean glass or plastic vial.		Lubricants may include condom lubricants in sexual assault cases or ordinate from oils and greases.
Firearms and Ammunition				
Live ammunition	Collect all available rounds.	Cushion within outer container using cotton wool or gauze to prevent movement, contact and marking. Outer container should be cardboard, wood or plastic.	State live ammunition and number of rounds.	Mark with investigator initials on the side of cartridge case.
Spent ammunition	Collect all available pieces, including fragments.	Cushion within outer container using cotton wool or gauze to prevent movement, contact and marking. Outer container should be cardboard, wood or plastic.		Mark with investigator initials on the base of bullet or side of cartridge case to preserve striations. Do not attempt to remove any material on the spent ammunition of fragments.

(Continued)

Evidence Type	Collection	Packaging	Labeling Notes	Miscellaneous
Firearms	Unload firearm and check chamber of semiautomatic. Note the position of all rounds in a revolver before removing and which is aligned with the barrel. Never insert any object into the barrel.	Attach tag and package in cardboard box. Live rounds may be placed in bag or envelope in box. Secure firearm to prevent movement in packaging.	Clearly identify contents on packaging and indicate direction of the barrel. Verify firearm is unloaded and clearly indicate this on packaging.	Document serial number, if visible. Firearms recovered from water should be kept from drying out.

Biological Evidence

Evidence Type	Collection	Packaging	Labeling Notes	Miscellaneous
Dried samples and stains	If object cannot be seized, collect as much of the stain as possible by swabbing or cutting. Submit entire stained object when feasible.	Package in paper not plastic once evidence is dry.	Label as biohazard. Cleary indicates location from which swabbings or cuttings are taken.	Use the least number of swabs possible. Air dry swabs completely before packaging. Never package in plastic.
Stained fabric items	Submit entire item when possible. Items can include clothing, leashes, blankets, etc.	Items should be packaged separately after air-drying.	Label as biohazard.	Stain patterns may be important and can only be assessed when entire item is available. If cuttings must be taken, the location from which they were taken should be clearly indicated.

(*Continued*)

Evidence Type	Collection	Packaging	Labeling Notes	Miscellaneous
		Packaging must be paper or cardboard and items should not be able to move around in packaging. Place in cardboard box or paper bags, packed to prevent shifting of contents. Placing card inside a garment can help.		
Cigarette butts	Submit entire item.	Package in paper or cardboard box. Do not package in plastic.	Label as biohazard. State location of recovery.	
Cans, bottles or cups	Submit entire item if possible. Alternatively swab drinking area with moistened sterile swab.	Package in paper or cardboard, never in plastic. Allow swab to air dry before packaging.	Label as biohazard. Indicate location swabbed.	
Envelopes	Submit entire item.	Package in paper.		Keep dry
Condoms	Submit entire item.	Freeze in leak-proof container	Label as biohazard	Ensure that inner and outer surfaces of condom as not cross-contaminated through careless handling. Suspect DNA will be located in interior of condom while victim DNA may be recovered from the exterior.

(*Continued*)

Evidence Type	Collection	Packaging	Labeling Notes	Miscellaneous
Touch DNA	Submit entire item when possible. Alternatively swab area of interest with moistened sterile swab.	Package in paper or cardboard, never plastic.	Indicate location of swabbing.	If swabbing, consider locations that are unlikely to have multiple sources of DNA to avoid complex mixtures. If submission is not to determine the wearer of an item, indicate the area likely to have been touched by a suspect.
Bite marks	Gently swab bite mark with moistened sterile swab.	Package in paper or cardboard, never plastic.	Indicate the location of bite mark.	Avoid swabbing areas with blood.
Teeth/bones	Collect entire item.	If dry, package in paper/ cardboard. If moist, place into leak-proof container and freeze.	Label as biohazard. Indicate location of recovery.	If part of a set of unidentified remains, include veterinarian's report, if applicable. Molars and long bones are preferred for DNA analysis.
Feces	Collect entire sample.	Package in leak-proof container and freeze.		
Toxicology samples	Consult veterinarian			
Drugs and Poisons				
Liquids	Collect at least 15 mL if possible, preferably more.	If container cannot be sealed, transfer liquid contents to leak-proof container.	Label with type of contents and mark fragile, if appropriate.	Use minimum sample necessary for field tests. Note any field testing results.

(Continued)

Evidence Type	Collection	Packaging	Labeling Notes	Miscellaneous
Powders/tablets/capsules (Nonprescription)	Collect all material.	Package in leak-proof container. If latent prints or analysis of package are necessary, package material and packaging separately.	Label with type of contents.	Use minimum sample necessary for field tests. Note any field testing results.
Plant material	Collect all material. If conducting a field test, use the smallest amount possible.	Place fully dry material in any container and seal. Material that is not fully dry should be placed in a paper bag and sealed.	Show the type of material and origin, if known.	Weight is very important; therefore all material should be collected. Material that is not fully dry should be loosely packed. Note any field testing results.
Paraphernalia	Use leak-proof packaging to prevent loss of any sample present on items. Package any material in items separately, e.g., liquids, powders or plant material	Use appropriate rigid containers for needles, razor blades and other sharp objects. If objects are glass, use a rigid package and cushion item.	Mark needles as biohazard and all sharp objects with a sharps label.	
Prescription medication	Keep in original container.	Place tamper evidence seal on container.		Check individual, human or animal, on prescription and who prescribed the drug. Note how much remains in container. If original container is not available, Merck index can be sued to tentatively identify the material.

(Continued)

Evidence Type	Collection	Packaging	Labeling Notes	Miscellaneous
Documents				
Handwritten/ printed, typewritten	Use suitably sized envelope to hold unfolded documents.			
Typewriter	Use sturdy packaging. Do not attempt to produce typewriter samples unless directed to do so.	Package securely to prevent damage.	Include serial number, make and model of typewriter	Seize typewriter ribbon and submit for examination and evidence of questioned document contents.
Charred	Carefully place onto card reinforcement to protect from further damage.			
Trace Evidence				
Hairs	Unknown hairs should be picked with forceps. Known hair samples should be pulled with the root, never cut.	Place in druggist fold and then into secure outer package such as plastic bag or envelope.	Location should be specified. Source of known hairs should be clearly identified.	Hairs form the same item may be kept together UNLESS they are from the interior and exterior of a garment or item.
Fibers	Fibers should be picked when possible, but may also be tape-lifted from an item.	Place in druggist fold and then into secure outer package such as plastic bag or envelope.	Location of fibers or tape lifts should be specified.	Known fabric samples should be chosen carefully as different parts of garments, e.g., sleeve versus collar, may have differences in dyes, etc.

(Continued)

Evidence Type	Collection	Packaging	Labeling Notes	Miscellaneous
Paint	Paint chips may be picked with forceps. Tape lifting should be avoided. Known paint samples should be removed with clean single edge razor blades. Known samples should be taken from the area of interest.	Place in druggist fold and then into secure outer package such as plastic bag or envelope.	Origin of known paint samples should be specified.	Razor blades used to obtain paint samples may be included in the package, but the labeling should state this.
Glass	Glass fragments should be picked with forceps. Tape-lifting should be avoided.	Place in druggist fold and then into secure outer package such as plastic bag or envelope. Larger pieces of glass should be reinforced with cardboard to prevent further breakage.		When physical match is possible, all broken glass should be collected; otherwise a representative sample is sufficient.
Soil	Collect carriers of soil when possible. Collect discrete pieces of soil, never vacuum. Known samples should be collected from suspected point of origin; collect multiple known samples, packaged separately, when necessary.	Package dry soil in leak-proof container. Wet soil may be air-dried or packaged in leak-proof container and frozen.	Origin of known samples should be specified.	

(*Continued*)

Evidence Type	Collection	Packaging	Labeling Notes	Miscellaneous
Building materials	Collect representative sample.	Use box or paper bag, seal to prevent leakage.		
Tape	Gently stick tape to plastic backing, never card or paper. Do not stick adhesive sides together.			Tape can hold important DNA or fingerprint evidence, as well as trace evidence.
Fingerprints				
Nonporous items (glass, tile, metal, plastic, etc.)	Handle in areas where prints are not likely to be present such as textured areas and edges. Minimize handling.	Package in boxes or paper bags. Secure in a manner to prevent movement of the item and smearing of areas of prints.	Label container. Items may be tagged, or initials should be written in areas where prints are not suspected.	Gloves must be worn
Porous items (paper and cardboard, unfinished wood)	Handle carefully using gloved hands. Avoid areas where prints are suspected.	Package in paper.	Label container. Initial item in location away from suspected prints.	Gloves must be worn
Lifts	Lifts should be secured to an appropriate backing material such as coated card (some come with the backing attached).	Package in sealed envelope.	Each lift should be clearly labeled on reverse of backing.	Multiple lifts can be packaged in a single envelope. Lifts are best when latent prints are developed with black powder and a white backing is used.
Adhesive tape	Handle carefully to avoid gloves sticking to adhesive. Avoid allowing adhesive sides to stick together.	If no prints suspected on adhesive, then tape may be placed adhesive side down on a plastic surface such as a page protector.	Label container or small area of tape where no prints suspected.	Fingerprints can be present on both the adhesive and backing side. Prints on adhesive are usually patent in nature.

(Continued)

Evidence Type	Collection	Packaging	Labeling Notes	Miscellaneous
		This should be packaged to avoid rubbing of backing side on container smearing prints that may be present.		
		If prints could be present on both sides, then the tape should be carefully secured to the bottom of a cardboard box backing side down. The tape must be secured to prevent rubbing against the container.		
Wet or submerged items (e.g., weapons)	Items should be kept wet/ submerged and should not be allowed to dry.	Package in plastic containers with tight-fitting lids.	Initial and label container.	Container can contain water to ensure item remains wet. If item is submerged in water, use water from that location.

Imprints/Impressions/Tool marks

Evidence Type	Collection	Packaging	Labeling Notes	Miscellaneous
Lifted	Use gel lifters of appropriate size, cut down if necessary.	Package in envelopes (reinforce with card to prevent bending or folding).	State location of lift.	

(Continued)

Evidence Type	Collection	Packaging	Labeling Notes	Miscellaneous
Cast	Cast with dental stone or plaster of paris. Reinforce with wooden sticks or wire.	Package in strong cardboard box and cushion to protect if necessary. Only package when completely dry.	Initial back of cast. State location and type of cast (tire, footwear). Mark package as fragile.	Ensure evidence-quality photographs are obtained prior to casting. Dental stone is preferred over plaster of paris. Do not attempt to brush off debris or clean in any other way.

Appendix B
Nonveterinary
Crime Scene Kit

Note that this listing is quite comprehensive, and most scenes will not require all of the components as many for specialized use are included. However, investigators who respond to crime scenes regularly should keep a well-stocked kit of basic items available at all times and have the ability to gather the others as needed. As items are consumed, they should be replaced as soon as possible after scene processing is complete. Any rechargeable batteries, such as camera and flash batteries, should be recharged immediately after use and checked for charge regularly between scenes.

Documentation

Notepad (spiral bound at top is best)
Clipboard
Forms (may be agency-specific or investigator-generated)
Premade standard diagrams (e.g., vehicle exterior and interior, animal projections)
Graph paper (useful for sketching)
Pencils
Pens
Sharpies or other permanent markers
Eraser
Ruler

Evidence Location and Documentation

Evidence cones and placards (or stiff colored card stock to create placards)
Scales
  White
  Gray
  Black

L-shaped scales
Disposable adhesive scales
Alternate light sources
    UV for trace evidence and biological fluid
    IR for gunshot residue/sooting and injuries
High-intensity visible light source/flashlight
Tape measures (some in extra-long lengths)
Laser measure
Thermometer
GPS (most cell phones have this feature)

Evidence Collection and Packaging

Paper bags (assorted sizes)
Coin envelopes
Plastic evidence bags (assorted sizes)
Metal cans and lids
Ointment tins
Glass vials and jars (jars may be used with alcohol to collect insect
    evidence)
Pieces of card (to stabilize fragile samples)
Plastic specimen containers
Sharpie or permanent marker
Tamper evident evidence tape
Regular strong packing tape
Cardboard boxes (optional, but useful to have some available)
GSR kits
Sterile swabs
Cuticle sticks (fingernail or claw scrapings)
Glassine pouches
White paper pad (for druggist folds, 5″×7″ is a good size)
Unused page protectors
Phosphate buffered saline or distilled water
Scalpel handle with blades (disposable scalpels are available)
Single-edge razor blades
Box cutter with disposable blades
Forceps (disposable are available but a pair of fine-point metal forceps
    is useful)
Large and small scissors
Trowel (for soil samples)

Fingerprint and large-size lifters
Trace evidence lifting tape
Butcher paper roll
Alcohol wipes (to sanitize forceps)

Photography

Camera
    35 mm with interchangeable lenses is best
    Wide-angle lens
    Macro lens (for taking close-up and 1:1 photographs)
    Normal lens
    Telephoto lens

Extra memory cards (as many as possible)
External flash
Spare batteries (plus charger if applicable)
Lens wipes and other cleaning devices
Flood light
Filters (for documentation with alternate light sources)
Tripod (for low light or for perpendicular shots)
Level or plumb line (when shots must be perpendicular)

Screening Tests

Field screening tests for common drugs (as budget permits)
    Blood screening reagents (phenolphthalein, o-tolidine, trimethyl benzi-
dine or hemastix per agency policy or personal preference)
    RSID (as budget permits, note not all animal biological fluids work with
these)

Fingerprint Enhancement

Powders
    Black
    White
    Fluorescent
    Magnetic and nonmagnetic (depending on brush preference)

Brushes (investigator preference)
  Magnabrush
  Feather
  Camel hair
  Fiberglass

Fingerprint tape (different sizes)
Backing cards (white and black)
Fingerprint lifters
Portable superglue fumer or cartridges

Casting

Dental stone
Plaster of paris
Mixing bowl
Spatula
Molds
Mikrosil
Tongue depressors (mixing and stabilization of cast)
Plastic bags
Plastic weigh boats
Chicken wire pieces (stabilization of casts)

Trajectory Measurements

Colored strings
Tripod
Laser (if available)
Protractors (different sizes)
Rods

Personal protective equipment (PPE)

Disposable gloves (multiple boxes)
Disposable masks
Disposable booties
Disposable hairnet and beard coverings
Tyvec® suits
Safety glasses

Miscellaneous

Kimwipes
Hand wipes and sanitizer
Hand tools (at some scenes, it may be necessary to dismantle or remove
    fixtures)
Digging implements (if burials are a possibility)
Sifters
Paint brushes
Stakes
String
Tarp
Bleach and alcohol for sanitizing purposes (alcohol may also be used for
    insect collection)
Biohazard bags
Sharps containers
Garbage bags
Manilla folders
Duct tape

Appendix C
Example Veterinary Forensic Forms

The forms and checklists that follow may be useful for note taking during clinical and postmortem exams. These forms and checklists would be considered work-product and can be subpoenaed in a court case. They should be maintained as part of the case file. Worksheets should not be considered final work product, as a veterinarian should produce a summary report of their opinion on accidental, natural illness or non-accidental injury or death (or undetermined as appropriate). These forms are illustrative, and each organization may want to draft their own, with the guidance of their own legal counsel.

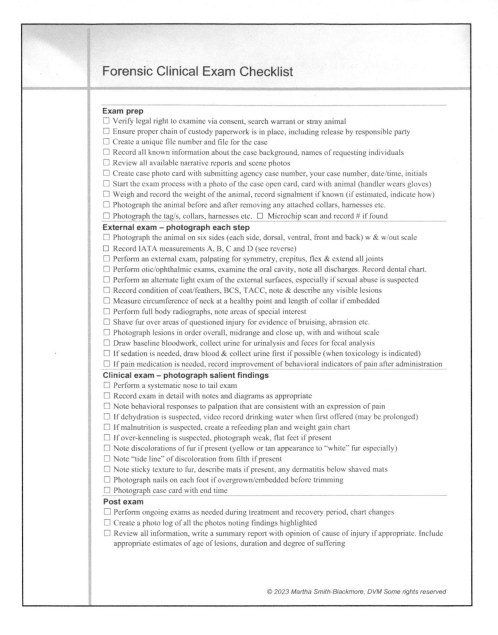

Forensic Clinical Exam Checklist

Exam prep
☐ Verify legal right to examine via consent, search warrant or stray animal
☐ Ensure proper chain of custody paperwork is in place, including release by responsible party
☐ Create a unique file number and file for the case
☐ Record all known information about the case background, names of requesting individuals
☐ Review all available narrative reports and scene photos
☐ Create case photo card with submitting agency case number, your case number, date/time, initials
☐ Start the exam process with a photo of the case open card, card with animal (handler wears gloves)
☐ Weigh and record the weight of the animal, record signalment if known (if estimated, indicate how)
☐ Photograph the animal before and after removing any attached collars, harnesses etc.
☐ Photograph the tag/s, collars, harnesses etc. ☐ Microchip scan and record # if found

External exam – photograph each step
☐ Photograph the animal on six sides (each side, dorsal, ventral, front and back) w & w/out scale
☐ Record IATA measurements A, B, C and D (see reverse)
☐ Perform an external exam, palpating for symmetry, crepitus, flex & extend all joints
☐ Perform otic/ophthalmic exams, examine the oral cavity, note all discharges. Record dental chart.
☐ Perform an alternate light exam of the external surfaces, especially if sexual abuse is suspected
☐ Record condition of coat/feathers, BCS, TACC, note & describe any visible lesions
☐ Measure circumference of neck at a healthy point and length of collar if embedded
☐ Perform full body radiographs, note areas of special interest
☐ Shave fur over areas of questioned injury for evidence of bruising, abrasion etc.
☐ Photograph lesions in order overall, midrange and close up, with and without scale
☐ Draw baseline bloodwork, collect urine for urinalysis and feces for fecal analysis
☐ If sedation is needed, draw blood & collect urine first if possible (when toxicology is indicated)
☐ If pain medication is needed, record improvement of behavioral indicators of pain after administration

Clinical exam – photograph salient findings
☐ Perform a systematic nose to tail exam
☐ Record exam in detail with notes and diagrams as appropriate
☐ Note behavioral responses to palpation that are consistent with an expression of pain
☐ If dehydration is suspected, video record drinking water when first offered (may be prolonged)
☐ If malnutrition is suspected, create a refeeding plan and weight gain chart
☐ If over-kenneling is suspected, photograph weak, flat feet if present
☐ Note discolorations of fur if present (yellow or tan appearance to "white" fur especially)
☐ Note "tide line" of discoloration from filth if present
☐ Note sticky texture to fur, describe mats if present, any dermatitis below shaved mats
☐ Photograph nails on each foot if overgrown/embedded before trimming
☐ Photograph case card with end time

Post exam
☐ Perform ongoing exams as needed during treatment and recovery period, chart changes
☐ Create a photo log of all the photos noting findings highlighted
☐ Review all information, write a summary report with opinion of cause of injury if appropriate. Include appropriate estimates of age of lesions, duration and degree of suffering

IATA measurements (a standardized scheme for measuring dogs)

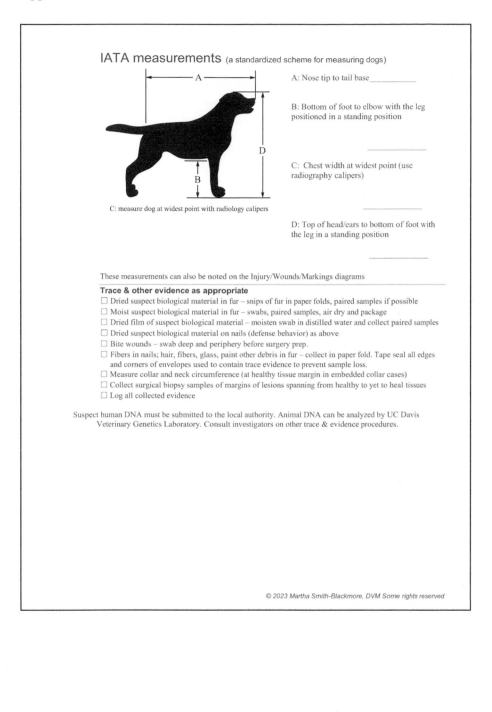

A: Nose tip to tail base_____

B: Bottom of foot to elbow with the leg positioned in a standing position

_____

C: Chest width at widest point (use radiography calipers)

_____

C: measure dog at widest point with radiology calipers

D: Top of head/ears to bottom of foot with the leg in a standing position

_____

These measurements can also be noted on the Injury/Wounds/Markings diagrams

Trace & other evidence as appropriate

☐ Dried suspect biological material in fur – snips of fur in paper folds, paired samples if possible

☐ Moist suspect biological material in fur – swabs, paired samples, air dry and package

☐ Dried film of suspect biological material – moisten swab in distilled water and collect paired samples

☐ Dried suspect biological material on nails (defense behavior) as above

☐ Bite wounds – swab deep and periphery before surgery prep.

☐ Fibers in nails; hair, fibers, glass, paint other debris in fur – collect in paper fold. Tape seal all edges and corners of envelopes used to contain trace evidence to prevent sample loss.

☐ Measure collar and neck circumference (at healthy tissue margin in embedded collar cases)

☐ Collect surgical biopsy samples of margins of lesions spanning from healthy to yet to heal tissues

☐ Log all collected evidence

Suspect human DNA must be submitted to the local authority. Animal DNA can be analyzed by UC Davis Veterinary Genetics Laboratory. Consult investigators on other trace & evidence procedures.

NECROPSY INTAKE CONSENT FORM

Examiner Case #: _____   Submitting entity case #_____

Submitting Officer: (Name/Town) _____

Address of incident: _____

Description of animal:_____

Owner's name/address (if known): _____

I understand that I am submitting the deceased animal described above to

_____for the purposes of a postmortem examination.
I understand that this necropsy exam will be thorough, and at the end of this
exam the animal's body will not be in a condition to be viewed. A postmortem
exam often determines the cause of death; however the exam does not
guarantee a diagnosis.

I understand if the cause of death appears to be from unnatural/non-
accidental causes, the suspicion of a crime will be reported to the appropriate
law enforcement department in the county, city or town where the incident is
suspected to have occurred (if law enforcement is not yet involved).

I understand if a crime is suspected to have occurred, the body should be
maintained as evidence for the duration of the judicial process. We are unable
to maintain frozen remains for a period of any longer than two weeks after the
conclusion of the postmortem exam.

By signing below, I certify that I am authorized to consent to a post-mortem
examination of this animal. I also agree that I will take possession of the frozen
remains within two weeks after the conclusion of the examination.

_____ Signed   Date_____

_____ Printed name

Forensic Necropsy Checklist

Necropsy prep
- ☐ Verify legal right to necropsy via consent, search warrant or found animal on public property
- ☐ Ensure proper chain of custody paperwork is in place, including release by responsible party
- ☐ Create a unique file number and file for the case
- ☐ Record all known information about the case background, names of requesting individuals
- ☐ Review all available narrative reports and scene photos
- ☐ Create case photo card with submitting agency case number, your case number, date/time, initials
- ☐ Start the necropsy process with a photo of the case open card, card with body bag (wear gloves)
- ☐ Photograph the tag/s, closure/s on the bag ☐ Microchip scan and record # if found
- ☐ Weigh and record the weight of the remains in the bag, record signalment if known
- ☐ Photograph the bag and remains as you enter the bag at each level

External exam – photograph each step
- ☐ Photograph the animal on six sides (each side, dorsal, ventral, front and back) w & w/out scale
- ☐ Record IATA measurements A, B, C and D (see reverse)
- ☐ Perform an external exam, palpating for symmetry, crepitus, flex & extend all joints
- ☐ Perform otic/ophthalmic exams, examine the oral cavity, note all discharges. Record dental chart.
- ☐ Perform an alternate light exam of the external surfaces, especially if sexual abuse is suspected
- ☐ Record condition of coat/feathers, BCS, TACC, note & describe any visible lesions
- ☐ Assess and describe general state of decomposition, note odor, staining of fur, material in fur etc
- ☐ Perform full body radiographs, note areas of special interest
- ☐ Shave the remains of fur, repeat all over photography with and without scales
- ☐ Number found lesions directly on the animal as appropriate with a permanent marker
- ☐ Photograph lesions in order overall, midrange and close up, with and without scale
- ☐ Describe lesion locations (distance from midline and other landmark) and size on note pages

Internal exam – photograph each step
- ☐ Reflect the skin and inspect the inner surface, paying special attention to areas with lesions
- ☐ Open and examine joints, open femur; preserve frozen bone marrow sample (starvation suspect)
- ☐ Left side down, open abdomen, note free fluids, feel diaphragm for negative pressure
- ☐ Open thorax, note fluids, photograph cavities before disrupting organs
- ☐ Examine each abdominal organ, describe & note findings, breadloaf solid organs, biopsy samples
- ☐ Open hollow organs, freeze ingesta (poisoning suspect), sieve/wash/describe stomach contents
- ☐ Describe, photograph lesions, parasites noted, save fecal sample for floatation (neglect cases)
- ☐ Estimate age based on dentition, eyes, body condition, joint condition, presence/absence of thymus, radiographs. Note intact vs. spayed/neutered
- ☐ Remove pluck, describe and sample organs. Open the heart, examine valves, chordae, papillae
- ☐ Remove & describe eyes
- ☐ Open skull, describe brain, breadloaf; open spinal column & remove cord if indicated
- ☐ Secure remains, retag and photograph
- ☐ Photograph case card with end time

Post necropsy
- ☐ Return bagged remains to storage (frozen, refrigerated or to submitting agency)
- ☐ Create a photo log of all the photos noting findings highlighted
- ☐ Review all information, write a summary report with opinion of death – natural, accidental, non-accidental, euthanasia, undetermined. Include appropriate estimates of age of lesions, duration and degree of suffering

IATA measurements (a standardized scheme for measuring dogs)

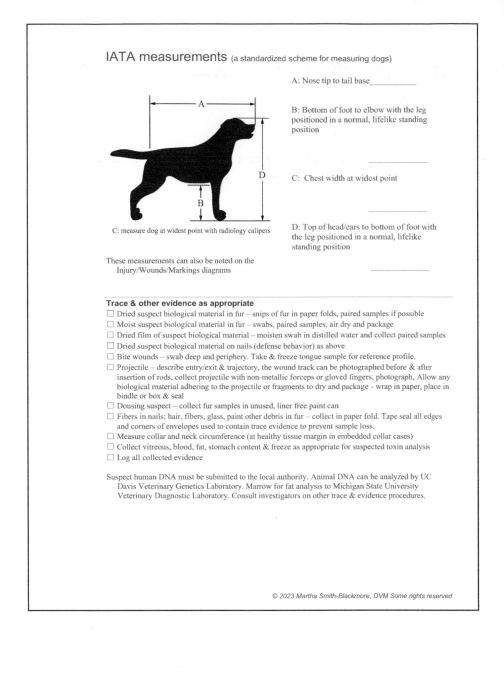

A: Nose tip to tail base_____

B: Bottom of foot to elbow with the leg positioned in a normal, lifelike standing position

_____

C: Chest width at widest point

_____

C: measure dog at widest point with radiology calipers

D: Top of head/ears to bottom of foot with the leg positioned in a normal, lifelike standing position

These measurements can also be noted on the Injury/Wounds/Markings diagrams

_____

Trace & other evidence as appropriate

☐ Dried suspect biological material in fur – snips of fur in paper folds, paired samples if possible
☐ Moist suspect biological material in fur – swabs, paired samples, air dry and package
☐ Dried film of suspect biological material – moisten swab in distilled water and collect paired samples
☐ Dried suspect biological material on nails (defense behavior) as above
☐ Bite wounds – swab deep and periphery. Take & freeze tongue sample for reference profile.
☐ Projectile – describe entry/exit & trajectory, the wound track can be photographed before & after insertion of rods, collect projectile with non-metallic forceps or gloved fingers, photograph, Allow any biological material adhering to the projectile or fragments to dry and package - wrap in paper, place in bindle or box & seal
☐ Dousing suspect – collect fur samples in unused, liner free paint can
☐ Fibers in nails; hair, fibers, glass, paint other debris in fur – collect in paper fold. Tape seal all edges and corners of envelopes used to contain trace evidence to prevent sample loss.
☐ Measure collar and neck circumference (at healthy tissue margin in embedded collar cases)
☐ Collect vitreous, blood, fat, stomach content & freeze as appropriate for suspected toxin analysis
☐ Log all collected evidence

Suspect human DNA must be submitted to the local authority. Animal DNA can be analyzed by UC Davis Veterinary Genetics Laboratory. Marrow for fat analysis to Michigan State University Veterinary Diagnostic Laboratory. Consult investigators on other trace & evidence procedures.

<u>**Gross Exam Worksheet - Necropsy**</u>

Examining DVM: Date & time: a.m. p.m.

GENERAL OBSERVATIONS: (Nutritional, physical care, signalment, state of decomposition)

Weight: _____ #/kg   Purina BCS _____ TACCS_____
Describe tissue abnormalities observed, color, texture, lesion distribution if seen.

EXTERNAL/SKIN: (haircoat, skin, pinna, feet, subcutaneous fat & subcutaneous bruising)

Separate sheet(s) attached for wound/injury and distribution: Yes   No

MUSCULOSKELETAL SYSTEM: (Bones, joints, ligaments, tendons, muscles)

Radiographs taken: Yes   No   **Microchip present:** Yes   No

                          Chip # if present & scanned_____

BODY CAVITIES: Fat stores, abnormal fluids, hydration (tissue moistness)

HEMOLYMPHATIC: (Spleen, lymph nodes, thymus)

RESPIRATORY SYSTEM: (Nasal cavity, larynx, trachea, lungs, bronchi, regional LNs)

CARDIOVASCULAR SYSTEM: (Heart, pericardium & great vessels)

1

Gross Exam Worksheet - Necropsy

Case #_____Date:_____ Examiner Initials_____

Describe tissue abnormalities observed, color, texture, lesion distribution if seen.

DIGESTIVE SYSTEM: (Oral structures, esophagus, stomach, GI tract, liver, gall bladder, pancreas, mesenteric lymph nodes)

GI contents_____

Collected: Yes No **Intestinal parasites observed?**   Yes   No

Feces submitted for ova and parasites? Yes No

URINARY SYSTEM: (Kidneys, ureters, urinary bladder, urethra)

REPRODUCTIVE SYSTEM: (Ovaries, uterus, vagina, mammary glands, placenta OR testes, scrotum, penis, prepuce, prostate)

ENDOCRINE SYSTEM: (Adrenals, thyroid, parathyroids, pituitary)

NERVOUS SYSTEM: (Brain, spinal cord & peripheral nerves)

SENSORY ORGANS: (Eyes, ears, nose, tongue)

LABORATORY STUDIES: (List tests submitted & results, if available)

2

Fixed Tissue Histology Checklist

Case #_____Date collected_____ Initials_____

Preserve tissues (no thicker than 1 cm) in 10 % buffered formalin, 1 part tissue to 10 parts formalin. Include sections of all lesions. Tissues collected below (check or circle).

__ **Salivary gland, Oral/pharyngeal mucosa, tonsil** - + any areas w/erosions, lesions.

__ **Tongue** - cross section near tip including both mucosal surfaces.

__ **Lung** - sections from several lobes including a major bronchus __ **Trachea**

__ **Thyroid/parathyroids**

__ **Lymph nodes** - cervical, mediastinal, bronchial, mesenteric, lumbar. Transect.

__ **Thymus** if present

__ **Heart** - Sections from both sides including valves

__ **Liver** - sections from 3 different areas including gall bladder

__ **Spleen** - Cross sections including capsule.

__ **GI Tract** - 3 cm long sections of: **Esophagus, Stomach** - multiple sections, **Intestines** - multiple sections from different areas
__ **Omentum** - ~3 cm square

__ **Pancreas** - sections from two areas

__ **Adrenals** - entire gland with transverse incision.

__ **Kidney** -cortex and medulla from each kidney

__ **Urinary bladder, ureters, urethra** – 2cm cross sections of each

__ **Reproductive tract** – Uterus, ovaries w/longitudinal cuts into lumens of horns. Both testes (trans cut) w/epididymis. Prostate transversely cut.
__ **Eye**

__ **Brain** - cut longitudinally along midline.

__ **Spinal cord** (if neurologic disease) - sections from cervical, thoracic and lumbar cord.

__ **Diaphragm and Skeletal muscle** - cross section of thigh muscles

__ **Opened rib or longitudinally sectioned femur** - marrow must be exposed for fixation

__ **Skin** - full thickness of abdominal skin, lip and ear pinna. If sampling a healing lesion or burn

include section from healthy tissue through healing edge into deepest area of wound

__ **Neonates: umbilical stump** - include surrounding tissues

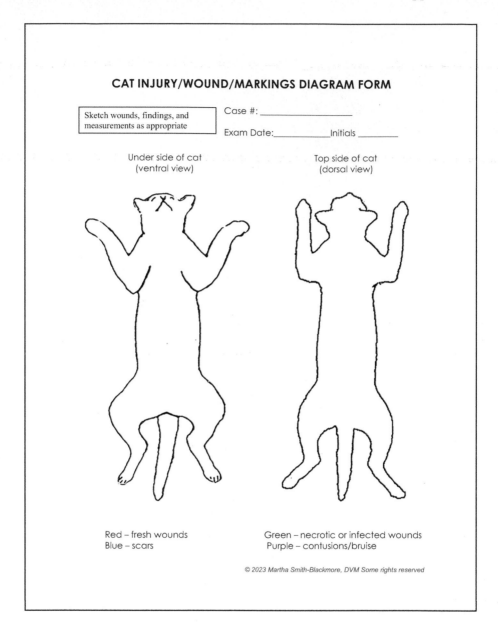

CAT INJURY/WOUND/MARKINGS DIAGRAM FORM

Sketch wounds, findings, and
measurements as appropriate

Case #: _____

Exam Date:_____Initials _____

Under side of cat
(ventral view)

Top side of cat
(dorsal view)

Red – fresh wounds
Blue – scars

Green – necrotic or infected wounds
Purple – contusions/bruise

Case #: _____ Exam Date:_____ Examiner's initials_____

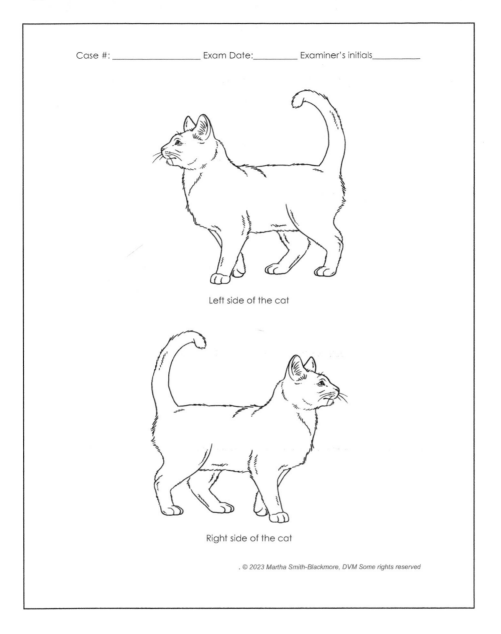

Left side of the cat

Right side of the cat

Case #: _____ Exam Date:_____ Examiner's initials_____

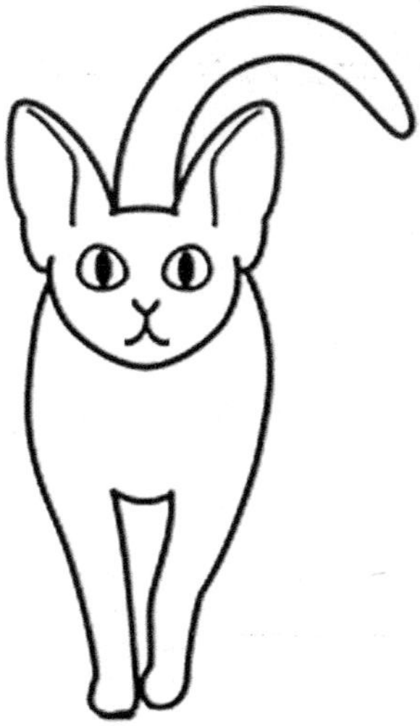

Front of cat 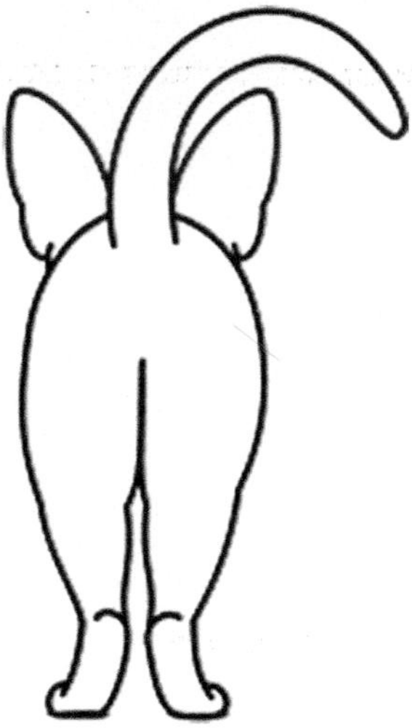   Rear of cat

Notes:_____

_____

_____

_____

Feline
BODY CONDITION/PHYSICAL/ENVIRONMENTAL/DECOMPOSITION SCORES

Case #_____   Date_____   Examiner initials _____

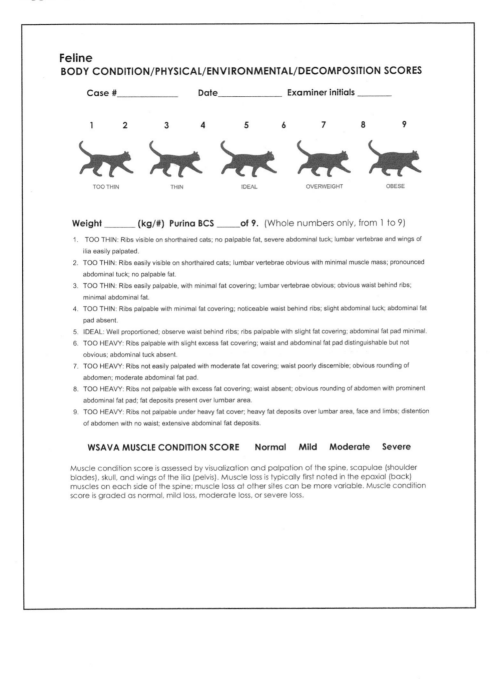

| 1 | 2 | 3 | 4 | 5 | 6 | 7 | 8 | 9 |

TOO THIN   THIN   IDEAL   OVERWEIGHT   OBESE

Weight _____ (kg/#) Purina BCS _____of 9. (Whole numbers only, from 1 to 9)

1. TOO THIN: Ribs visible on shorthaired cats; no palpable fat, severe abdominal tuck; lumbar vertebrae and wings of ilia easily palpated.
2. TOO THIN: Ribs easily visible on shorthaired cats; lumbar vertebrae obvious with minimal muscle mass; pronounced abdominal tuck; no palpable fat.
3. TOO THIN: Ribs easily palpable, with minimal fat covering; lumbar vertebrae obvious; obvious waist behind ribs; minimal abdominal fat.
4. TOO THIN: Ribs palpable with minimal fat covering; noticeable waist behind ribs; slight abdominal tuck; abdominal fat pad absent.
5. IDEAL: Well proportioned; observe waist behind ribs; ribs palpable with slight fat covering; abdominal fat pad minimal.
6. TOO HEAVY: Ribs palpable with slight excess fat covering; waist and abdominal fat pad distinguishable but not obvious; abdominal tuck absent.
7. TOO HEAVY: Ribs not easily palpated with moderate fat covering; waist poorly discernible; obvious rounding of abdomen; moderate abdominal fat pad.
8. TOO HEAVY: Ribs not palpable with excess fat covering; waist absent; obvious rounding of abdomen with prominent abdominal fat pad; fat deposits present over lumbar area.
9. TOO HEAVY: Ribs not palpable under heavy fat cover; heavy fat deposits over lumbar area, face and limbs; distention of abdomen with no waist; extensive abdominal fat deposits.

WSAVA MUSCLE CONDITION SCORE   Normal   Mild   Moderate   Severe

Muscle condition score is assessed by visualization and palpation of the spine, scapulae (shoulder blades), skull, and wings of the ilia (pelvis). Muscle loss is typically first noted in the epaxial (back) muscles on each side of the spine; muscle loss at other sites can be more variable. Muscle condition score is graded as normal, mild loss, moderate loss, or severe loss.

Case #: _____ Date:_____ Examiner's initials_____

TUFTS ANIMAL CARE AND CONDITION (TACC) Physical Care Score _____ of 5.

5 Terrible Extremely matted haircoat, prevents normal motion, interferes with vision, perineal areas irritated from soiling with trapped urine and feces. Hair coat essentially a single mat. Cat cannot be groomed without complete clipdown. Foreign material trapped in matted hair. Nails extremely overgrown, may be penetrating pads, causing pain and make normal walking very difficult or uncomfortable. Collar, if present, may be embedded in cat's neck.

4 Poor Substantial matting in haircoat, large chunks of hair matted together that cannot be separated with a comb or brush. Occasional foreign material embedded in mats. Much of the hair will need to be clipped to remove mats. Long nails force feet into abnormal position and interfere with normal gait. Perineal soiling or irritation likely. Collar, if present, may be extremely tight, abrading skin.

3 Borderline Numerous mats present in hair, but cat can still be groomed without a total clip down. No significant perineal soiling or irritation from waste caught in matted hair. Nails are overdue for a trim and long enough to cause cat to alter gait when he or she walks. Collar, if present, may be snug and rubbing off hair.

2 Lapsed Haircoat may be somewhat dirty or have a few mats present that are easily removed. Remainder of coat can easily be brushed or combed. Nails in need of a trim. Collar, if present, fits comfortably.

1 Adequate Clean, hair of normal length for the breed, and hair can easily be brushed or combed. Nails do not make contact with toe pads. Collar, if present, fits comfortably.

TUFTS ANIMAL CARE AND CONDITION (TACC) Environmental Health Scale _____ of 5.

5 Filthy Many days to weeks of accumulation of feces and / or urine. Overwhelming odor, air may be difficult to breathe. Large amount of trash, garbage, or debris present; inhibits comfortable rest, normal postures, or movement and / or poses a danger to the animal. Very difficult or impossible for animal to escape contact with feces, urine, mud, or standing water. Food and / or drinking water contaminated.

4 Very unsanitary Many days of accumulation of feces and / or urine. Difficult for animal to avoid contact with waste matter. Moderate amount of trash, garbage, or clutter present that may inhibit comfortable rest and/or movement of the animal. Potential injury from sharp edges or glass. Significant odor makes breathing unpleasant. Standing water or mud difficult to avoid.

3 Unsanitary Several days of accumulation of feces and urine in animal's environment. Animal is able to avoid contact with waste matter. Moderate odor present. Trash, garbage, and other debris cluttering animal's environment but does not prohibit comfortable rest or normal posture. Clutter may interfere with normal movement or allow cat to become entangled, but no sharp edges or broken glass that could injure cat. Cat able to avoid mud or water if present.

2 Marginal As in #1, except may be somewhat less sanitary. No more than 1-2 days' accumulation of feces and urine in animal's environment. Slight clutter may be present.

1 Acceptable Environment is dry and free of accumulated feces. No contamination of food or water. No debris or garbage present to clutter environment and inhibit comfortable rest, normal posture and range of movement or pose a danger to or entangle the animal.

"Environment" refers to the kennel, pen, yard, cage, barn, room, tie-out or other enclosure or area where the animal is confined or spends the majority of its time. All of the listed conditions do not need to be present in order to include a cat in a specific category. The user should determine which category best describes a particular cat's condition.

Case #: _____ Date:_____ Examiner's initials_____

FOR POSTMORTEM SPECIMENS:

☐ **Check if previously stored frozen and thawed for examination**

Fresh: no discoloration or insect activity, able to shave fur

Early decomposition: gray to green discoloration, bloating, post-bloating rupture, cannot shave due to skin slippage, hair loss

Advanced decomposition: moist decomposition of tissues, sagging of flesh, caving in of abdomen, extensive insect activity, bone exposure of less than half of the skeleton, mummification

Skeletonization: bones with some body fluids present or tissue covering less than half of the skeleton, dry bones

Extreme decomposition: skeletonization with bleaching or exfoliation or metaphyseal loss or cancellous exposure (6 months to >3 years)

Notes:_____

_____

_____

_____

_____

_____

_____

_____

_____

_____

_____

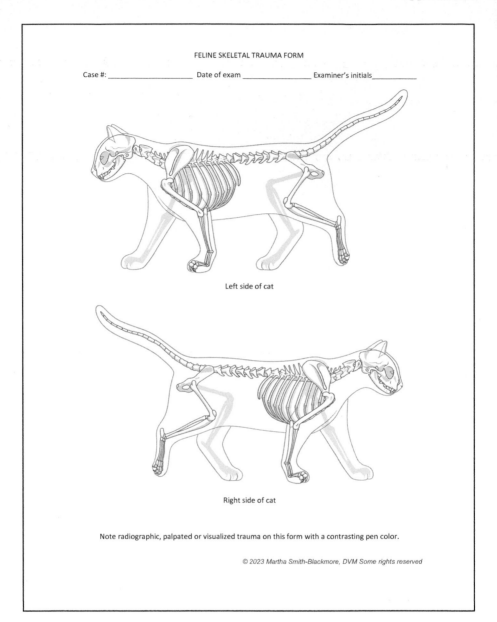

FELINE SKELETAL TRAUMA FORM

Case #: _____ Date of exam _____ Examiner's initials_____

Left side of cat

Right side of cat

Note radiographic, palpated or visualized trauma on this form with a contrasting pen color.

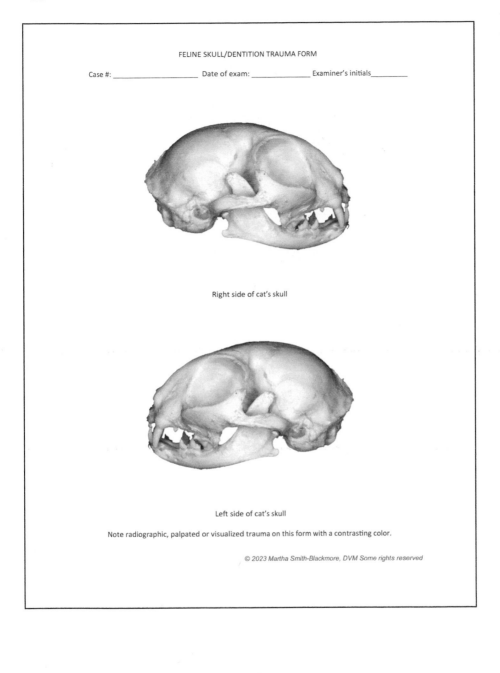

FELINE SKULL/DENTITION TRAUMA FORM

Case #: _____ Date of exam: _____ Examiner's initials_____

Right side of cat's skull

Left side of cat's skull

Note radiographic, palpated or visualized trauma on this form with a contrasting color.

FELINE SKULL/DENTITION TRAUMA FORM

Case #: _____ Date of exam: _____ Examiner's initials_____

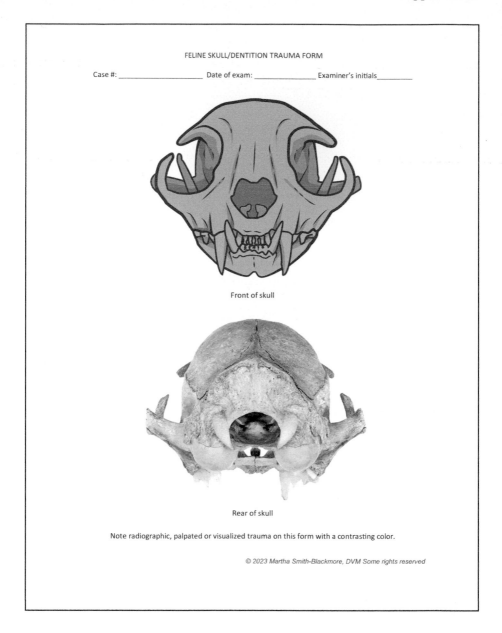

Front of skull

Rear of skull

Note radiographic, palpated or visualized trauma on this form with a contrasting color.

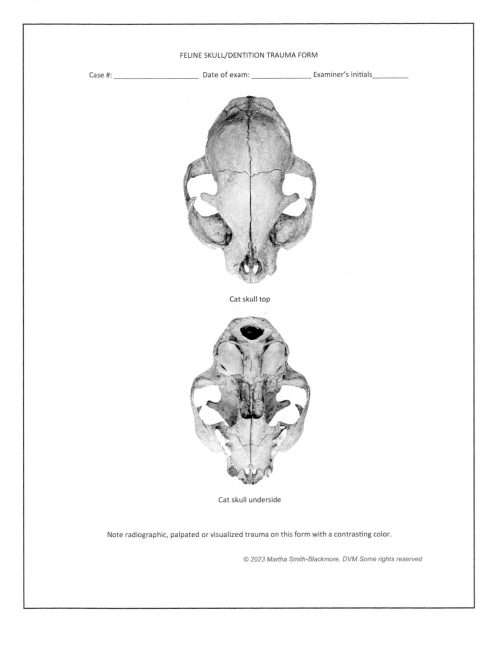

FELINE SKULL/DENTITION TRAUMA FORM

Case #: _____ Date of exam: _____ Examiner's initials_____

Cat skull top

Cat skull underside

Note radiographic, palpated or visualized trauma on this form with a contrasting color.

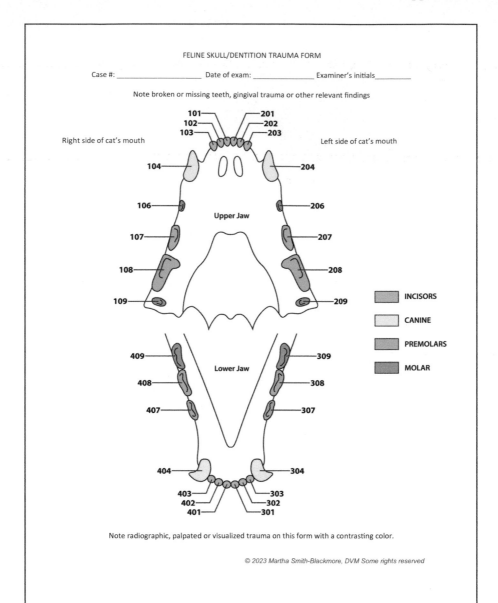

FELINE SKULL/DENTITION TRAUMA FORM

Case #: _____ Date of exam: _____ Examiner's initials_____

Note broken or missing teeth, gingival trauma or other relevant findings

Right side of cat's mouth

Left side of cat's mouth

101
102
103
201
202
203

104 — 204

Upper Jaw

106 — 206
107 — 207
108 — 208
109 — 209

INCISORS

CANINE

PREMOLARS

MOLAR

Lower Jaw

409 — 309
408 — 308
407 — 307

404 — 304
403 — 303
402 — 302
401 — 301

Note radiographic, palpated or visualized trauma on this form with a contrasting color.

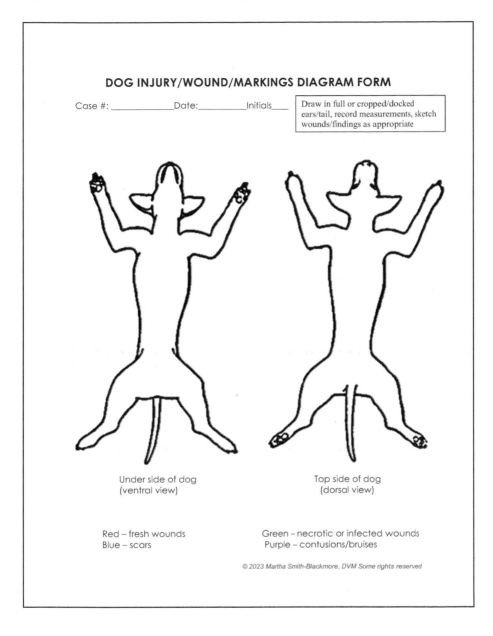

DOG INJURY/WOUND/MARKINGS DIAGRAM FORM

Case #: _____ Date:_____ Initials____

Draw in full or cropped/docked ears/tail, record measurements, sketch wounds/findings as appropriate

Under side of dog
(ventral view)

Top side of dog
(dorsal view)

Red – fresh wounds
Blue – scars

Green – necrotic or infected wounds
Purple – contusions/bruises

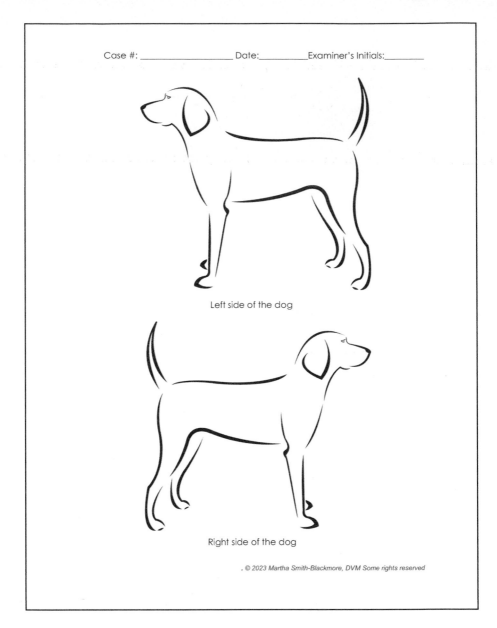

Case #: _____ Date:_____Examiner's Initials:_____

Left side of the dog

Right side of the dog

Case #: _____ Date:_____Examiner's Initials:_____

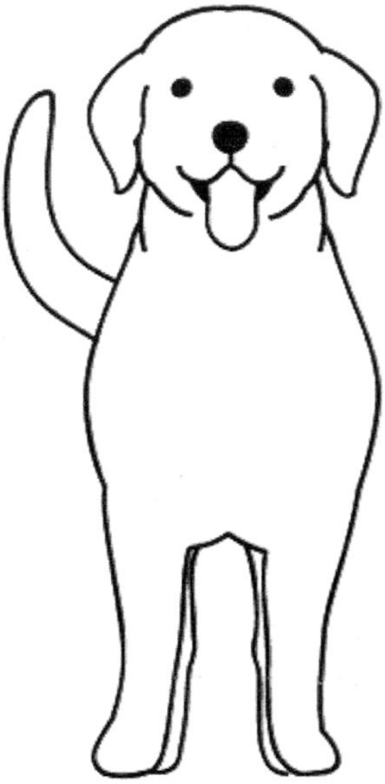

Front side of the dog

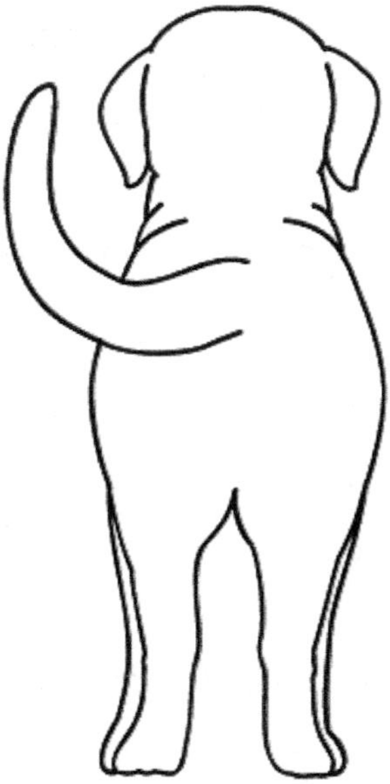

Rear side of the dog

Notes:_____

_____

_____

_____

Canine
DOG BODY CONDITION/PHYSICAL/ENVIRONMENTAL DECOMPOSITION SCORES

Case #_____ Date_____ Examiner initials _____

Weight _____(#/kg/) **PURINA BCS** _____of 9. (Whole numbers only, from to 9)

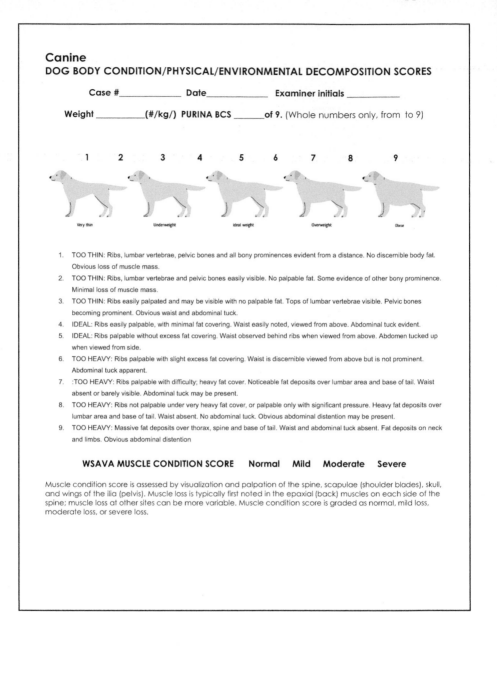

1. TOO THIN: Ribs, lumbar vertebrae, pelvic bones and all bony prominences evident from a distance. No discernible body fat. Obvious loss of muscle mass.
2. TOO THIN: Ribs, lumbar vertebrae and pelvic bones easily visible. No palpable fat. Some evidence of other bony prominence. Minimal loss of muscle mass.
3. TOO THIN: Ribs easily palpated and may be visible with no palpable fat. Tops of lumbar vertebrae visible. Pelvic bones becoming prominent. Obvious waist and abdominal tuck.
4. IDEAL: Ribs easily palpable, with minimal fat covering. Waist easily noted, viewed from above. Abdominal tuck evident.
5. IDEAL: Ribs palpable without excess fat covering. Waist observed behind ribs when viewed from above. Abdomen tucked up when viewed from side.
6. TOO HEAVY: Ribs palpable with slight excess fat covering. Waist is discernible viewed from above but is not prominent. Abdominal tuck apparent.
7. :TOO HEAVY: Ribs palpable with difficulty; heavy fat cover. Noticeable fat deposits over lumbar area and base of tail. Waist absent or barely visible. Abdominal tuck may be present.
8. TOO HEAVY: Ribs not palpable under very heavy fat cover, or palpable only with significant pressure. Heavy fat deposits over lumbar area and base of tail. Waist absent. No abdominal tuck. Obvious abdominal distention may be present.
9. TOO HEAVY: Massive fat deposits over thorax, spine and base of tail. Waist and abdominal tuck absent. Fat deposits on neck and limbs. Obvious abdominal distention

WSAVA MUSCLE CONDITION SCORE   Normal   Mild   Moderate   Severe

Muscle condition score is assessed by visualization and palpation of the spine, scapulae (shoulder blades), skull, and wings of the ilia (pelvis). Muscle loss is typically first noted in the epaxial (back) muscles on each side of the spine; muscle loss at other sites can be more variable. Muscle condition score is graded as normal, mild loss, moderate loss, or severe loss.

Case #: _____ Date:_____ Examiner's initials_____

TUFTS ANIMAL CARE AND CONDITION Physical Care Score _____ of 5.

5 Terrible Extremely matted haircoat, prevents normal motion, interferes with vision, perineal areas irritated from soiling with trapped urine and feces. Hair coat essentially a single mat. Dog cannot be groomed without complete clipdown. Foreign material trapped in matted hair. Nails extremely overgrown into circles, may be penetrating pads, causing abnormal position of feet and make normal walking very difficult or uncomfortable. Collar or chain, if present, may be embedded in dog's neck.

4 Poor Substantial matting in haircoat, large chunks of hair matted together that cannot be separated with a comb or brush. Occasional foreign material embedded in mats. Much of the hair will need to be clipped to remove mats. Long nails force feet into abnormal position and interfere with normal gait. Perineal soiling or irritation likely. Collar or chain, if present, may be extremely tight, abrading skin.

3 Borderline Numerous mats present in hair, but dog can still be groomed without a total clip down. No significant perineal soiling or irritation from waste caught in matted hair. Nails are overdue for a trim and long enough to cause dog to alter gait when it walks. Collar or chain, if present, may be snug and rubbing off neck hair.

2 Lapsed Haircoat may be somewhat dirty or have a few mats present that are easily removed. Remainder of coat can easily be brushed or combed. Nails in need of a trim. Collar or chain, if present, fits comfortably.

1 Adequate Dog clean, hair of normal length for the breed, and hair can easily be brushed or combed. Nails do not touch the floor, or barely contact the floor. Collar or chain, if present, fits comfortably.

TUFTS ANIMAL CARE AND CONDITION Environmental Health Scale _____of 5.

5 Filthy Many days to weeks of accumulation of feces and / or urine. Overwhelming odor, air may be difficult to breathe. Large amount of trash, garbage, or debris present; inhibits comfortable rest, normal postures, or movement and / or poses a danger to the animal. Very difficult or impossible for animal to escape contact with feces, urine, mud, or standing water. Food and / or drinking water contaminated.

4 Very unsanitary Many days of accumulation of feces and / or urine. Difficult for animal to avoid contact with waste matter. Moderate amount of trash, garbage, or clutter present that may inhibit comfortable rest and/or movement of the animal. Potential injury from sharp edges or glass. Significant odor makes breathing unpleasant. Standing water or mud difficult to avoid.

3 Unsanitary Several days of accumulation of feces and urine in animal's environment. Animal is able to avoid contact with waste matter. Moderate odor present. Trash, garbage, and other debris cluttering animal's environment but does not prohibit comfortable rest or normal posture. Clutter may interfere with normal movement or allow dog to become entangled, but no sharp edges or broken glass that could injure dog. Dog able to avoid mud or water if present.

2 Marginal As in #1, except may be somewhat less sanitary. No more than 1-2 days' accumulation of feces and urine in animal's environment. Slight clutter may be present.

1 Acceptable Environment is dry and free of accumulated feces. No contamination of food or water. No debris or garbage present to clutter environment and inhibit comfortable rest, normal posture and range of movement or pose a danger to or entangle the animal.

"Environment" refers to the kennel, pen, yard, cage, barn, room, tie-out or other enclosure or area where the animal is confined or spends the majority of its time. All of the listed conditions do not need to be present in order to include a dog in a specific category. The user should determine which category best describes a particular dog's condition.

Case #: _____ Date:_____ Examiner's initials_____

FOR POSTMORTEM SPECIMENS:

☐ **Check if previously stored frozen and thawed for examination**

Fresh: no discoloration or insect activity, able to shave fur

Early decomposition: gray to green discoloration, bloating, post-bloating rupture, cannot shave due to skin slippage, hair loss

Advanced decomposition: moist decomposition of tissues, sagging of flesh, caving in of abdomen, extensive insect activity, bone exposure of less than half of the skeleton, mummification

Skeletonization: bones with some body fluids present or tissue covering less than half of the skeleton, dry bones

Extreme decomposition: skeletonization with bleaching or exfoliation or metaphyseal loss or cancellous exposure (6 months to >3 years)

Notes:_____

_____

_____

_____

_____

_____

_____

_____

_____

_____

_____

CANINE SKELETAL TRAUMA FORM

Case #: _____ Date of exam _____ Initials_____

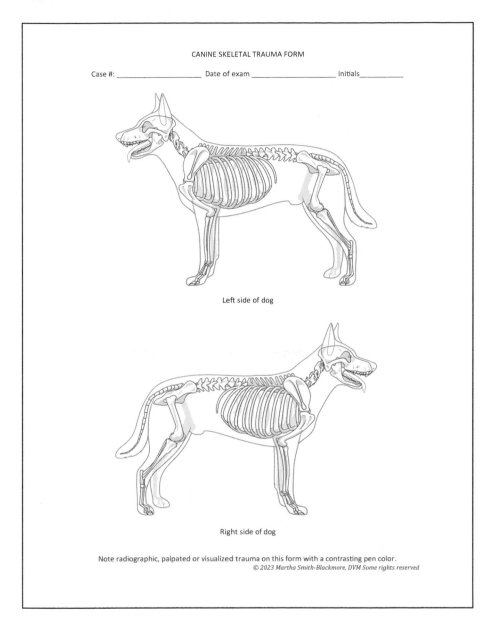

Left side of dog

Right side of dog

Note radiographic, palpated or visualized trauma on this form with a contrasting pen color.

CANINE SKULL/DENTITION TRAUMA FORM

Case #: _____ Date of exam: _____ Examiner's initials _____

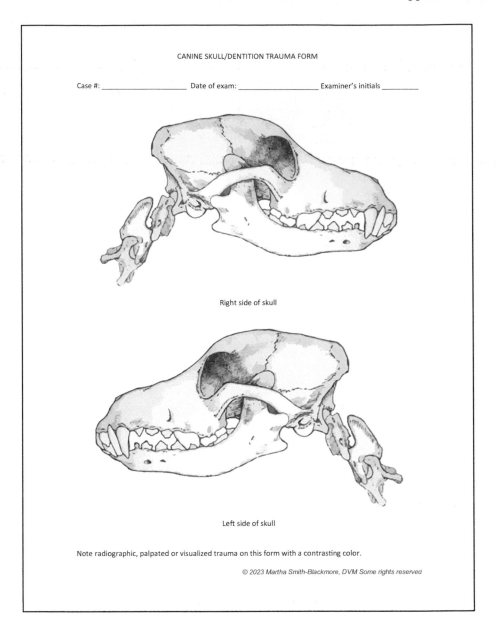

Right side of skull

Left side of skull

Note radiographic, palpated or visualized trauma on this form with a contrasting color.

CANINE SKULL/DENTITION TRAUMA FORM

Case #: _____ Date of exam: _____ Examiner's initials _____

Right maxillary teeth   Left maxillary teeth   Left mandibular teeth   Right mandibular teeth

100 quadrant   200 quadrant   300 quadrant   400 quadrant

Teeth of upper jaw (maxilla)   Teeth of lower jaw (mandible)

Note radiographic, palpated or visualized trauma on this form with a contrasting color.

CANINE SKULL/DENTITION TRAUMA FORM

Case #: _____ Date of exam: _____ Examiner's initials _____

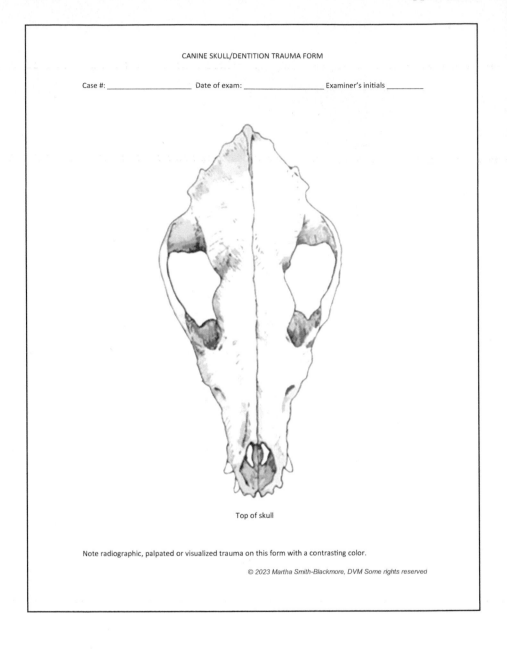

Top of skull

Note radiographic, palpated or visualized trauma on this form with a contrasting color.

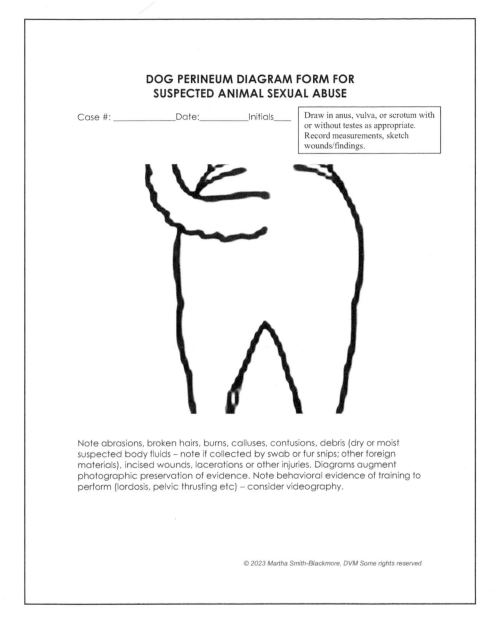

**DOG PERINEUM DIAGRAM FORM FOR
SUSPECTED ANIMAL SEXUAL ABUSE**

Case #: _____Date:_____Initials____

Draw in anus, vulva, or scrotum with
or without testes as appropriate.
Record measurements, sketch
wounds/findings.

Note abrasions, broken hairs, burns, calluses, contusions, debris (dry or moist
suspected body fluids – note if collected by swab or fur snips; other foreign
materials), incised wounds, lacerations or other injuries. Diagrams augment
photographic preservation of evidence. Note behavioral evidence of training to
perform (lordosis, pelvic thrusting etc) – consider videography.

Case #: _____ Date:_____Examiner's Initials:_____

> Draw in vulva, penis/prepuce, or scrotum with or without testes as appropriate. Record measurements, sketch wounds/findings.

Note measurements and findings in contrasting colors.

Remember that evidence of ASA may include toxicology, oral swabs, evidence of binding or muzzling for restraint, head trauma or other non-accidental injury inflicted as part of or to enable the sexual abuse.

Notes:_____

_____

_____

_____

Index

Note: **Bold** page numbers refer to tables and *italic* page numbers refer to figures.

351

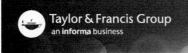